Handbook of Perioperative and Procedural Patient Safety

Handbook of Perioperative and Procedural Patient Safety

Edited by

Juan A. Sanchez

Group Vice President, Graduate Medical Education HCA Healthcare
Nashville, TN, United States

Robert S. D. Higgins

President, Brigham and Women's Hospital, Executive Vice President,
Mass General Brigham, Brigham and Women's Hospital, Boston,
Massachusetts, United States

Paula S. Kent

Johns Hopkins Armstrong Institute for Patient Safety and Quality,
Baltimore, MD, United States
Johns Hopkins University School of Nursing,
Baltimore, MD, United States
Johns Hopkins Bloomberg School of Public Health,
Baltimore, MD, United States

ELSEVIER

Publisher: Mica H. Haley
Acquisitions Editor: John G. Vassallo
Editorial Project Manager: Sam Young
Production Project Manager: Kiruthika Govindaraju
Cover Designer: Vicky Pearson Esser

3251 Riverport Lane
St. Louis, Missouri 63043

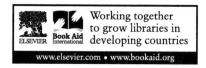

Working together to grow libraries in developing countries

www.elsevier.com • www.bookaid.org

This book is dedicated to all the patients and families who entrust us to protect them from preventable adverse events daily. We hope this book contributes to eliminating these events in all surgical and procedural areas and is instrumental in creating safe healthcare environments. It is also dedicated to all the healthcare professionals who provided safe, compassionate care at enormous personal risk during the recent worldwide pandemic and to the families who support them.

Contents

CHAPTER 13   Occupational well-being, resilience, burnout, and job satisfaction of surgical teams 205

Vera Meeusen, PhD, CHM, MA, RN, FACPAN, AFACHSM, Stephen Paul Gatt, MD, FANZCA, FRCA, FACHSM, FCICM, AFRCMA, et alii, et eundem, Paul Barach, B.Med.Sci, MD, MPH, Maj (ret.), AUA and André Van Zundert, MD, PhD, FRCA, EDRA, FANZCA

CHAPTER 14   Redesigning the operating room for safety 231

Marius Fassbinder, MD and James H. Abernathy, III, MD, MPH

Contributors

Ephrem Abebe, MS, MPHARM, PhD
Department of Pharmacy Practice, College of Pharmacy, Purdue University, West Lafayette, IN, United States; Regenstrief Center for Healthcare Engineering, Purdue University, West Lafayette, IN, United States

James H. Abernathy, III, MD, MPH
Interim Executive Vice Chair, ACCM, Chief, Division of Cardiac Anesthesiology, Core Faculty, Armstrong Institute of Patient Safety, Department of Anesthesiology & Critical Care Medicine, Johns Hopkins University, Baltimore, MD, United States

Diane Alejo, BA
Division of Cardiac Surgery, Johns Hopkins University School of Medicine, Baltimore, MD, United States

Paul Barach, B.Med.Sci, MD, MPH, Maj (ret.), AUA
Thomas Jefferson University School of Medicine, Philadelphia, PA, United States; Honorary Professor, Faculty of Medicine, The University of Queensland, Brisbane, QLD, Australia; Honorary Professor, University of Birmingham, Birmingham, United Kingdom; Professor, Sigmund Freud University, Vienna, Austria

Cheryl Connors, DNP, RN, NEA-BC
Johns Hopkins University, Baltimore, MD, United States

R. Lebron Cooper, MD
Department of Anesthesiology, Indiana University Health Arnett Hospital, Lafayette, IN, United States

Steven C. Cunningham, MD, FACS
Division of Pancreatic and Hepatobiliary Surgery, Ascension Saint Agnes Hospital Center and Cancer Institute, Baltimore, MD, United States

Dan Degnan, PharmD, MS, CPPS, FASHP
Department of Pharmacy Practice, College of Pharmacy, Purdue University, West Lafayette, IN, United States; Regenstrief Center for Healthcare Engineering, Purdue University, West Lafayette, IN, United States

Poching DeLaurentis, PhD
Regenstrief Center for Healthcare Engineering, Purdue University, West Lafayette, IN, United States

Hanan H. Edrees, DrPH, MHSA
Advisor, Public Health Authority, Riyadh, Kingdom of Saudi Arabia; Associate Faculty, Johns Hopkins University: Bloomberg School of Public Health, Baltimore, MD, United States

John C. Evanko, MD MBA
Executive Vice President & Chief Medical Officer, MCIC Vermont, LLC, New York, NY, United States

Marius Fassbinder, MD
Assistant Professor, Department of Anesthesiology, George Washington University, Washington, DC, United States

Stephen Paul Gatt, MD, FANZCA, FRCA, FACHSM, FCICM, AFRCMA, et alii, et eundem
Professor of Anesthesiology & Reanimation, University of Udayana, Denpasar, Bali, Indonesia; Associate Professor, University of New South Wales, Sydney, NSW, Australia

Michael C. Grant, MD, MSE
Associate Professor, Department of Anesthesiology and Critical Care Medicine and Surgery, Johns Hopkins University School of Medicine, Baltimore, MD, United States; Armstrong Institute of Patient Safety and Quality, The Johns Hopkins Medical Institutions, Baltimore, MD, United States

Brendan L. Grant, MSE
General Dynamics Advanced Information Systems, Fairfax, VA, United States

Conrad J. Grant, MS
APL Chief Engineer, The Johns Hopkins Applied Physics Laboratories, Laurel, MD, United States

Elliott R. Haut, MD, PhD, FACS
Department of Surgery, Department of Anesthesiology and Critical Care Medicine, Department of Emergency Medicine, The Johns Hopkins University School of Medicine, Baltimore, MD, United States; The Armstrong Institute for Patient Safety and Quality, Johns Hopkins Medicine, Baltimore, MD, United States; Department of Health Policy and Management, The Johns Hopkins Bloomberg School of Public Health, Baltimore, MD, United States

Robert Higgins, MD MSHA
President, Brigham and Women's Hospital, Executive Vice President, Mass General Brigham, Brigham and Women's Hospital, Boston, MA, United States

Julie Johnson, MSPH, PhD
Department of Surgery, Feinberg School of Medicine, Northwestern University, Chicago, IL, United States

Paula S. Kent, DrPH, MSN, MBA, RN, CPPS
Patient Safety Specialist, Johns Hopkins Armstrong Institute for Patient Safety and Quality, Baltimore, MD, United States; Adjunct Faculty, Johns Hopkins University School of Nursing, Baltimore, MD, United States; Associate Faculty, Johns Hopkins Bloomberg School of Public Health, Baltimore, MD, United States; Johns Hopkins University, Baltimore, MD, United States

Shankar Kurra, MD, MBA
Sentara Virginia Beach General, Virginia Beach, VA, United States

Thomas L. Matthew, MD, MS
Cardiothoracic Surgery, Johns Hopkins School of Medicine, Director Johns Hopkins Cardiothoracic Surgery at Suburban Hospital, Bethesda, MD, United States

Vera Meeusen, PhD, CHM, MA, RN, FACPAN, AFACHSM
CNC Endoscopy Unit, Princess Alexandra Hospital, Woolloongabba, QLD, Australia; Associate Professor, Faculty of Medicine, The University of Queensland, Brisbane, QLD, Australia; Clinical Nurse Consultant, Princess Alexandra Hospital, Brisbane, QLD, Australia

Dave Patrishkoff, MA
Dr Patel College of Osteopathic Medicine, Nova Southeastern University, Fort Lauderdale, FL, United States

Edward Popovich, PhD
Dr Koran C Patel, College of Osteopathic Medicine, Nova Southeastern University, Fort Lauderdale, FL, United States

Paul Risner, JD
President, Paul E. Risner, P.A.

Juan A. Sanchez, MD, MPA, FACS
Group Vice President for Graduate Medical Education, HCA Healthcare, Nashville, TN, United States

Artem Shmelev, MD
Department of Surgery, Columbia University Medical Center, New York, NY, United States

Becky Southern, RN
Caldwell Butler Associates

Jerry Stonemetz, MD
Medical Director, Perioperative Services, Anesthesia & Critical Care Medicine, Johns Hopkins University, Baltimore, MD, United States

Sanda A. Tan, MD, PhD, FACS, FASCRS
Program Director in General Surgery Residency, UCF/HCA Florida West Hospital, Pensacola, FL, United States; Professor, University of Central Florida, College of Medicine, Orlando, FL, United States

André van Zundert, MD, PhD, FRCA, EDRA, FANZCA
Professor & Chair Anesthesiology, Faculty of Medicine, The University of Queensland, Brisbane, QLD, Australia; Department of Anaesthesia and Perioperative Medicine, Royal Brisbane and Women's Hospital, Herston, QLD, Australia

Katherine G. Verdi, MD
Resident, Department of Surgery, Johns Hopkins School of Medicine, Baltimore, MD, United States

Kristen L.W. Webster, PhD
Department of Patient Safety, Regulatory, and Accreditation, Cincinnati Children's Hospital Medical Center, Cincinnati, OH, United States

Hadley K. Wesson, MD MPH
Assistant Professor, Department of Surgery, Johns Hopkins School of Medicine, Baltimore, MD, United States

Hal Wiggin, PhD
Dr Koran C Patel College of Osteopathic Medicine, Health Informatics Department, Nova Southeastern University, Fort Lauderdale, FL, United States

Richard J. Zink, BA, MBA
Regenstrief Center for Healthcare Engineering, Purdue University, West Lafayette, IN, United States

Preface

Since the early 1990s, when the veterans administration's efforts to assess and improve outcomes were published, quality assessment and process improvement initiatives have become the cornerstone of patient care in the daily operations of health care enterprises. In 1994, the National Veteran's Affairs Surgical Quality Improvement Program (VASQIP) was established across all VA hospitals with a primary focus on improving surgical outcomes.[1] Khuri et al. presented the first national validated outcomes-based risk-adjusted report in 1998 outlining the structure, data collection, analysis, and reporting of clinical outcomes following surgery. Validation of this process improvement effort over the past several decades suggests that continuous quality assessment and improvement universally enhances *"the patient care culture"*.[2]

So, what is a patient safety culture? The Agency for Healthcare Research and Quality (AHRQ) defines patient safety culture as *the extent to which an organization's culture supports, promotes, and improves patient safety. It refers to a set of values, beliefs, and norms that are shared by healthcare practitioners and other staff throughout the organization that influence their actions and their behaviors.* They further suggest that the values, norms, beliefs, and behaviors related to keeping patients safe from preventable harm can be rewarded, supported, expected, and accepted in any healthcare delivery setting. An organization's culture permeates every level of the organization from the unit level to the department to the organization to the health system (Figure 1). As such, a culture of safety is fundamental to improving healthcare outcomes and protecting patients from unintended events during the delivery of their care.

In this **Handbook of Perioperative and Procedural Patient Safety**, the authors have embarked upon a comprehensive review of patient safety from the assessment of risk to the safe conduct of anesthesia, procedural sedation, and the prevention of healthcare-associated infections, to name a few of the key topics. Many of these chapters outline effective approaches to patient safety activities with an emphasis on improving the safety climate of surgical areas. By stressing ways to promote patient safety, including how interprofessional teams work and learn together, this book can guide surgical personnel in developing practices, habits, and routines that make the surgical environment safe for patients.

This book aims to complement and expand the scope of current activities to protect patients from preventable adverse events by covering fundamental and emerging concepts in safety science from a broad perspective. It is intended to be a useful resource, not only for front-line clinicians but also for those involved in managing clinical areas and making resource allocation decisions. The ultimate goal of the **Handbook** is to help establish a culture of surgical safety and continuous improvement that systematically ensures that all providers *"strive to not only improve outcomes but to get the right care to the right patient at the right time, every time."*

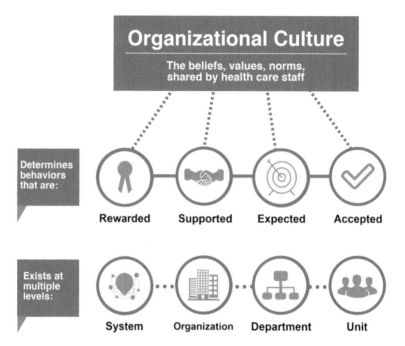

FIGURE 1

Organizational culture.[3]

Sources

1. Grover F, Johnson RR, Shroyer AL, Marshall G, Hammermeister KE. The Veterans Affairs continuous improvement in cardiac surgery study. *Ann Thorac Surg* 1994;**58**(6): 1845–51.
2. Khuri SF, Daley J, Henderson W, Hur K, et al. The Department of Veteran's Affairs the first national, validated, outcome-based, risk-adjusted, and peer-controlled program for the measurement and enhancement of the quality of surgical care. National VA Surgical Quality Improvement Program. *Ann Surg* 1998;**228**(4):491–507.
3. What is patient safety culture? Agency for Healthcare Research and Quality. Content last reviewed March 2022. Rockville, MD: Agency for Healthcare Research and Quality. https://www.ahrq.gov/sops/about/patient-safety-culture.html.

The science of human error

Cheryl Connors, DNP, RN, NEA-BC, Paula S. Kent, DrPH, MSN, MBA, RN, CPPS

Johns Hopkins University, Baltimore, MD, United States

What is human error?

Human error is inescapable simply because we are human. Human error is an act that is not intended, may happen at random, and may not be fully preventable.[1] Some words that may be used to describe human error include but are not limited to inadvertent, slip, lapse, mistake, or accident. The outcome that results from human error is usually undesirable and sometimes outside of acceptable limits. Most importantly, true human error is a deviation from intention.[2]

There are various definitions of human error that share a common theme—an unintended act. And there are many different types of errors described: errors of omission (not doing something that should be done), errors of commission (doing the wrong thing), technical errors (failure related to human—technical interface), organizational errors (system set-ups), and near-miss errors which don't reach the patient but could cause harm if they did.[3] However, understanding human error may simply be acknowledging and accepting that humans are not perfect. Humans are fallible and a part of a sociological existence. We may even argue that there is no science to human error. Human error may be a part of social work.[4]

Human error has earned the spotlight in healthcare for 2 decades now. It was in 1999 when the Institute of Medicine (IOM), now known as the National Academy of Medicine (NAM), released "To Err is Human," a publication that identified as many as 98,000 patient deaths resulted from medical error in the United States.[5] Since this initial effort to understand the magnitude of medical error, more recent studies conclude that much larger proportions of patient death and harm result from error. Medical error may be the third leading cause of death in the United States.[6]

Human error and healthcare

Healthcare meets the definition criteria as a complex system for humans to work in, composed of "many interacting parts where it is difficult, if not impossible, to predict the behavior of the system based on knowledge of its component parts."[7] The demanding macrosystem (container that holds micro- and mesosystems together) of healthcare is made up of microsystems (smallest part of the system that provides

Handbook of Perioperative and Procedural Patient Safety. https://doi.org/10.1016/B978-0-323-66179-9.00014-2

care to the patient (i.e., a clinical unit)) and a variety of mesosystems (glue linking microsystems) which contribute to the care and safety of our patients and families).[8] When estimating the number of staff involved in one patient's care for one shift, it seems that there can be various numbers at each microsystem.

Microsystems involved to care for one acutely ill patient in one 12 hour shift:

Microsystem 1: Pharmacy (technicians and pharmacists).

Microsystem 2: Blood bank (technicians, nurses, and doctors).

Microsystem 3: Radiology (techs and doctors).

Microsystem 4: Emergency department (techs, nurses, and doctors).

Microsystem 5: ICU (nurses and doctors).

Since our complex systems are not perfected and to err is human,[5] medical error has been of great concern. Data clearly show that the healthcare system has grown to be more complex, with more acute patient needs and slim resources requiring nationwide efforts to improve patient safety and to implement safer systems within healthcare.[9] With a lack of highly reliable principles in place on a consistent basis, our healthcare system will continue to allow human error.

Person approach versus the system approach [9]

Contributing factors to human error include but are not limited to stress, fatigue, hunger, emotional state, communication, teamwork, leadership, situational awareness or lack thereof, etc.[10] Given the complex nature of healthcare, it is no wonder these factors play a significant role in the healthcare system.

Once error is identified, there are two approaches to understanding the nature of how the error occurred: first, the person approach where the organization typically blames the individual for the error. Cases such as Eric Cropp, PharmD,[11] and Kimberly Hiatt, RN,[12] are examples where people were blamed for mistakes that occurred under their watch. The person approach might suggest the healthcare provider was careless, negligent, or inattentive.[9] Unfortunately, the healthcare provider likely suffers consequences that impact them personally and professionally, such as in the two cases mentioned above. The impact of the person approach may not be a system that is safer, rather a relief on the organizations' responsibility for patient safety and a punitive culture.[13]

Examples: Person approach

Eric Cropp (2006)

Pharmacist working in an Ohio hospital.

Only pharmacist on staff for whole hospital.

Approves chemo that was mixed by the pharmacy tech.

Chemo administered to patient.

Patient dies from chemo concentration.

Eric is dismissed from job and criminally charged.

> **Examples: Person approach—cont'd**
>
> **Kimberly Hiatt (2010)**
>
> Nurse working in a Seattle hospital.
> Makes a medication error—10-fold overdose.
> Nurse reports mistake immediately.
> Patient suffers complications, ultimately dies.
> Nurse dismissed from job.
> Kimberly commits suicide months later.

The system approach recognizes system factors that influence how the healthcare provider operates, acknowledging the conditions which may have set the healthcare provider up for error.[9] Some examples include staffing models, workload, policies, technical reliance, and the basic environment in which they work. Addressing system issues and applying interventions that will improve the safety of the system will reduce the possibility of the error reoccurring.[14]

> **Example. System approach**
>
> A medication error reaches a patient. The multidisciplinary team (doctor, nurse, tech, pharmacist, pharmacy tech, safety officer, and unit leader) gather to analyze why the error occurred. A detailed description of what happened and why it happened was presented. The medication was in a pharmacy bin that was identical to the ordered medication. The pharmacy tech inadvertently chose the wrong medication. The pharmacist approved the medication and labeled it as ordered. The nurses administered the correctly labeled medication. The intervention was to change the bin colors, locations, and labels in the pharmacy and eventually use bar coding for medication preparation.

In healthcare, both the person and system approaches must be considered if high reliability and "just culture" are considered goals of achievement.[15]

Swiss cheese model

The famous Swiss cheese model based on Reason's model of accident causation (1990) has been used to depict how holes in our microsystems can lead to error. The illustration describes our microsystems as layers of defense, like humans mostly not perfect which is illustrated by the holes. When a failure slips through a hole, we rely on the next layer of defense to catch it. When each layer of defense fails, the error often reaches the patient.

One consideration described in the Swiss cheese model is latent conditions (Fig. 1.1). Latent conditions are those decisions made by organizational leaders that create the conditions in which healthcare providers work.[16] An example of a latent condition is when a safety concern that is a system flaw has surfaced and has been brought to the decision-maker's attention. The decision-maker decides that the current condition is suffice because of budgetary constraints despite the potential risk for poor patient outcomes. Healthcare providers (aka humans) continue to work under these suboptimal conditions in an already complex environment. Eventually a catastrophic event reaches the patient because of the system flaw which has not been addressed.[10]

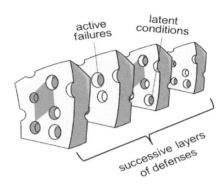

FIGURE 1.1

Diagram of Reason's Swiss cheese model.[9]

Active failures include attitudes and/or actions of people at delivery of care.[10] The path of choice to act can be influenced by the culture of the surrounding team or environment with no intent to do harm, a human error. Harm does not need to be catastrophic to be a major concern. Sometimes, active failures, those that reach the patient, are simply the result of latent conditions.

Example: Latent condition

Organizational policy states "Use blue emergency crash carts for all emergency situations."

Clinical staff identify that items are difficult to find; cart is not easy to open or use and not intuitive; there have been many incidents where staff felt confused between the pediatric and adult carts. Delays to care during emergencies are reported frequently for both pediatric and adult emergency situations.

Staff identify a newly designed cart that would better meet their needs. They conduct time trial to show evidence that the new cart saves 4 min during an emergency. Staff present findings to leadership.

Since the new cart would cost a lot of money, leadership prefers to continue using the current blue cart as there have not been any poor outcomes that we can link to the cart.

Staff continue to struggle with the current cart and often use workarounds that are inefficient to care for patients during emergencies.

Example: Active failure

An emergency is called for a patient. A nurse brings the blue cart to the patient's room. The nurse shuffles through four drawers to locate the correct endotracheal tube. After 3 min, he runs to the emergency supply server down the hall which is a back-up supply that staff created since staff struggle with the blue cart. Another 5 min pass as he cannot find the endotracheal tube. The patient deteriorates and now requires an emergency cricothyrotomy. The nurse does not report the incident as he has submitted several in the past and feels that "no one is listening and nothing will be done anyway."

The number of errors has not decreased since the IOM report in 1999, and in fact they have increased tremendously.[6] It is believed that reporting culture has improved and it is known that patient safety research and publications have skyrocketed.[17] Our work is far from complete as healthcare has not yet achieved a state of high reliability.

Case study

A 63-year-old female is highly suspicious for lung cancer. The immediate plan of care is to complete a right upper lobectomy. The day prior to surgery, she receives a pre-op call and is questioned about which lung. The patient says "right lung." The pre-op nurse is clearly confused because her paper says left lung. By the end of the 20 min conversation, the patient feels confused and scared. She thought the pre-op nurse was testing her. Luckily the patient had an advocate upon whom she called. They reviewed all scans together to confirm that it was in fact the right lung.

Upon arrival to surgery, the patient's surgeon met with the patient and family. He acknowledged that there was a posting error and she was originally posted for the left lung. Surgery was successful and the patient went home 3 days post-op.

The patient was supposed to receive home care visits that were arranged before discharge. Day 8 post-op arrived, but no home care visits occurred as discussed. The patient was restless overnight, experiencing increased pain and swelling in her back. At 9 a.m., the patient called the office to describe her symptoms. The receptionist told her that a nurse would call her back shortly.

At 12:30 p.m., the symptoms were worse and the patient had not yet received a call from the nurse. The patient called again to describe worsening symptoms. Thirty minutes later the nurse returned the call. The nurse didn't express an understanding or concern and requested a picture be sent. One hour later, the nurse called the patient to say this doesn't look urgent, "take some pain medicine and get some rest, we cannot see you today." The patient's advocate told the patient to go to urgent care for assessment. The urgent care doctor detected a large pneumothorax and massive subcutaneous emphysema, suggesting emergency treatment. The advocate called the on-call doctor as the clinic nurse/office closed at 4:15 p.m. Three calls to the on-call resident and 3 hours passed before contact was made. The patient was told to come to the hospital for direct admit.

At 9 p.m., the patient was admitted. Soon thereafter, a chest tube was inserted at the bedside. The advocate noted that the floor was very dirty in the room and requested housekeeping.

The patient remained stable yet continued to be inpatient. The surgeon was asked for the pathology report. The patient and patient's family were told "it was cancer." Since other areas of the scan illuminated areas of concern out of the lung, the family had a lot of questions. The surgeon said "it was cancer, I took it out. Nothing else is needed." He left the room.

For the reminder of the stay, several medical team members came to see the patient without washing their hands, wearing gloves, and touching the patient after touching various pieces of equipment in the room, including a trash can. The nursing staff was constantly interrupted by staff Ascom phones during patient care, answering the phones with gloves on and replacing phones in their pockets.

At 14 days post-op, the patient was released from the hospital 5 days after the readmission. On day 16, the patient had a fever and was diagnosed with an infection. The patient was readmitted to the hospital for treatment. This is now the second readmission in less than 3 weeks.

After thorough investigation, the following factors were identified as contributors to poor outcomes for this patient.

Active failures and latent conditions

Wrong site posting: This was a clerical error entered by the surgeon's nurse. She completed the posting while being interrupted approximately three times by other staff members.

Lack of home visits: Case manager was overtasked on the day she met the patient and forgot to add her to the home visit list as promised.

Phone triage for complication: Clinic was short staffed and the nurse who took the call doesn't usually take patient calls. The nurse could not contact the surgeon because he was in a long surgery and the clinic was full for the day. The nurse reports having personal issues that affected her emotional state.

Delay in call back for complication: The resident was told not to call back by a senior surgeon because this patient already spoke to the nurse in the clinic; resident was responsible for covering three other services.

Dirty floor on admission: Room was cleaned at shift change, hand-off regarding the floor not being cleaned failed to happen between housekeepers. Housekeeping was short staffed.

Inadequate hand hygiene: Competencies not complete regarding "in room" hand hygiene. The residents were rushing due to work overload. Ascom phones are required for timely communication.

Brief/curt communication: The surgeon had been in the operating room (OR) for 16 hours and was exhausted.

Post-op infection: Hospital charged with responsibility based on care reported, actual source unknown—potentially lack of hand hygiene practices.

Undesirable outcomes for the patient and hospital:

Longer than expected recovery for patient.
Patient dissatisfied with care.
Ten additional inpatient nights.
Hospital was charged with expenses for hospital acquired infection.
Hospital was held accountable for readmission within 30 days.

Although simple human error was a factor in this case study, latent conditions and system issues influenced the actions of the healthcare providers. Fortunately, this patient is alive and well. However, she chose to seek the continuation of her care elsewhere.

Surgery may be one of the more complex arenas in healthcare. Some control exists when patients are relatively stable and the procedures can be scheduled, yet the coordination required to move the patient safely through pre-op, the OR, and post-op care can certainly be challenging. The various individuals involved in these areas of care require stellar communication and teamwork to foster a culture of safety. According to Molina et al., there is an association perception of OR safety of surgical practice and hospital-level 30-day patient death rates.[18]

Summary

Human error will likely continue in healthcare. Healthcare organizations should make efforts to understand errors from a systems perspective and implement changes that will prevent reoccurrence and minimize the risks.[7] Creating a healthy reporting culture and a nonpunitive "just culture" environment may help detect potential and actual errors.[1] Engaging the frontline staff can promote a better understanding of how errors happen so that strong, targeted interventions can be implemented.[14]

References

1. Marx D. Retrieved on November 22, 2019 from, https://www.unmc.edu/patient-safety/_documents/patient-safety-and-the-just-culture.pdf; 2007.
2. Reason J. *Human error.* New York, NY: Cambridge University Press; 1990.
3. Ilan, Fowler. *Brief history of patient safety and science.* 2005.
4. Wallace B, Ross A. *Beyond human error, taxonomies and safety science.* Taylor & Francis Group; 2006.
5. Kohn LT, Corrigan JM, Donaldson MS. *(Institute of Medicine) To err is human: building a safer health system.* Washington, DC: National Academy Press; 2000.
6. Makary MA, Daniel M. Medical error—the third leading cause of death in the US. *BMJ* 2016;**353**:i2139.
7. World Health Organization (WHO). Retrieved on November 8, 2019 from, https://www.who.int/patientsafety/education/curriculum/course3_handout.pdf; 2012.
8. Likosky DS. Clinical microsystems: a critical framework for crossing the quality chasm. *J Extra-Corpor Technol* 2014;**46**(1):33.
9. Reason J. Human error: models and management. *BMJ* 2000;**320**:768–70.
10. Brennan PA, Mitchell DA, Holmes S, Plint S, Parry D. Good people who try their best can have problems: recognition of human factors and how to minimise error. *Br J Oral Maxillofac Surg* 2016;**54**(1):3–7.

11. Institute for Safe Medication Practices (ISMP). *Eric cropp weighs in on the error that sent him to prison*. Retrieved on October 24, 2019 from, https://www.ismp.org/resources/eric-cropp-weighs-error-sent-him-prison.

12. Institute for Safe Medication Practices (ISMP). Too many abandon the "second victims" after medical errors 2011;**16**(14).

13. Moncilovich M. Verdict marks an end to the nonpunitive culture. *Am J Health Syst Pharm* 2010;**67**(3):177—8.

14. Timmel J, Kent PS, Holzmueller CG, Paine L, Schulick RD, Pronovost PJ. Impact of the Comprehensive Unit-based Safety Program (CUSP) on safety culture in a surgical inpatient unit. *Jt Comm J Qual Patient Saf* 2010;**36**(6):252—60.

15. Tsao K, Browne M. Culture of safety: a foundation for patient care. *Seminars in pediatric surgery* 2015, December;**24**(6):283—7. WB Saunders.

16. Day RM, Demski RJ, Pronovost PJ, Sutcliffe KM, Kasda EM, Maragakis LL, et al. Operating management system for high reliability: Leadership, accountability, learning and innovation in healthcare. *J Patient Safety Risk Manag* 2018;**23**(4):155—66.

17. Stelfox HT, Palmisani S, Scurlock C, Orav EJ, Bates DW. The "To Err is Human" report and the patient safety literature. *Qual Saf Health Care* 2006;**15**(3):174—8. https://doi.org/10.1136/qshc.2006.017947.

18. Molina G, Berry WR, Lipsitz SR, Edmondson L, Li Z, Neville BA, Moonan AT, Gibbons LR, Gawande AA, Singer SJ, Haynes AB. *Ann Surg* 2017 Oct;**266**(4): 658—66. https://doi.org/10.1097/SLA.0000000000002378.

Further reading

1. Florence Nightingale. *Notes on hospitals*. 3rd edition 1863.

The scope and prevalence of perioperative harm

Hanan H. Edrees, DrPH, MHSA [1,2]

[1]*Advisor, Public Health Authority, Riyadh, Kingdom of Saudi Arabia;* [2]*Associate Faculty, Johns Hopkins University: Bloomberg School of Public Health, Baltimore, MD, United States*

It is no doubt that perioperative harm is frequent.

Surgery has been identified as the source of many unavoidable medical errors and deaths.[1] However, recent studies have proved that many of these adverse events are preventable.[2,3] The success of clear processes and guidelines, effective communication and teamwork, improved collaboration, and the reduction of distractions have helped in identifying and improving current challenges in surgical care. The aim of this chapter is to provide an overview on the scope and prevalence of perioperative patient harm.

The scope of perioperative care

Perioperative care includes the evaluation and care management during three periods: the preoperative, the peroperative (or intraoperative), and the postoperative stage. In particular, the perioperative period begins when the patient is admitted, undergoes anesthesia and surgery, and then ends when the patient is discharged.[4] The objective of perioperative medicine is to deliver the best care in each of these three periods in order to meet the needs of patients undergoing major surgery.[5] This can be accomplished by adopting evidence-based care pathways and safe surgery checklists.

1. Preoperative Phase

   This initial phase starts with the patient's decision to undergo surgery and ends when the patient is entering the operating room.[6] During the preoperative period, the healthcare provider prepares the patient physically (medical history, physical examination, and medication review) and psychologically for the surgery.[7]

   The goal of the preoperative phase is to actively promote patient engagement and shared decision-making.[8] Although healthcare providers generally make decisions based on evidence and the patient's health, it is essential: to assess the patient's current medical status and history, to provide a clinical risk profile, and to provide patient recommendations for the entire perioperative period. Some of these recommendations include informed decisions on whether to proceed with

Handbook of Perioperative and Procedural Patient Safety. https://doi.org/10.1016/B978-0-323-66179-9.00007-5

the surgery, the choice of surgery, and the identification of risk factors and patient conditions that might require additional care or longer term care. This preparation can take place over a long period of time where the patient may be required to fast, undergo tests, wait for the availability of an organ for transplant, or lose weight. On the other hand, this phase can be very short where the patient is in need of an emergency surgical procedure or is facing acute trauma.

Undergoing a surgical procedure can be a difficult and traumatic time for patients. In an effort to carefully monitor the patient's condition throughout the perioperative phases, some healthcare providers have embraced the enhanced recovery after surgery (ERAS) protocols, which are multimodal perioperative care pathways designed to achieve quick recovery after surgery.[9] The ERAS protocols include patient education, preoperative counseling, early mobilization, oral intake of fluid, nutrition optimization, and ambulation.

In addition to examining the clinical risks the patient may undergo, it is essential to manage the patient's anxiety levels that may result due to the long wait period before the surgery takes place or due to the sudden trauma the patient has faced. This type of anxiety can be effectively managed with constant interaction with the healthcare team, particularly the physician, surgeon, or nurse.

2. Peroperative Phase

The peroperative or intraoperative phase includes the surgery or surgical procedure being performed. During this phase, the patient is monitored, transferred to the operating room, and prepped and undergoes anesthesia. This can include general anesthesia for complete unconsciousness, regional anesthesia, or local anesthesia to prevent pain while the patient is awake. Peroperative radiation therapy or blood salvage may also take place. This phase ends when the patient is transferred to the postanesthesia care unit also known as PACU.

When the surgery commences, the healthcare team composed of the surgeon, the anesthesiologist, nurse, and others will closely monitor the patient's vital signs, assist the surgeon, adhere to clinical guidelines, and focus on safety procedures associated with infection prevention.

3. Postoperative Phase

This phase begins immediately after the surgery has ended and where the patient has been transferred to the PACU. This period can either be brief or can take place over several months where the patient requires additional treatment or undergoes rehabilitation.

The goal of this phase is to monitor and manage the patient's physical and psychological health postsurgery. The postsurgery recovery stage can include monitoring of infections, pain, temperature maintenance, mobility, urination/bowel movements, nutrition, and hydration (Table 2.1).

Table 2.1 The scope of perioperative care.[7]

Steps in perioperative care	Brief description
1. Preoperative basic health assessment and medication review	Health assessment includes: **1.** Medical history: indication for surgical procedure; allergies and intolerances to medications, anesthesia, or other agents; known medical problems; surgical history; trauma; current medications; focused review of issues pertinent to the planned procedure **2.** Physical examination: weight, height, and body mass index; vital signs—blood pressure, pulse (rate and regularity), respiratory rate, cardiac pulmonary, other pertinent exam
2. Medical conditions	Cardiovascular disease, sleep apnea, diabetes mellitus, chronic medication use, nicotine cessation
3. Antibiotic management	Antibiotic selection, prevention of Endocarditis, procedures in patients with previous total joint replacement, colorectal surgery, antibiotic administration
4. Patient education and communication	- Understanding patient's reading level, potential visual impairments, and learning barriers - Preoperative showering and shaving, preoperative fasting recommendations
5. Patient, procedure, and site verification	Preprocedure planning and preparation, scheduling
6. Surgical site marking with initials	Site marking by surgeon
7. Regional anesthesia techniques and verification process	Obtaining informed consent from the patient
8. Patient transported to intraoperative area using checklist (reverify patient identification)	- Final verification *This is the last step in the preoperative area before the patient is transferred to the operating/procedure room
9. Verify site marking/position patient/skin preparation/clipping	Skin preparation and hair removal
10. Prior to incision—active verbal time-out	- Time-out is performed after surgeon scrubbed and gowned and just prior to beginning the procedure - Each time-out includes the following elements: patient name, procedure to be performed, site of procedure, patient position

Continued

Table 2.1 The scope of perioperative care.[7]—cont'd

Steps in perioperative care	Brief description
11. Discrepancies	If a discrepancy is identified, the surgery will not take place until the discrepancy is resolved
12. Hard stop	If any part of the verification process was not followed or a discrepancy was identified, then the procedure will not continue until all steps of the verification process are completed and until the discrepancies have been resolved. The procedure may also be canceled and rescheduled
13. Reverify/pause if internal laterality/implants/ spine level	If procedure involves internal laterality, implants, or spine level, an intraoperative pause will be conducted
14. Safe site implementation	The time-out is best followed with a particular person/role has the responsibility to call the time-out. The surgeon should be the one to take the lead on initiating the time-out
15. Communication	Briefing, structured handoff for any surgical personnel changes, structured handoff process
16. Never events	Retained foreign objects—baseline count, if counts not reconciled then perform postoperative follow-up and perform delayed wound closure/open packing, final count; and retained foreign object prevention process, patient returns to operating/procedure room for final wound closure, hard stop—perform reconciliation process, imaging if counts not reconciled, close wound
17. Environmental	Normothermia planning and management, preventing fires in the OR/procedure room, general environmental concerns, environmental controls: operating/ procedure room survey
18. Follow-up appointments	Patients should be encouraged to schedule and keep all follow-up appointments with their surgeon and primary clinician

The prevalence of perioperative harm

Some studies have indicated that almost half of all adverse events are associated with surgeries.[10,11] In 2004, data collected from 56 countries indicated that the annual volume of major surgeries was estimated at 187−281 million operations.[12] In 2008, over 230 million operations were performed globally.[12] The Hospital Episode Statistics (HES) estimated that there were 11 million primary surgical procedures that were performed in the National Health System in 2015.[13]

The WHO predicted that significant surgical complications in industrialized countries were estimated at 3%−22% of surgeries, whereas the death rate was determined to be 0.4%−0.8%.[13−15] More than half of these adverse events were indicated to be preventable.[11,16] Recent studies in developing countries determine that the death rate in surgical care is anywhere from 5% to 10%.[17−19] Additionally, the rate of mortality associated with anesthesia can be as high as 1 in 150.[20] Furthermore, the WHO predicted that a 3% perioperative adverse event rate and a 0.5% mortality rate at the global level will yield to about 7 million patients with surgical complications and 1 million mortalities annually.[21]

Additionally, anesthesia complications continue to be one of the main causes of death globally. Almost 30 years ago, patients undergoing general anesthesia had an estimated 1 in 5000 chance of dying from anesthesia complications.[22] By implementing safe surgery best practices, the risk has decreased to 1 in 200,000 in industrialized countries. Unfortunately, the risk of anesthesia complications is 100 to 1000 times in developing countries, with mortality rates ranging from 1:3000 in Zimbabwe[23] to 1:500 in Malawi[24] (Table 2.2).

Patient safety initiatives to reduce perioperative harm

According to the Joint Commission on Accreditation of Healthcare Organizations, communication is the most common root cause of sentinel events.[25] Regardless of the numerous efforts that have been introduced to reduce and eliminate perioperative harm globally, there continues to be a gap in current clinical practices and evidence-based practices.

Many organizations have addressed miscommunication issues among their surgical teams by creating checklists and care pathways, while others have implemented new policies and prioritized the importance of open communication and reporting of adverse events throughout the perioperative period. However, in order for these patient safety initiatives to succeed, leadership must create a positive safety climate or culture in surgical departments.[26]

Delayed or inaccurate communication between healthcare providers negatively impacts patient care and ultimately leads to adverse events or medical errors. Evidence suggests that the timely transfer of accurate and relevant patient data, such as test results, complications, or consultations, can happen using handover/handoff tools.

Table 2.2 Prevalence rates for perioperative harm from the literature.

Study	Setting/ population	Findings	Lessons learned
Ghaferi AA, Birkmeyer JD, Dimick JB. Variation in hospital mortality associated with inpatient surgery. *N Engl J Med* 2009;**361**(14): 1368–75.	Data from American College of Surgeons National Surgical Quality Improvement Program include 84,730 patients undergone inpatient general and vascular surgery (2005–07)	- Hospital death rates: 3.5%–6.9% - Overall hospital complication rates: 24.6%–26.9% - Major complication rates in hospitals: 16.2%–18.2% - Mortality rates in hospitals: 12.5% –21.4%	- Essential to implement evidence-based practices to prevent complications - Critical to collaborate with intensive care unit (ICU) setting given that patients with high complications get transferred to the ICU - Timely recognition and management of patient complications - Importance of utilizing patient safety tools, such as checklists - Significance of understanding structural and organizational factors that lead to complications
Panagioti M, Khan K, Keers RN, Abuzour A, Phipps D, Kontopantelis E, et al. Prevalence, severity, and nature of preventable patient harm across medical care settings: systematic review and meta-analysis. *BMJ* 2019;**366**: l4185.	Systematic review and meta-analysis for certain databases from 2000 to 2019. 70 studies involving 337,025 patients were included in the meta-analysis	- Around 1 in 20 patients are exposed to preventable harm in medical care - One of highest pooled prevalence estimates of: (a) preventable patient harm reported in surgery (10%, 7%–13%) and (b) overall harm in surgery (20%, 14%–27%) (n = 6 studies)	- Preventable patient harm is a problem across all medical care settings - Essential to place a greater focus on advanced medical specialties, such as surgical units and ICUs, given that harm is immediate, serious, or has a cumulative impact on patients

Table 2.2 Prevalence rates for perioperative harm from the literature.—*cont'd*

Study	Setting/ population	Findings	Lessons learned
			- Important to build evidence across subspecialties, vulnerable populations, developing countries, and others - Strategies for avoiding preventable harm include identifying individual and organizational contributors to harm, technology utilized, clinical and administrative tasks associated with perioperative care - Essential to improve assessment and reporting standards to prevent harm
Anderson O, Davis R, Hanna GB, Vincent CA. Surgical adverse events: a systematic review. *Am J Surg* 2013; **206**(2):253−62.	Systematic review to quantify patient harm in surgery includes 14 studies with 16,424 surgical patients	- Adverse events occurred in 14.4% (12.5%−20.1%) of patients - Preventable adverse events occurred in 5.2% (4.2%−7.0%) - Consequences of 3.6% (3.1%−4.4%) of adverse events were fatal, of 34.2% (29.2%−39.2%) were moderate, and of 52.5% (49.8%−55.3%) were minor	- Errors in nonoperative management caused more frequent adverse events in comparison to errors that took place in surgical techniques

Continued

Table 2.2 Prevalence rates for perioperative harm from the literature.—*cont'd*

Study	Setting/ population	Findings	Lessons learned
Pearse RM, Moreno RP, Bauer P, Pelosi P, Metnitz P, Spies C, et al. Mortality after surgery in Europe: a 7 day cohort study. *Lancet* 2012;**380**:1059 −65.	- The European Surgical Outcomes Study (EuSOS) conducted a 7-day cohort period in 28 European countries in April 2011 with 46,539 patients - The objective of the study was to describe mortality rates and patterns of critical care resource use for noncardiac surgical patients	- Mean surgical mortality has reached 4% (n = 1855) - Mortality rates varied widely between countries: Iceland 21.5%, Latvia 16.9% −26.2%, the United Kingdom 0.44%, Finland 6.92%, and Poland 2.37% −20.27% - Poland, Latvia, Romania, and Ireland had higher mortality rates when compared to the United Kingdom—the country with the largest database (n = 10,630 patients) - 73% of patients who died were not admitted to critical care after surgery	- Wide variations in country mortality data indicate the need for strong and effective national and international strategies to improve care for surgical patients
Wang Y, Eldridge N, Metersky ML, Verzier NR, Meehan TP, Pandolfi MM, et al. National trends in patient safety for four common conditions, 2005 −11. *N Engl J Med* 2014;**370**(4): 341−51.	- Data extracted from medicare patient safety monitoring system (medical records) for 21 adverse events in 4372 hospitals across the United States from 2005 to 2011 - Total of 61,523 patients, with 16,481 patients requiring surgery	- Rates of in-hospital adverse events increased among the population requiring surgery	- Existing challenges with addressing harm in surgery - The need for more targeted patient safety interventions among surgical patients to reduce adverse events
Rutberg H, Risberg MB, Sjödahl R, Nordqvist P, Valter L, Nilsson L.	650-bed university hospital in Sweden—total of 960 medical records from 2009	- 271 adverse events identified in 197 patients - Adverse events were more	- Strengthen adverse event reporting systems - Healthcare systems should

Table 2.2 Prevalence rates for perioperative harm from the literature.—*cont'd*

Study	Setting/population	Findings	Lessons learned
Characterisations of adverse events detected in a university hospital: a 4-year study using the Global Trigger Tool method. *BMJ Open* 2014;**4**(5): e004879.	to 2012, where 48% were surgical cases	common in surgical care in comparison to medical care - 26% of patients who underwent surgical care had at least one adverse event - The most common type of adverse events was postoperative wound infections (40%)	adopt a portfolio of tools to prevent patient harm. Some include incident reporting and medical record review and analysis of patient claims
Macarthur DC, Nixon SJ, Aitken RJ. Avoidable deaths still occur after large bowel surgery. *Br J Surg* 1998;**85**:80–3	- Assessment of in-hospital deaths following large bowel surgery in Southeast Scotland (Royal College of Surgeons of Edinburgh)	- 187 deaths - Adverse events in 78 patients (42%) - 26 deaths (14%) following an anastomotic leak - 43 deaths (23%) occurred because surgery was delayed, initial diagnosis was delayed - Half of the patients who died in the study had identifiable deficiencies in their management	- The importance for greater consultant involvement with patients
Wanzel KR, Jamieson CG, Bohnen JM. Complications on a general surgery service: incidence and reporting. *Can J Surg* 2000;**43**: 113–7	- Complications for all patients admitted to the general surgery service at Wellesley Central Hospital (university-affiliated teaching hospitals) over a 2-month period	- 192 general surgery inpatients over 1277 patient-days from June 1996 to August 1996 - 75 patients (39%) suffered a total of 144 complications—2 complications were fatal, 10 were life threatening, 90 were moderate	- Surgical complications are common and underreported - Preventing complications is critical to improve quality of care and reduce costs - Hospitals should develop strategies to improve the recording and

Continued

Table 2.2 Prevalence rates for perioperative harm from the literature.—*cont'd*

Study	Setting/ population	Findings	Lessons learned
		severity, 42 were trivial - Of the 144 complications, 26 potentially led to a medical error - 112 of complications occurred during or after the surgery - 9 complications were not documented in progress notes, 115 were not presented at weekly M&M rounds, 95 were not documented	reporting of complications
McGuire HH, Horsley JS, Salter DR, Sobel M. Measuring and managing quality of surgery: statistical versus incidental approaches. *Arch Surg* 1992;**127**: 733–8	Retrospective study from 1977 to 1990 at the surgical service of the McGuire Veterans Affairs Medical Center, Richmond, VA; residents and surgeons who provided surgical care	- 44,603 major operations - 2428 patients suffered 2797 complications (6.3%) and 749 patients (1.7%) died - List of 48 common procedures with associated complication rates	- Reporting surgical complications and hospital infection rates is necessary to reduce patient harm - Multidisciplinary staff should discuss complications, hospital infections, and ways to detect/ anticipate patient diseases - Critical to review every case in which a patient has suffered any complication

Given that surgeries generally take place in hospitals, freestanding surgical centers, or healthcare providers' private clinics, successful perioperative care requires effective teamwork and communication between the surgeon, anesthesiologist, primary care physician, nurses, consultant, and other key members of the healthcare team. Open communication promotes learning within institution and improves patient outcomes, patient satisfaction, and patient safety culture. It allows healthcare providers within the surgical team to raise concerns, reflect, analyze, and collaborate to form guidelines and preventive measures.

The following list includes examples of communication tools that have been widely used in the perioperative process:

1. ERAS protocols
   The aim of ERAS pathways is to reduce the stress response to surgery and enable rapid patient recovery. Some studies have found that implementing ERAS protocols has reduced the length of stay and surgical complications after surgery.[27]
2. Standardized handoff communication tools
   A. Examples from other industries
      Several handoff tools have been developed by surgical teams to be used within the surgical department and in communicating with other departments, including intensive care. One organization has borrowed examples from aviation and racing through discussion with aviation captains and the Formula 1 motor racing teams.[28] As a result of implementing these handover tools, the number of technical errors was significantly reduced.
   B. SBAR Tool: Situation-Background-Assessment-Recommendation
      The SBAR tool has originally been developed for communication on submarines and has been adapted in healthcare by Kaiser Permanente of Colorado.[29] It provides a framework for communication among healthcare providers about the patient's condition. *Situation* offers a brief statement of the problem; *Background* provides information related to the problem and overall situation; *Assessment* includes an analysis of options for treatment; and *Recommendation* provides the action requested or recommendation for detailed treatment plan.
   C. Discharge Summary
      According to the Joint Commission on Accreditation of Healthcare Organizations, discharge summaries should be completed within 30 days and include the following elements: "the reason for hospitalization; significant findings; procedures performed and care, treatment, and services provided; the patient's condition at discharge; and information provided to the patient and family, as appropriate.[30]"
3. The World Health Organization (WHO) Surgical Safety Checklist[31]
   Evidence suggests that communication and teamwork failures are common in surgery. The use of a surgical safety checklist may help prevent errors, adverse events, and surgical complications. This checklist was created as part of the *Safe*

Surgery Saves Lives Program and aimed to ensure that 'never-events' will not occur in surgery. The goal of this 19-item checklist is to decrease medical errors and adverse events as well as increase teamwork and communication. Although the checklist has been effectively used by surgical teams globally and has shown a significant reduction in morbidity and mortality, some healthcare providers have been using the checklist to 'check the box' rather than being consistent and compliant. Hence, compliance with the checklist yields improved patient outcomes.

4. Medical Team Training (MTT)

   Some institutions have enrolled their staff in MTT as a result of the poor communication between surgeons, anesthesiologists, and nurses.[32] The MTT is a dedicated training session that includes didactic instruction, interactive participation, role-play, training films, and clinical vignettes.

Recommendations to advance perioperative practice

Although several global efforts have aimed to reduce perioperative harm, the problem continues to exist. Reducing patient harm in surgery will initially require implementing and closely monitoring an international patient safety agenda. The following list provides additional recommendations to reduce harm and advance surgical practice:

a. Reporting adverse events and medical errors that have occurred throughout the perioperative process is key to reducing patient harm. Many organizations have implemented electronic clinical safety reporting systems (CSRS), such as Safety Reporting System (SRS), UHC's Patient Safety Net (PSN), and others, that have captured a range of errors—from near misses to sentinel events. In order for complications to be accurately captured into these systems, leadership must create a strong organizational patient safety climate that empowers staff to speak up when errors occur.

b. National and global surveillance on morbidity and mortality rates in each of the perioperative phases is essential. The availability of surgical data and complication rates in both developed and developing countries is limited. Implementing surveillance systems will allow healthcare leaders and providers to identify and monitor system failures to reduce patient harm. Although some studies and organizations have attempted to collect surgical data, many of the data collection methods have not been standardized, which yields to a wide variation in results.

c. There should be a clear focus on communication and teamwork among the surgical team to avoid and reduce patient harm. Utilizing standardized and evidence-based communication tools will promote cooperation and collaboration among the team.

d. Surgical teams should support by leadership to develop and implement cost-effective and evidence-based strategies that could improve the quality of perioperative care and management.

e. While the adoption of new technologies (including drugs, devices, processes of care, procedures, or techniques) and computerized programs has helped healthcare providers to coordinate surgical care and document patient progress, there continues to be a gap in fully adopting these programs. In an effort to reduce patient harm, the surgical team should consider the best possible care for the patient, regardless of the technology being adopted. Moreover, it is essential for surgeons and institutions to fully assess the technology for efficacy and intended patient outcomes.[33]

f. It is critical for the entire surgical team to understand the full scope of each member, including the core knowledge, skills, and experience, expected of healthcare providers involved in perioperative care.[34] This will lead to improved communication, further collaboration, and transparency among all healthcare providers involved.

g. In order to reduce patient harm during the perioperative period, it will be beneficial for all healthcare providers involved to update and include new standards of care with a focus on long-term benefits associated with each surgical procedure.

h. Non-healthcare industries have shown that evidence of process improvements and the promotion of safety culture have a significant impact on an industry's safety records.[2] Establishing surgical protocols and checklists can improve the standards of training, practice, and perioperative surgical care.

i. The cost of surgical care is high, which can lead to challenges for some institutions and developing countries with limited resources, poor infrastructure and equipment, limited supply of experienced healthcare staff, and unreliable services. A global and national agenda that solely focuses on surgical care will help in addressing some of the costs associated with surgical care.

Although surgery can save many lives, there continues to be substantial harm in conducting surgical procedures. The following chapters will focus on raising the standards in surgical care, adopting patient safety strategies to reduce perioperative harm, and engaging leadership in eliminating patient harm.

References

1. Vincent C, Amalberti R. *Safer healthcare.* Cham: Springer International Publishing; 2016.
2. Calland JF, Guerlain S, Adams RB, Tribble CG, Foley E, Chekan EG. A systems approach to surgical safety. *Surg Endosc Other Interv Tech* 2002;**16**(6):1005−14.

3. Vincent C, Moorthy K, Sarker SK, Chang A, Darzi AW. Systems approaches to surgical quality and safety: from concept to measurement. *Ann Surg* 2004;**239**(4):475−82.
4. National Institute for Health and Care Excellence. NICE Guideline. *Perioperative care in adults final scope.* www.nice.org.uk/guidance.
5. Pearse RM, Holt PJ, Grocott MP. Managing perioperative risk in patients undergoing elective non-cardiac surgery. *Br Med J* 2011;**343**:d5759.
6. Spry C. *Essentials of perioperative nursing.* 3rd ed. Jones & Bartlett Publishers; 2005.
7. Card R, Sawyer M, Degnan B, Harder K, Kemper J, Marshall M, et al. Institute for clinical systems improvement. Perioperative protocol. Updated March 2014.
8. Grocott MP, Plumb JO, Edwards M, Fecher-Jones I, Levett DZ. Re-designing the pathway to surgery: better care and added value. *Perioper Med* 2017;**6**(1):9.
9. Melnyk M, Casey RG, Black P, Koupparis AJ. Enhanced recovery after surgery (ERAS) protocols: time to change practice? *Can Urol Assoc J* 2011;**5**(5):342.
10. Gawande AA, Zinner MJ, Studdert DM, Brennan TA. Analysis of errors reported by surgeons at three teaching hospitals. *Surgery* 2003;**133**(6):614−21.
11. Leape LL, Brennan TA, Laird N, Lawthers AG, Localio AR, Barnes BA, et al. The nature of adverse events in hospitalised patients. Results of the Harvard Medical Practice Study II. *N Engl J Med* 1991;**324**(6):277−384.
12. Weiser TG, Regenbogen SE, Thompson KD, Haynes AB, Lipsitz SR, Berry WR, Gawande AA. An estimation of the global volume of surgery: a modelling strategy based on available data. *Lancet* 2008;**372**(9633):139−44.
13. Gawande AA, Thomas EJ, Zinner MJ, Brennan TA. The incidence and nature of surgical adverse events in Colorado and Utah in 1992. *Surgery* 1999;**126**:66−75.
14. WHO Team. Integrated Health Services. In: *WHO guidelines for safe surgery.* 1st ed. Geneva: World Health Organization; 2008.
15. Kable AK, Gibberd RW, Spigelman AD. Adverse events in surgical patients in Australia. *Int J Qual Health Care* 2002;**14**:269−76.
16. Brennan TA, Leape LL, Laird NM, Hebert L, Localio AR, Lawthers AG, et al. Incidence of adverse events and negligence in hospitalized patients. Results of the Harvard Medical Practice Study I. *N Engl J Med* 1991;**324**:370−6.
17. Bickler SW, Sanno-Duanda B. Epidemiology of paediatric surgical admissions to a government referral hospital in the Gambia. *Bull World Health Organ* 2000;**78**:1330−6.
18. Yii MK, Ng KJ. Risk-adjusted surgical audit with the POSSUM scoring system in a developing country. *Br J Surg* 2002;**89**:110−3.
19. McConkey SJ. Case series of acute abdominal surgery in rural Sierra Leone. *World J Surg* 2002;**26**:509−13.
20. Ouro-Bang'na Maman AF, Tomta K, Ahouangbevi S, Chobli M. Deaths associated with anaesthesia in Togo, West Africa. *Trop Doct* 2005;**35**:220−2.
21. World Health Organization. *WHO guidelines for safe surgery 2009: safe surgery saves lives.* 2009. https://apps.who.int/iris/bitstream/handle/10665/44185/9789241598552_eng.pdf;jsessionid=0F49DC5B92C53C8BD18991C29958F78C?sequence=1. [Accessed March 2019].
22. Leape L. Error in medicine. *J Am Med Assoc* 1994;**272**:1851−7.
23. McKenzie AG. Mortality associated with anaesthesia at Zimbabwean teaching hospitals. *S Afr Med J* 1996;**86**:338−42.
24. Hansen D, Gausi SC, Merikebu M. Anaesthesia in Malawi: complications and deaths. *Trop Doct* 2000;**30**:146−9.

25. Joint Commission on Accreditation of Healthcare Organizations. *Sentinel events: Evaluating cause and planning improvement.* Oakbrook Terrace, IL: Joint Commission on Accreditation of Healthcare Organizations; 1998.
26. Makary MA, Sexton JB, Freischlag JA, Millman EA, Pryor D, Holzmueller C, Pronovost PJ. Patient safety in surgery. *Ann Surg* 2006;**243**(5):628.
27. Varadhan KK, Neal KR, Dejong CH, Fearon KC, Ljungqvist O, Lobo DN. The enhanced recovery after surgery (ERAS) pathway for patients undergoing major elective open colorectal surgery: a meta-analysis of randomized controlled trials. *Clin Nutr* 2010;**29**(4):434–40.
28. Catchpole KR, De Leval MR, McEwan A, Pigott N, Elliott MJ, McQuillan A, et al. Patient handover from surgery to intensive care: using Formula 1 pit-stop and aviation models to improve safety and quality. *Pediatr Anesth* 2007;**17**(5):470–8.
29. Kaiser Permanente of Colorado. *SBAR technique for communication: a situational briefing model.* 14 September 2005. http://www.ihi.org/IHI/Topics/PatientSafety/SafetyGeneral/Tools/SBARTechniqueforCommunicationASituationalBriefingModel.htm.
30. The Joint Commission. *Standard IM.6.10: hospital accreditation standards.* Oakbrook Terrace, IL: Joint Commission on Accreditation of Healthcare Organizations; 2006. p. 338–40.
31. WHO Surgical Safety Checklist. https://www.who.int/patientsafety/safesurgery/checklist/en/; 2009.
32. Awad SS, Fagan SP, Bellows C, Albo D, Green-Rashad B, De La Garza M, Berger DH. Bridging the communication gap in the operating room with medical team training. *Am J Surg* 2005;**190**(5):770–4.
33. Wilson CB. Adoption of new surgical technology. *BMJ* 2006;**332**(7533):112–4.
34. Grocott MPW, Pearse RM. Perioperative medicine: the future of anaesthesia? *Br J Anaesth* 2012;**108**:723–6.

Systems thinking in the operating room

3

Michael C. Grant, MD, MSE[1,2], Brendan L. Grant, MSE[3], Conrad J. Grant, MS[4]

[1]*Associate Professor, Department of Anesthesiology and Critical Care Medicine and Surgery, Johns Hopkins University School of Medicine, Baltimore, MD, United States;* [2]*Armstrong Institute of Patient Safety and Quality, The Johns Hopkins Medical Institutions, Baltimore, MD, United States;* [3]*General Dynamics Advanced Information Systems, Fairfax, VA, United States;* [4]*APL Chief Engineer, The Johns Hopkins Applied Physics Laboratories, Laurel, MD, United States*

Introduction

Background

The gap between the current and desired states of healthcare has been increasingly well established. There are a number of sobering statistics offered to illustrate that healthcare delivery falls short of proposed standards. Providing adequate (much less exceptional) healthcare poses an incredible challenge, not only due to the ever-increasing complexity of the patients and pathophysiology involved but also due to the mounting intricacy of the financial, infrastructural, and bureaucratic conditions that have been established along the way. In the early 2000s, the National Academy of Engineering and the Institute of Medicine (now known as the National Academy of Medicine) issued a joint report that called for broader application of engineering principles, shown to revolutionize other areas of industry, to the healthcare landscape.[1] This was followed more than a decade later by statements from both the President's Council of Advisors on Science and Technology and the Royal Academy of Engineering that recommended stronger collaboration between engineering and medicine to leverage expertise and experience in both disciplines to address deficiencies in healthcare delivery.[2,3] Unfortunately, meaningful applications that align engineers and medical professionals are still relatively uncommon in medicine.

Systems engineering and the operating room

Systems Engineering (SE) represents an opportunity to enhance interdisciplinary collaboration and improve upon the delivery of medical care.[4] SE involves the prospective design, implementation, integration, validation, management, and iteration of a system. In order to best illustrate how SE can be readily applied to medicine, we must first define a "system." The International Council of Systems Engineering provides the following definition[5]:

A system is a construct or collection of different elements that together produce results not obtainable by the elements alone. The elements, or parts, can include people, hardware, software, facilities, policies, and documents; that is, all things required to produce systems-level results. The results include system-level quali- ties, properties, characteristics, functions, behavior, and performance. The value added by the system as a whole, beyond that contributed independently by the parts, is primarily created by the relationship among the parts; that is, how they are interconnected.

Based upon this definition, a system is defined not only by its constituent parts (i.e., components) but also by the relationship that exists between those parts. Kos- siakoff and colleagues, in their text entitled *Systems Engineering Principles and Practice*, offer a more distilled version and state that a system is "a set of interrelated components working together toward some common objective."[6]

Traditionally, the term *system* has been applied to machines and/or technologies that require complex engineering to create an operational unit. This is evident in the case of a motor vehicle that requires hardware (i.e., vehicle frame, dashboard, bumper, wheels) to interact with one another through the supply of fuel, electricity, software, and human interface in order to achieve the outcome of transportation, among other functions. Importantly, the term is not limited to highly technological systems but can also reference organizational, procedural, or computational sce- narios. Based upon this latter consideration, numerous complex medical examples may apply, including patient-care pathways, perioperative programs, or even oper- ating rooms. An operating room is, in fact, a highly complex system in that it in- volves people (i.e., surgeons, nurses, anesthesiologists, patients), hardware (i.e., mechanical ventilator, monitors, surveillance equipment, computers), software, in- terfaces (i.e., screens, cameras, keyboards, microphones), and intricate processes (i.e., checklists, policies) that are interrelated and share a set of common objectives. In this fashion, much like SE can be leveraged to improve upon the design and implementation of a motor vehicle, the approach can provide a useful strategy to optimize the efficiency, functionality, and ultimately the outcome of an operating room as well. Simply stated, SE guides the creation of complex systems and can therefore be applied to the operating room to address a host of problems.

Systems engineering drivers

There are two primary drivers for redesigning an existing system: a deficiency in the performance of the current design, and/or the availability of new technology or methodology that can significantly improve outcomes when incorporated into the design. In the operating room context these drivers manifest themselves as follows:

1. *Deficiency in performance*—Perceived or realized the gap between current and desired system outcomes. This may refer to a system that fails to consistently meet certain standards or operates inefficiently (i.e., excessive cost or time). In

the operating room, this is represented by regular delays in procedure starts or room turnover times, failure to comply with performance standards such as sterilization or barrier technique, or even increased incidence of healthcare-associated conditions (i.e., surgical site infection, central line–associated bloodstream infection). Regardless, the existing system is unable to consistently achieve the established practice standards.

2. *Technological opportunity*—The development of new or updated technology is anticipated to improve existing performance. Examples in the operating room are plentiful in this regard and include new version anesthesia machines, echocardiography equipment, laparoscopic/robotic devices, alternate monitoring solutions, or an upgraded electronic medical record. The new technology provides the heightened capability to augment existing processes, improve diagnostic accuracy, or target a therapeutic window compared to that which is currently available.

Whether identifying a current deficiency or anticipating a future opportunity, the implication of utilizing SE to design the system is that the problem is highly complex and the solution will require some sensitivity and consideration for the impact on the entire system.[7] Certainly, no well-intentioned provider sets out to underperform and it is not uncommon for outcomes to be predetermined by the poor design of existing systems. Conversely, providers often expect that a new technology (i.e., electronic medical record) will immediately narrow performance gaps only to experience issues with poor integration into practice or negative impacts on the workflow that only exacerbate existing inefficiencies. It is in these scenarios that the use of SE can serve to optimize medical care by identifying these issues ahead of time and mitigating them through the prospective system design.

Systems approach

The Systems Approach, which has been recently described by Ravitz et al. in their manuscript entitled The Future of Healthcare through a Systems Approach, recommends collaboration between healthcare professionals and systems engineers to optimally design and implement healthcare systems solutions.[8] It contends that large, complex problems should be solved prospectively and systematically (as opposed to in a reactive and/or ad hoc fashion). As the authors state, this allows for a holistic, rather than a reductionist approach to complex problem-solving. Essentially, in order to develop a solution to a system problem, the whole system, instead of a narrow aspect of it, should be formally evaluated, redesigned, and validated.

To illustrate this point, consider a common problem for the operating room setting: lengthy operating room "turnover times," or excessive time between the conclusion of one procedure and the start of a subsequent one. Such delays are costly, contribute to poor provider morale, and can even impact the safety and quality of patient care. When evaluating the cause of such a delay, it is easy for an individual, depending upon their own limited perspective, to reflexively attribute the inefficiency to a specific provider, staff member, or even the patient himself or herself. As a result, it is common for solutions to require individuals to simply work harder, maintain a greater degree of vigilance, or complete assigned tasks more quickly.

The Systems Approach would prescribe an altogether different strategy for evaluating these delays. Aside from key bedside providers (i.e., nurses, physicians, advanced provider staff), assessment would be expanded to include less obvious participants in the care spectrum, including transport services, the preanesthesia holding area, patient registration, operating room environmental services, and more. Beyond personnel, existing workflow would be evaluated, along with unit and operating room policy, consent procedures, and interprovider communication patterns. The physical infrastructure, equipment, laboratory, monitoring resources, and information technology footprint would all potentially be incorporated into the analysis. At the end, the solution to delayed turnover would likely represent a composite of several (or numerous) systems interventions—which are likely underappreciated or go unnoticed altogether by a single individual without applying a Systems Approach to the solution.

Application of the Systems Approach, ultimately, is represented by: (a) Systems Thinking, a philosophical viewpoint, coupled with the (b) System Development Lifecycle, a framework for the development and implementation of system design/intervention.

Systems thinking

Systems Thinking suggests that complex problems and their associated solutions lay at the intersection between three systems-level dimensions: workflow, culture, and technology. This perspective recognizes that each operational environment incorporates a unique combination of these dimensions, and solutions that fail to account for each one of them are likely to be insufficient. Unfortunately, healthcare is replete with example solutions where at least one arm of the Systems Thinking triad is unaddressed.

Consider the following scenario, which illustrates some of the considerations incorporated into Systems Thinking. Recent advancements in technology have led to the development of noninvasive hemodynamic monitors. These monitors theoretically allow a provider to assess a patient's volume status using representative pressure waveforms derived from noninvasive blood pressure and plethysmography. The breakthrough technology allows for the differentiation between etiologies of blood pressure derangements, provides a point-of-care assessment and management, and potentially eliminates the need for invasive alternatives such as the use of arterial, central venous, or pulmonary catheterization. Based on these theoretical benefits, a reflexive response to the availability of such technology would be to deploy a full fleet of these monitors across a given operating room suite. However, there are a number of potential limitations to this response:

a. *Technology:* Whereas the monitor may represent a technological advancement, it also introduces additional challenges. These include the necessary integration of the monitor—either through automated or provider-based transcription—with the electronic medical record, surveillance and security of sensitive healthcare data, and mitigation of any discordance of monitor data with existing data and technologies (i.e., urine output, laboratory data, echocardiography). In this manner, the decision to insert a new technological "widget" is not an isolated decision and almost certainly impacts technologies/processes already set in place.

b. *Workflow:* This area is probably most clearly impacted by the introduction of a new technology. Aside from the necessary formal education of providers and staff, the supply chain must be assessed and updated to ensure for proper stocking, cleansing, servicing, and disposal of equipment. The operating room should be evaluated to ensure the monitor could be incorporated based on ergonomics and available physical space. Further, provider and staff will be directly impacted, whether positively through the rapid assessment and management of complex hemodynamics issues, or negatively by increasing the tasks to initiate/conclude procedures, troubleshoot the device, or divided/competing attention among other necessary workflow tasks.

c. *Culture:* Although less well defined than its counterparts, this dimension may well underpin success or failure to the greatest degree. Replacement of existing clinical norms is challenging unless facilitated by enthusiasm and acceptance by providers, staff, and administration. This is particularly true when current practice is familiar, easy to apply in the existing environment, and perceived to be superior to the alternative.

Therefore, a multifaceted implementation strategy centered on education, cost—benefit analysis, and sensitivity to existing norms is necessary.

Systems Thinking provides a perspective where solution teams recognize that systems solutions are successful when accounting for all three dimensions of the operational environment.

System development lifecycle

The theory behind Systems Engineering, particularly as it applies to healthcare, is that successful solutions to complex problems originate from teams who employ Systems Thinking as an overarching philosophical perspective and couple the approach with a systematic framework for the design and implementation of the system solution. This framework is referred to as the System Development Lifecycle (SDLC). As shown in Fig. 3.1, the SDLC is initiated when a key SE driver is identified, operating within the context of Systems Thinking. One might consider the SDLC to provide a "playbook" for the development and implementation of a

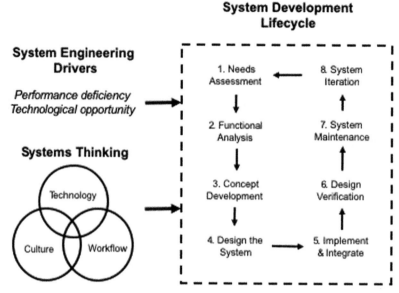

Schematic of the drivers, considerations and overview of the stages of development of solution systems.

complex solution (i.e., new system) to a given problem. The SDLC is comprised of a number of steps designed to facilitate the assessment of the problem, analysis of the existing system, design and implementation of a requisite solution, validation of the results, and eventual program iteration. Below, each phase of the SDLC is delineated, along with a brief synopsis of an individual SE tool commonly utilized to assist in that phase of development (Table 3.1).

Needs assessment

Based upon the initial SE driver, whether a performance deficiency or technological opportunity, the initial phase of the SDLC requires that you perform a baseline needs assessment. This phase is characterized by: (a) identifying the specific area(s) for desired improvement and (b) establishing the metrics for success. Essentially, it calls for the assessment of the current system and awareness of the desired one. In order to design system solutions, a needs assessment will identify the system metrics. Put simply, this step establishes the specific requirements that must be achieved in order to determine that the new system performs as it is intended.

Available Tools: A "gap analysis" compares and contrasts the current system with the desired one and quantifies the gap between the two. To aide in gap analysis, it is common to establish measures of performance (MOPs). These can include a host of potential measures in the operating room, including first case start times, case turnover rates, surgical block time utilization, overtime expenses, patient

Table 3.1 Phases of the system development lifecycle.

Phase	Description	Representative tool
Needs assessment	Identify areas of desired system improvement and establish metrics of performance for program/system success.	Measures of performance (MOP)
Functional analysis	Identify the resources, expertise, structure, and processes available in the current system and determine the functions necessary to meet the chosen system metrics.	Concept of operations (CONOPs)
Concept development	Assess a variety of alternative system designs and explore, define, and conceptualize the overall system solution.	Trade studies
Design the system	Define and articulate the functions, physical architecture, processes, and interfaces of the final system design. These are derived from knowledge gained from the initial phases of the SDLC.	Context diagrams
Implement and integrate	Incorporate new components, functions, and processes into the existing system. Integration should be sensitive to current culture, workflow, and any physical constraints.	N-squared (N^2) diagram
Design verification	Test and evaluation phase, whereby system performance is assessed using established metrics. Successful verification is contingent upon achieving desired results.	Prototyping
System maintenance	Scheduled and/or ad hoc maintenance to system components or processes. Assumes that systems require continuous upgrades and improvements to optimize efficiency and performance.	Run chart—dashboarding
System iteration	Repetitive process whereby the system is redesigned, reimplemented, and reassessed in a continuous or cyclical fashion. Assumes that there are always opportunities for improvement.	System development lifecycle

outcomes, etc. *These measures can serve as obvious and immediate metrics for success. Your team should intentionally select the MOPs upon which to base the new or updated system. As we will outline going forward, the remainder of the system design and implementation is informed by which metrics are initially selected.*

Functional analysis

Once a team has identified the key metrics or desired capabilities of the intended system, they need to perform a formal assessment of their current system functionality. The functional analysis phase determines what resources, expertise, structure, and processes are available and can be leveraged in the new system design. In addition, the functional analysis phase is an opportunity for the system design team to determine which functions are necessary to ultimately meet the metrics identified in the needs assessment phase. Per our previous example, if one desires to improve turnover efficiency, that metric must be broken down into its constituent parts. Case turnover includes safely transporting the patient from the operating room, collecting and storing case equipment, sterilizing the operating room, restocking necessary supplies and medications, accessioning subsequent case equipment, and so on. Each of these individual functions must be addressed in subsequent system solution in order to meet the desired metric of reducing turnover time. A solution that fails to address any one of these functions is, therefore, unlikely to succeed.

Available Tool: Traditional systems engineers often employ a Concept of Operations (CONOPs) to help articulate this phase.[9] A CONOPs is a conceptual drawing or schematic used to outline the basic functionality of the overall system based upon a given perspective. For example, a CONOPs of the operating room could outline the basics of case starts from the perspective of an anesthesiologist. It details, often through illustration, the steps necessary to bring a patient into an operating room and induce the anesthetic. This tool helps to provide appropriate context to the overall operations in place as well as emphasize their perspective in the setting. CONOPs often serve to identify key measures of performance that might be important to a specific participant role.

Concept development

Concept development, as the name describes, is where teams begin to explore, define, and conceptualize the overall system solution. Based upon the results of the needs assessment and functional analysis, there are a number of potential components that might be incorporated into the system design. Systems engineers will assess a variety of alternatives and select the individual aspects that are most likely to address the necessary requirements of the system. In essence, they are beginning the process of selecting the preferred system concept.

Available Tool: It is quite common for teams to utilize Trade Studies to compare and contrast various system components. Trade Studies break down components into individual characteristics and then assign them weights. For example, if you are interested in purchasing a certain type of vitals monitor for the operating room, you may assess the quality of the visual display, the tone and amplitude of the alarms, the interface characteristics, the power requirements, and its ability to integrate with your other hardware. Based upon your assessment of these individual characteristics and the emphasis (i.e., weight) you place on each characteristic, it is likely that one specific kind of monitor will outperform another. This comparison exercise is an example of a Trade Study. It helps to quantify and organize the assessment of potential components within your ultimate system design.

Design the system

At this stage, it is time to officially design the system. Based upon baseline requirements (i.e., measures of performance), existing functionality (i.e., concept of operations), and the results of conceptual development (i.e., trade studies), the actual system design can be derived. Here, you make final selection of individual components, define the processes through which they interact, and determine the overall system output. For the first time in the process, there is a clear sense of the appearance and functionality of the new system.

Available Tool: It is within this phase of the SDLC that context diagrams can be helpful. Context diagrams aide in the high-level design of systems by providing structure and articulating the constraints of the system design. Context diagrams are like "blue prints" in that they can show the physical interaction between parts of the system (i.e., the monitor attaches directly with the anesthesia machine) or they can inform the functional interactions (i.e., the monitor interfaces electronically with the anesthesia machine and captures relevant patient vitals data). Context diagrams help to provide, at a glance, a sense of system scope. They depict the entirely of the system and provide a mechanism for communication and more intricate system design.

Implement and integrate

Anyone who has attempted to transcribe the conceptual design into a fully realized product has encountered perhaps the most challenging phase of the SDLC. Implementation and integration of the updated system is a multifaceted exercise whereby new components of the system are integrated with existing ones. Often, this is realized through trial and error, whereby the updated system—derived from the system design phase—is deployed and tested to determine if it functions as intended. A classic example of system implementation and integration in healthcare is in the deployment of a new electronic health record (EHR). The EHR serves as a repository for patient health data, including laboratory data, images, and documentation, and it must therefore not only be integrated into all of the available provider terminals but also communicate with existing electronic financial, administration, and clinical infrastructure. It should integrate with available hardware, operate fluidly to capture real-time data in an increasingly dynamic clinical environment, and interface ergonomically enough to support (rather than impede) provider workflow. Each of these elements should be quantified and individually addressed during the implementation and integration of a novel EHR solution.

Available Tool: Integration challenges tend to stem from failure to recognize the challenges associated with interfaces between components. Whether those interfaces are physical (i.e., the mounting of a device on a piece of equipment), functional (i.e., how moisture, heat, and sound can impact the ability of a widget to operate properly), or process-based (i.e., one task cannot proceed without the complete of another), acknowledgment of interfaces is paramount to overall system success. The N-squared diagram, originally utilized the US space program, is a document that schematically articulates how individual subsystems/components interface with one another. It specifically outlines the nature of the interface and can even list the requirements necessary to achieve an optimal interface.

Design verification

This phase, also called Test and Evaluation, provides an opportunity to validate or assess the system solution. Metrics identified in the initial phases of development serve as a natural point of reference. Simply stated, the system is considered a success if it achieves the desired metrics. If the system was designed and implemented appropriately, then it should narrow the gap between desired and realized performance. Medicine is replete with a host of examples of design verification, including administrative measures such as length of stay, mortality, and cost or clinical outcomes such as healthcare-associated conditions, morbidity metrics, and quality of life. Any or all of these provide adequate footing for the assessment of the resulting system.

Available Tool: Although uncommon in healthcare, more traditional systems engineers in industry tend to utilize prototyping to verify aspects of their system design. Prototypes represent early models that share physical, functional, or operational characteristics with the final component. Prototypes can be incorporated into the system as a means to test components without requiring the final production to occur beforehand. This is advantageous because failures can lead to key modifications in design or prevent mass production of deficient components. This is also an opportunity for the practitioners to "test drive" the system in the presence of the development engineers to tailor it for its intended use and eliminate the risk of unintended impediments.

System maintenance

The SDLC is not complete at the point of design verification. A successful system cannot remain successful without ongoing system maintenance. This can be performed in either a scheduled or ad hoc basis. Scheduled maintenance requires that interval assessment be performed to determine that the system continues to perform at desired levels and that individual components meet their individual specifications. It is not uncommon for technology to become "outdated" or for new performance gaps to be identified. Regular interval maintenance is necessary to ensure a fully updated and functional system. In certain circumstances, an ad hoc maintenance is necessary. Individual components may malfunction (i.e., software glitch, wear and tear from mishandling) and require immediate maintenance to ensure the entire system functions properly. It is often the case that the majority of a system's lifecycle is spent in the maintenance phase with either scheduled or ad hoc improvements made to ensure a fully functional product.

Available Tool: It is commonplace in healthcare, particularly when discussing quality and patient safety, to assess data using a Run Chart. Essentially, a run chart expresses a data value plotted over time. A series of run charts, whereby individual endpoints (i.e., outcomes, length of stay, mortality) are expressed over time, can provide a dashboard to highlight relative successes and failures of a given program. It also allows for temporal relationships to be drawn from the data because points of inflection can be correlated with other system-level stressors/interactors (i.e., leadership changes, adoption of new policy, shift in patient payor mix).

System iteration

Regardless of the degree of system success, it is well understood that no solution is final. Systems do not exist in a vacuum, and therefore, additional performance deficiencies or new technology opportunities are constantly identified. Systems development is expressed as a lifecycle because consistent verification, assessment, and iteration are necessary to allow systems to remain relevant as constraints, resources, expertise, and policy evolve. Iteration is a repetitive process whereby the system is redesigned, reimplemented, and reassessed in a continuous fashion to ensure optimal performance and efficiency. This feedback loop is achieved by beginning the SDLC anew (Fig. 3.1).

Systems engineering through enhanced recovery programs

Although SE in healthcare remains in its relative infancy, there are several examples of perioperative solutions that stem from applying the SE conceptual framework. Enhanced Recovery Programs (ERPs) are one such example.[10] ERPs are bundled, evidence-based multifaceted care models that span the perioperative continuum.[11] These programs establish multidisciplinary teams, identify areas of poor clinical performance, select measures of clinical success, derive interventions from evidence-based literature, and systematically apply elements to improve the quality and safety of care.[12] When properly designed and implemented, ERPs are useful surrogates to the SE Approach and may provide an adequate point of reference for healthcare providers and SE experts to apply SE principles in the perioperative environment. As shown in Table 3.2, providers can utilize the SDLC to establish a

Table 3.2 Enhanced recovery programs and the system development lifecycle.

Phase	Example within enhanced recovery programs
Needs assessment	Institutions often adopt an ERP in response to underperforming on some key perioperative metric. Selected metrics include healthcare costs, major organ injury, or postoperative recovery times.
Functional analysis	ERPs will leverage existing resources including laparoscopic equipment, regional anesthesia, acute pain services, physical and respiratory therapy personnel, and nursing to outfit a formal program. In certain circumstances, recognition that these services or expertise are unavailable or underrepresented can help identify where to invest in program development.
Concept development	Providers utilize evidence-based guidelines to determine which care elements or interventions are included in a formal ERP. The decision to select a given medication or intervention is weighed against formulary restrictions, financial considerations, or other systems factors.

Continued

Table 3.2 Enhanced recovery programs and the system development lifecycle.—*cont'd*

Phase	Example within enhanced recovery programs
Design the system	After selecting the various interventions to include in an ERP, teams must organize the infrastructure (i.e., locations, people, processes, protocols) necessary to provide the key preoperative, intraoperative, and postoperative elements to outfit the program.
Implement and integrate	Certain facets of ERPs are subject to trial and error. Formulary restrictions, nursing workflow, electronic medical record issues, and more can impact the ability to perform any given pathway intervention. It may require redesigning, removal, or substitution of certain elements to fully integrate an ERP.
Design verification	After full implementation, program success is determined through the interval review of selected metrics. Reports in the form of dashboards can be helpful to inform ERP teams on overall progress.
System maintenance	ERPs are evolving programs that require regular evaluation. Updated evidence is made available through trial data, local practice patterns evolve, and unit protocols updates may require aspects of the program to be concomitantly updated.
System iteration	The goal of an ERP is to achieve its intended metric. At that point, subsequent performance deficiencies or technological opportunities inform ERP iteration.

system-level solution through the installation of an ERP for major surgery. ERPs are increasingly popular across the United States as a model for reducing unwanted variability in care, maximizing return on investment, hastening patient recovery, and mitigating the potentially harmful effects of inpatient care.

Conclusion

Medicine tends to select well-meaning, gifted providers who are trained in differential diagnosis, surgical intervention, and comparative science to address physical illness. The operating room represents a complex healthcare environment where care is often dictated by systems-level constraints that are regulatory, economic, technological, and procedural in nature. This poses a significant challenge to developing meaningful prospective solutions to deficient care. This chapter is written to introduce the healthcare provider to the basic vernacular and framework applied by systems engineers to methodically solve similarly complex problems. By recognizing that large-scale problems require a Systems Approach, multidisciplinary teams of healthcare providers—armed with skillsets derived from the field of—can apply Systems Thinking through the SDLC in collaboration with the systems engineers to achieve durable systems solutions.

References

1. National Academy of Engineering and Institute of Medicine. *Building a better delivery system: a new engineering/health care partnership*. Washington, DC: The National Academies Press; 2005. https://doi.org/10.17226/11378.

2. President's Council of Advisors on Science and Technology. *Report to the president—better health care and lower costs: accelerating improvement through systems engineering*. Executive Office of the President of the United State; 2014. https://obamawhitehouse.archives.gov/sites/default/files/microsites/ostp/PCAST/pcast_systems_engineering_in_health care_-_May_2014.pdf.

3. Royal Academy of Engineering. *Engineering better care: a systems approach to health and care design and continuous improvement*. 2017. London, https://www.raeng.org.uk/publications/reports/engineering-better-care.

4. Kopach-Konrad R, Lawley M, Criswell M, et al. Applying systems engineering principles in improving health care delivery. *J Gen Intern Med* 2007;**22**(Suppl. 3):431—7. https://doi.org/10.1007/s11606-007-0292-3.

5. https://www.incose.org/systems-engineering (accessed 08/January/2022).

6. Kossiakoff A, Sweet WN, Seymour SJ, Biemer SM. *Systems engineering principles and practice*. 2nd ed. Hoboken: Wiley-Interscience; 2011.

7. Tropello SP, Ravitz AD, Romig M, Pronovost PJ, Sapirstein A. Enhancing the quality of care in the intensive care unit: a systems engineering approach. *Crit Care Clin* 2013;**29**(1):113—24. https://doi.org/10.1016/j.ccc.2012.10.009.

8. Ravitz A, Grant MC, Grant C. The future of healthcare through a systems approach. *Syst Syst Eng* 2018;**8428781**:527—34.

9. Romig M, Tropello SP, Dwyer C, et al. Developing a comprehensive model of intensive care unit processes: concept of operations. *J Patient Saf* 2018;**14**(4):187—92. https://doi.org/10.1097/PTS.0000000000000189.

10. Grant MC, Galante D, Hobson D, Lavezza A, Friedman M, Wu CL, Wick EC. Optimizing an enhanced recovery program: development of a post-implementation audit tool and strategy. *Joint Comm J Qual Saf* 2017;**43**:524—33.

11. Grant MC, Isada T, Ruzankin P, Whitman G, Lawton JS, Dodd-o J, et al. Results from an enhanced recovery program for cardiac surgery. *J Thorac Cardiovasc Surg* 2020;**159**(4):1393—402 [Epub ahead of print].

12. Grant MC, PioRoda C, Canner J, Galante DJ, Sommer P, Hobson D, Gearhart S, Wu CL, Wick EC. The impact of anesthesia influenced process measure compliance on length of stay: results from an enhanced recovery after surgery (ERAS) for colorectal surgery cohort. *Anesth Analg* 2019;**128**:68—74.

Culture of safety

4

Paula S. Kent, DrPH, MSN, MBA, RN, CPPS

Patient Safety Specialist, Johns Hopkins Armstrong Institute for Patient Safety and Quality, Baltimore, MD, United States; Adjunct Faculty, Johns Hopkins, University School of Nursing, Baltimore, MD, United States; Associate Faculty, Johns Hopkins Bloomberg School of Public Health, Baltimore, MD, United States

Background

The concept of a healthy patient safety culture in the perioperative setting embraces a number of critical concepts for healthcare practitioners including: recognition of organizational vulnerability in the provision and sustainability of safe patient care; acknowledgment that reporting of patient safety events and near misses relies on a supportive environment; support for staff at all levels to work through identification and analysis of defects, as well as development of system fixes; and organizational support for the infrastructure and resources to address safety events and culture (AHRQ online).[1] These cross many facets of healthcare including perioperative, inpatient, ambulatory, and critical care settings.

When *To Err is Human* was published in 2000 by the Institute of Medicine (IOM), now the National Academy of Medicine, it was the first time that the number of deaths associated with medical error was actually quantified. Healthcare leaders and researchers were confronted with the glaring dilemma of how 44,000–98,000 deaths per year could happen as a result of apparently preventable adverse events.[2] Improving the culture of safety is no longer optional but a focus of many well-established healthcare organizations in the United States. In 2009, the Joint Commission (JC) published a white paper describing leadership standards addressed by the JC. Leadership Standard LD.03.01.01 states that "leaders create and maintain a culture of safety and quality throughout the hospital." A particular element of performance addresses that leaders must evaluate the culture of safety and quality using valid and reliable tools."[3]

Several tools used to assess clician perceptions of safety culture are available in the public domain, including the Safety Attitudes Questionnaire (SAQ) and the Hospital Survey on Patient Safety (HSOPS).[4,5] In 2010, the National Quality Forum published a paper presenting 34 practices that demonstrate effectiveness in reducing the occurrence of adverse healthcare events. Safe Practice #2 addresses culture measurement, feedback, and intervention (Fig. 4.1).[6]

Safe Practice	Practice Statement
Safe Practice #2: Culture Measurement, Feedback, and Intervention	Healthcare organizations must measure their culture, provide feedback to the leadership and staff, and undertake interventions that will reduce patient safety risk

FIGURE 4.1

Safe Practice #2. National Quality Forum Safe practices for better healthcare—2010 update. 2010.

Retrieved from https://www.jointcommission.org/assets/1/18/WP_Leadership_Standards.pdf.

In 2015, the National Patient Safety Foundation issued a report examining patient safety over the years since the IOM published *To Err is Human*.[2] This report calls for a systems approach to achieve patient safety and a culture of safety in order to combat this significant area of concern. Recommendations in this report include support for the healthcare workforce and assurance that leaders would establish and sustain a safety culture.[2] We now have established requirements that leaders will measure, evaluate, and sustain a culture of safety, in addition to providing feedback and implementing action plans that are intended to reduce harm and risk. The JC has further identified 11 tenets that reflect the significance of safety culture and how patient harm is prevented (The Joint Commission—see Table 4.1).[7]

Definitions

Before we discuss these safety culture tenets, let's review several of the notable safety culture definitions. Safety culture in healthcare has been defined and studied as patient safety has evolved as a field in healthcare. The Association of periOperative Registered Nurses (AORN) believes that all healthcare personnel should strive toward a culture of safety. The AORN Guidance Statement defines safety culture as "a mindset centering on shared values, attitudes, or beliefs within an organization" and references communication, team, trust, resiliency, work flow, informed culture, and strong surgical team member relationships.[8] Edgar Schein, a much quoted leader in organizational culture and development, and a former professor at the MIT Sloan School of Management, has devoted much time and focus to work in organizational culture and the various subcultures. This work has supported his definition of culture as "a pattern of shared basic assumptions learned by a group as it solved its problems of external adaptation and internal integration ...." It can also be described as a "product of joint learning."[9] Pellegrini describes safety culture is the sum of what an organization does to provide optimal patient care.[10] The Patient Safety Systems (PS) chapter of The Joint Commission accreditation manuals defines safety culture as "the product of individual and group beliefs, values, attitudes, perceptions, competencies, and patterns of behavior that determine the organization's commitment to quality and patient safety."[1]

Table 4.1 11 tenets of a safety culture.

Number	Tenets
#1	Apply a transparent, nonpunitive approach to reporting and learning from adverse events, close calls, and unsafe conditions.
#2	Use clear, just, and transparent risk-based processes for recognizing and distinguishing human errors and system errors from unsafe, blameworthy actions.
#3	CEOs and all leaders adopt and model appropriate behaviors and champion efforts to eradicate intimidating behaviors.
#4	Policies support safety culture and the reporting of adverse events, close calls, and unsafe conditions. These policies are enforced and communicated to all team members.
#5	Recognize care team members who report adverse events and close calls, who identify unsafe conditions, or who have good suggestions for safety improvements. Share these "free lessons" with all team members (i.e., feedback loop).
#6	Determine an organizational baseline measure on safety culture performance using a validated tool.
#7	Analyze safety culture survey results from across the organization to find opportunities for quality and safety improvement.
#8	Use information from safety assessments and/or surveys to develop and implement unit-based quality and safety improvement initiatives designed to improve the culture of safety.
#9	Embed safety culture team training into quality improvement projects and organizational processes to strengthen safety systems.
#10	Proactively assess system strengths and vulnerabilities, and prioritize them for enhancement or improvement.
#11	Repeat organizational assessment of safety culture every 18–24 months to review progress and sustain improvement.

- The Joint Commission
- See Sentinel Event Alert Issue 57, "The essential role of leadership in developing a safety culture," for more information, resources, and references.

I really like the use of a definition of culture previously used by the Health and Safety Commission (HSE) in Great Britain (1993).[3] The HSE defined safety culture as "the product of individual and group values, attitudes, perceptions, competencies, and patterns of behavior that determine the commitment to, and the style and proficiency of, an organization's health and safety management." We now know that culture signals organizational priorities, defines behavioral norms, and influences employee attitudes and perceptions. We also know that safety culture shapes behaviors, attitudes, and motivation on the job. Safety culture can also be referred to as the importance of safety relative to other goals. The HSE further reported that organizations with a positive safety culture are based on mutual trust and shared perceptions of the importance of patient safety. Research has proven this over time.

Establishing a perioperative culture of safety is important, and research has demonstrated positive associations with clinical outcomes. Evidence shows that there are both improved clinical outcomes such as decreased central line—associated infections and human resource outcomes such as decreased nursing turnover rates, when there are improved teamwork and safety climate scores.[3,6,11–17] In many cases, research has found that when central line—associated blood stream infections, ventilator-associated pneumonia in the intensive care unit, and surgical site infections decrease, then the overall length of stay and mortality are reduced. Assessing the culture of safety and generating data and reports are certainly important for our staff and leadership in perioperative work settings. However, while data are valuable, the debriefing process transforms data into information. Debriefing is also known to accelerate improvement. Vigorito et al.[18] found that units using a semistructured debriefing of the safety culture assessment survey achieved a 10.2% reduction in infection rates, while units who did not debrief survey results accomplished only a 2.2% reduction. Work settings that leverage their strengths and focus on improvement efforts with culture check-ups will generally demonstrate sustainable culture score improvements in subsequent survey administrations. Any perioperative setting would welcome the opportunity to maintain a healthy patient safety culture and demonstrate improvements between each survey administration.

Although we have reviewed a number of safety culture definitions, a common definition is "the set of norms, values, perceptions and beliefs that govern behavior and ultimately outcomes."[19–21] Dov Zohar et al. defined the concept of safety climate as "representing shared employee perceptions of the priority of safety at their unit and the organization at large, especially in situations where safety competes with other performance facets such as care speed or its quality."[19] Paine et al. (2010) described the measurement of culture through long-term observations by anthropologists, and the measurement of climate by employee assessments of work-related norms. Many refer to climate when referring to patient safety survey results.[22]

Tenets of safety culture

Let's review the 11 tenets of safety culture defined by the JC with a focus on the perioperative setting (Table 4.1).[7] The first tenet we will address is "Apply a transparent, nonpunitive approach to reporting and learning from adverse events, close calls and unsafe conditions." This is particularly valuable in the perioperative setting. When OR staff—nurses, providers, and surgical technicians—are encouraged to report adverse and almost events, organizational leadership may be optimistic that both actual and almost events will be captured by the event reporting system. However, even with transparency and a nonpunitive approach, event reporting is voluntary and cannot be used to measure patient safety or error rates.[10] In the ideal safety world, the event reporting system should be accessible to everyone in the perioperative setting with nonpunitive support by all levels of personnel including providers, nurses, surgical techs, and associates. Leadership support of patient safety event reporting is an essential component of a healthy safety culture. The healthiest safety cultures recognize the value of identifying safety defects and proactively working toward prevention of harm. In some organizational cultures, however, it remains difficult to report errors and almost events without encountering sensitivity or fear of reprisal.

Another tenet of safety culture identified by the JC is the use of "clear processes to recognize and distinguish human errors and system errors from unsafe and blameworthy actions." Perioperative settings are frequently challenged by this tenet due to the complexity of care delivery in and around the operating rooms. Adverse events in any environment are difficult to identify in real time and distinguishing between human error and system error requires detail, a defined process, and consistency. Staff need to feel confident that reporting patient events is supported and leadership needs to have a clear definition of accountability. In many healthcare settings, this atmosphere has established a new focus on just culture. In 2010, the American Nurses Association published a white paper on the Just Culture concept and its application in healthcare. The Just Culture model requires establishing managerial competencies that hold individuals accountable for their mistakes and investigates the behavior that led to the mistake being made.[23,24]

A third tenet of a safety culture relies on confirmation of organizational trust and the modeling of appropriate behaviors throughout the organization, including leaders and CEOs. In this tenet, "CEOs and all leaders adopt and model appropriate behaviors and champion efforts to eradicate intimidating behaviors." Disruptive behavior, for example disrespectful communication in the operating rooms, has been found to inhibit essential elements of teamwork with a negative patient impact. When leadership models and sustains the expected staff behaviors of respect and trust, frontline perioperative staff are much better positioned to expect and demonstrate the same behaviors. Some breakdowns are known to occur when leadership claims to talk the talk, but fails to walk the walk. One critically important outgrowth of perioperative safety culture improvement has been the recognition of safety-related feedback and maintaining accountability for our culture.

A fourth tenet of safety culture is the consistent communication and enforcement of all organization policies that support patient safety culture and adverse event reporting. This should not be limited to simply "perioperative policies" but should embrace organization policies including any work setting where patients and families may connect to the perioperative arena or other aspects of the care delivery system. Patients and families alike identify that they feel the impact of and fully recognize the number of transitions of care their loved ones are transferred through every day. They also feel the stress, just as we do as care providers, when these transitions are not smooth or adequately supported. Our perioperative policies must support a safety culture and the reporting of adverse events.

A fifth tenet of safety culture is the recognition of healthcare team members who report adverse events, whether they are significant, near misses, simply unsafe condition accounts, or offer suggestions for safety improvements. In the "good catch" category where adverse events are avoided, leaders are encouraged to share lessons learned with all team members, closing the loop, and spreading the learning. There are a number of ways that safety issues can be shared with those who have taken the effort to report them including:

(1) A "close the loop" feature of the event reporting system
(2) All staff meetings (often weekly or monthly)
(3) Huddles (often at the beginning of the shift or OR case)
(4) Bulletin or Communication Boards (often in the break room or location with less visibility for patients and families, but accessible to staff and faculty)

The Joint Commission Center for Transforming Healthcare's Safety Culture project found that staff continued reporting events and making suggestions when they were recognized and experienced shared follow-up.

A sixth tenet of safety culture covers the determination of a baseline measure on safety culture for the organization and individual work settings or units. These surveys query staff and providers to rate the safety culture in their perioperative setting and in the organization as a whole, following a series of questions that can be grouped into five to eight themes, such as teamwork within units and transitions of care. Although there are a number of tools that will measure safety culture performance, two validated tools in the public domain are widely used:

(1) Hospital Survey on Patient Safety Culture (HSOPS)
(2) Safety Attitudes Questionnaire (SAQ)

In measuring safety culture, it is important to determine the appropriate work setting groupings for the survey administration. Any change in organizational culture is noted first at the local level for individual work settings, not at the overall organization score. In fact, in the perioperative setting, it is particularly important to distinguish between specialized OR and perioperative settings, given those cultures are likely to be uniquely different in the makeup of staff and demonstrated culture results. These factors should help leadership to identify all staff in that setting that would be administered the survey so it reflects the culture of that perioperative area.

A seventh tenet describes the importance of analyzing safety culture survey results from across the organization focusing on opportunities for quality and safety improvement. As critically important it is to analyze data at the local level, it is also important to look at the big picture across the organization and perioperative settings. Once the survey results have been reported back to leadership, it is helpful to consider these next steps listed in Table 4.2. Data must be debriefed at all levels of the organization to be of value. Often times, the significant aspects of the culture have changed between one survey administration and the next, since they may be as far apart as every 18—24 months. The debriefing process should take place soon after the results are available, allowing for time then to develop an action plan and implement or influence needed changes. This will be critical in providing an opportunity for staff to effect a change in culture, taking place at the local level of an organization, prior to the next survey administration.

Table 4.2 Safety culture debriefing steps.

Steps	Safety culture debriefing
#1	Review data at the organization and local work setting levels. Consider whether there are any trends or trajectories up or down, and if any are consistent or being sustained over time.
#2	Share data with local leadership. Ensure that any historical trends are also identified.
#3	Support processes for frontline staff at the local level to validate the reported results and identify areas of concern. These staff are generally the subject matter experts (SMEs) and simply need guidance and support in determining next steps.
#4	Set expectations. The culture assessment survey should be completed by as many staff as possible, within each work setting. Most organizations aim for unit level and organization wide response rates of 50%–80%. This number is likely to provide results that are considered representative of the staff. Set expectations also for the outcomes expected for the work setting debriefings, action plans, and improvement efforts.
#5	Share survey results with all levels of staff, including anyone who took the time to complete the survey. Debriefing of the results helps direct the data into information that can be used for patient safety improvement efforts.
#6	Support processes for frontline staff at the local level to validate the reported results and identify areas of concern. These staff are generally the SMEs and simply need guidance and support in determining next steps.
#7	Analyze safety culture survey results from across the organization to find opportunities for quality and safety improvement.
#8	Work setting—specific action plans should be supported and led by organization leaders.

An eighth tenet of safety culture is the development of work setting—specific patient safety and quality improvement action plans designed to improve the culture of safety. These may be aligned with organization mission and priorities but should focus on the areas that frontline staff identify as their priority and primary areas of concern. Examples are described in Table 4.2. One of the most important ways an organizations can affect a change in culture is to focus on themes that are important to the frontline staff and can actually impact a culture change over time. Even something as simple as communicating results of the survey for all staff involved, once they are available for dissemination, are important to ensure take place.

The ninth tenet of patient safety addresses the need to embed safety culture team training into our organizational quality improvement projects and organizational processes to strengthen safety systems already in place. Evidence shows that team training derived from evidence-based work, such as the TeamSTEPPS program supported by the Agency for Healthcare Research and Quality, has been successful in the improvement of team performance, particularly in areas of high acuity or stress.[25] Many work areas such as the organization's operating rooms, perioperative settings, and emergency departments can benefit from developing team performance for our established work teams and those created for emergency response or intervention. We benefit as staff and as patients when our perioperative teams become more patient focused with support from their team members. This will inherently lead to improved team performance in almost every situation.

A proactive assessment can be instrumental in preventing harm in the perioperative work setting, and most would agree, in any work setting throughout healthcare. This is the 10th tenet of safety culture and utilized by many disciplines in healthcare including risk management, patient safety, pharmacy, medicine, and nursing.[25] The JC has embraced a theoretical framework that establishes safety culture as one of the keys to high reliability. This framework holds "safety culture, leadership, and robust process improvement as three domains that are critical to high reliability within a heath care organization."[26] The proactive assessment is value-added when the team considers strengths and areas of high risk and establishes a priority for further investigation, and development of an improvement plan that can be supported or sustained by the organization.

The 11th and final feature in our list of safety culture tenets is the support of administering a safety culture assessment every 18–24 months in order to assess culture, analyze trends, review progress, and determine whether improvements have been sustained over time. Some critical components in this tenet of safety culture include the following:

(1) Assessments should be made at the local work setting level. In the perioperative department, this may include individual OR services, prep, and recovery areas being established as specific work settings. This could be a challenge since many staff including surgical faculty, attending physicians, nurses, and technicians may work across service lines and support OR services in multiple areas of the OR.

(2) Assessments must include the follow-up described in Table 4.2. If we fail to look at how the data are presented, showing where a particular OR service was 2 years ago, and the significant strides they have made in the past year, we may lose the opportunity to highlight a best practice or showcase an intervention that worked for patient safety improvement. Our work teams need to have data reported back for their local setting, be provided with the opportunity to validate the results, and be encouraged to develop an action item that will support an improvement based on their local culture. It is in this way, that their data become information with value.

In summary, perioperative leadership can work toward a safety culture of high reliability when staff are respected as clinical experts and there is a core attribute of trust. The JC has a framework that embraces safety culture, leadership, and robust process improvement as three areas critical to high reliability.[26] When survey data are shared and validated by staff and the team develops an action plan to affect a change toward patient safety improvement, staff respect the process (see Table 4.3 for examples of perioperative quality and safety improvement initiatives). This level

Table 4.3 Examples of perioperative quality and safety improvement initiatives.

Perioperative safety issue	Patient safety improvement initiative
#1—Communication issue	When a new process or concept is introduced, it will be communicated to staff in a number of different ways including: (1) staff meeting, (2) shift huddles, (3) individual meetings, and (4) posted on Communication Board. Measurement will be assessed by anecdotal evidence and improvement in Patient Safety Culture Assessment in the next survey. Anecdotal evidence will include staff explaining what they heard, describing the expectations, and interpreting their understanding of the new concept or process.
#2—Handoffs and transitions	The team will focus on Handoffs and Communication by creating a standardized readiness tool for prep to use for patients going to the OR. The team will also develop and implement a standardized OR to PACU handoff tool. Both tools will be piloted. The team will also review posting opportunities for necessary surgical equipment postings.
#3—Teamwork and a lack of coordination issue	Our team will work with nursing leadership to pair junior residents with OR nurses for a week at a time so that they work together in the OR for the entire week. We think this will help build relationships between our residents and the nurses in the OR, foster collegiality and a spirit of teamwork, and help improve patient safety by making everyone feel comfortable speaking up if they have a concern.
#4—Exhaustion	We plan to update new hire preceptor roles to help increase support for new staff. This will need to include an equipment day of training for new staff to help them learn equipment before going to units. We will also consider adding staff for high need hours on nights.
#5—Handoffs and transitions	We must implement a briefing at the end of a case: (1) determine as a group the minimum standardized handoff content relevant to facilitating care to the next phase to include items such as procedure completed, specimens, local administration, etc. (2) To trial/implement this tool to improve handoffs during transitions of care.

of trust is supported when organizations use their safety culture data for prevention of harm and team members are respected for their input and contributions to care. High reliability is a desired state in our perioperative culture, just as it is in the aviation industry. Perioperative hospital settings can establish a culture of safety and make significant progress toward high reliability by assuming these tenets of safety culture. Leadership is clearly essential in determining these priorities and clearly communicating these messages with staff at all levels.

References

1. AHRQ, Retrieved from https://psnet.ahrq.gov/primers/primer/5/Culture-of-Safety.
2. Kohn LT, Corrigan JM, Donaldson MS, editors. *To err is human: building a safer health system: the Institute of Medicine Report.* Washington, D.C.: National Academy Press; 2000.
3. The Joint Commission. *Leadership in healthcare organizations, a guide to joint commission leadership standards.* A Governance Institute White Paper; 2009. Retrieved from: https://www.jointcommission.org/assets/1/18/WP_Leadership_Standards.pdf.
4. Sexton JB, Helmreich RL, Neilands TB, Rowan K, Vella K, Boyden J, Roberts PR, Thomas EJ. The safety attitudes questionnaire: psychometric properties, benchmarking data, and emerging research. *BMC Health Serv Res* 2006. Retrieved from, https://bmchealthservres.biomedcentral.com/articles/10.1186/1472-6963-6-44.
5. Etchegaray JM, Thomas EJ. Comparing two safety culture surveys: safety attitudes questionnaire and hospital survey on patient safety. *BMJ Qual Saf* 2012. Retrieved from, https://www.ncbi.nlm.nih.gov/pubmed/22495098.
6. National Quality Forum. *Safe practices for better healthcare—2010 update.* 2010. Retrieved from, https://www.jointcommission.org/assets/1/18/WP_Leadership_Standards.pdf.
7. The Joint Commission. *Sentinel event alert, the essential role of leadership in developing a safety culture, issue 57.* 2017.
8. AORN. AORN guidance statement: creating a patient safety culture. *AORN J: Off Voice Perioperative Nurs* 2006;**83**(4). Retrieved from, https://aornjournal.onlinelibrary.wiley.com/doi/full/10.1016/S0001-2092(06)60012-4?sid=nlm:pubmed.
9. Kent P, Outten K. *Publication in progress.* 2019.
10. Pellegrini CA. Leadership is crucial to establishing safety culture, reducing adverse events. In: *Bulletin of the American College of Surgeons*; 2017. Retrieved from, http://bulletin.facs.org/2017/05/leadership-is-crucial-to-establishing-safety-culture-reducing-adverse-events/.
11. Pronovost P, Needham D, Berenholtz S, et al. An intervention to decrease catheter-related blood stream infections in the ICU. *N Engl J Med* 2006;**355**:2725−32.
12. Pronovost PJ, Goeschel CA, Colantuoni E, et al. Sustaining reductions in catheter-related bloodstream infections in Michigan intensive care units: an observational study. *Br Med J* 2010;**340**:c309.
13. Berenholtz SM, Pham JC, Thompson DA, et al. An intervention to reduce ventilator-associated pneumonia in the ICU. *Infect Control Hosp Epidemiol* 2011;**32**(4):305−14.
14. Lipitz-Snyderman A, Steinwachs D, Needham DM, et al. Impact of a statewide intensive care unit quality improvement initiative on hospital mortality and length of stay: retrospective comparative analysis. *Br Med J* 2011;**342**:d219. https://doi.org/10.1136/bmj.d219.
15. AHRQ. AHRQ patient safety project reduces bloodstream infections by 40 percent. Retrieved January 29, 2013 from http://www.ahrq.gov/news/press/pr2012/pspclabsipr.htm.
16. Waters HR, Korn Jr R, Colantuoni E, et al. The business case for quality: economic analysis of the Michigan Keystone Patient Safety Program in ICUs. *Am J Med Qual* 2011;**26**(5):333−9.

17. Wick EC, Hobson D, Bennett J, et al. Implementation of a surgical comprehensive unit-based safety program (CUSP) to reduce surgical site infections. *J Am Coll Surg* 2012;**215**(2):193−200.
18. Vigorito MC, McNicoll L, Adams L, Sexton B. Improving safety culture results in Rhode Island ICUs: lessons learned from the development of action-oriented plans. *Joint Comm J Qual Patient Saf* 2011;**37**(11):509−14.
19. Zohar, et al. Healthcare climate: a framework for measuring and improving patient safety. *Crit Care Med* 2007;**35**(4):1312−7.
20. Singer S, Lin S, Falwell A, et al. Relationship of safety climate and safety performance in hospitals. *Health Serv Res* 2009;**44**:399−421.
21. Schein EH. *Organizational culture and leadership: a dynamic view*. San Francisco: Jossey-Bass; 1992.
22. Paine LA, et al. Assessing and improving safety culture throughout an Academic Medical Centre: a prospective cohort study. *BMJ Qual Saf Healthc* 2010;**19**:547−54.
23. Marx D. Patient safety and the "just culture": a primer for healthcare executives. In: *"Prepared by David Marx, JD, for Columbia University under a grant provided by the National Heart, Lung, and blood Institute"*; 2001.
24. ANA Congress on Nursing Practice and Economics and the Board of Directors. *Position statement on just culture*. 2010. p. 1−7.
25. Thomas L, Galla C. Building a culture of safety through team training and engagement. *BMJ Qual Saf* 2013;**22**:425−34.
26. Chassin MR, Loeb JM. High-reliability health care: getting there from here. *Milbank Q* 2013;**91**(3):459−90.

Further reading

1. Schein, E., Retrieved from https://thehypertextual.com/2013/01/17/edgar-schein-organizational-culture-and-leadership/.
2. Timmel J, Kent PS, Holzmueller CG, et al. Impact of the comprehensive unit-based safety program (CUSP) on safety culture in a surgical inpatient unit. *Joint Comm J Qual Patient Saf* 2010;**36**(6):252−60.
3. Pham JC, Girard T, Pronovost PJ. What to do with healthcare incident reporting systems. *J Public Health Res* 2013;**2**(3):e27. Retrieved from, https://www.ncbi.nlm.nih.gov/pmc/articles/PMC4147750/pdf/jphr-2013-3-e27.pdf.

Dynamics of surgical teams

5

Thomas L. Matthew, MD, MS [1], Diane Alejo, BA [2]

[1]*Cardiothoracic Surgery, Johns Hopkins School of Medicine. Director Johns Hopkins Cardiothoracic Surgery at Suburban Hospital, Bethesda, MD, United States;* [2]*Division of Cardiac Surgery, Johns Hopkins University School of Medicine, Baltimore, MD, United States*

This important topic is evolving daily in operating rooms (ORs) around the world. Patients are living longer because of complex operations performed on a routine basis. Older and sicker patients are being treated. The margin for error to achieve excellent outcomes is smaller than ever before. Yet results are good and improving. This is largely due to teams working in a unified and coordinated fashion year after year.

There is evidence that surgical outcomes including quality and safety are largely related to teamwork including nontechnical skills of communication, collaboration, and coordination of care. Better teamwork is associated with fewer errors.[1,2]

Surgery is a team sport with outcomes depending on multiple players performing their roles both independently and in unison. A smooth operation means fewer postoperative problems and better outcomes. This includes morbidity and mortality.

As primarily a cardiac surgeon, I will use examples from cardiovascular surgery to discuss the dynamics of surgical teams. Cardiac surgery is particularly dependent on teamwork. It is a highly precise group of processes with many steps, and steps within steps. It requires decision-making and action with little margin for error. All of this is done under significant time constraint.

The cardiopulmonary bypass circuit used to maintain perfusion has fewer deleterious effects with shorter pump times. The longer the pump run, the greater the negative consequences. This puts all cardiac surgeons on a time clock to perform highly skilled intricate processes.

Teamwork makes efficiency and safety possible. Under time constraint a well-practiced team will perform complex processes more efficiently. Cardiac surgery often looks like a dance with many people moving in concert. Minor workflow disruptions are common. Most do not affect the outcome. However, as minor disruptions increase in frequency, operative performance is reduced, increasing the operative duration. In addition, the accumulation of minor problems also reduces the surgical team's ability to compensate for major errors. It is said that "little things matter."[3]

Teamwork reduces the number and mitigates the consequences of minor disruptions. In this way teamwork enhances safety. A well-trained team can see a cardiac surgical procedure from many angles. There are many trained eyes watching for problems. There are many minds available to anticipate and avoid problems. Team familiarity prevents minor problems as there is smooth communication at each step.

The University of Michigan studied 460,000 doctors caring for 251,000 heart bypass patients. They reported that a 25% increase in teamwork was associated with 17 fewer readmissions for every 1000 patients treated. "Our findings show that physician teamwork influences patient outcomes, even more than some measures of comorbid illness," John Hollingsworth, MD, MS.[4]

The importance of developing specialized and experienced teams in cardiac surgery have been shown around the world to make an impact on survival. Having a cardiac surgery team available for emergency cardiopulmonary bypass in place saved the lives of drowning victims in Switzerland. After many unsuccessful attempts it was found that giving emergency medical services the ability to call to mobilize a cardiac surgery team greatly improved the outcomes.[5] Outcomes had been poor until the dedicated team was built, having the right people together at the right time with proper communication created the ability to improve outcomes and save lives.

Most will agree that in general teamwork is a good idea. It seems obvious to anyone asked about the subject. Yet there is a large gap between a good idea and execution of an excellent performance. An example of this is the reduction of central line infections by Dr. Peter Pronovost in the intensive care unit (ICU) at the Johns Hopkins Hospital and later in ICUs in the state of Michigan. Everyone thought that everything was being done well to avoid line infections. Yet the problem persisted. It was only when permission was given for any team member to call out deviations from standardized practice was there an improvement in outcomes.[5] This principle of "nontechnical teamwork skills" applies to surgical teams as well. Unlike an ICU procedure, OR procedures involve multiple people in specific roles over a longer period of time. Surgical quality depends upon the effective interaction of these team members (Fig. 5.1).

Team components and responsibilities

Surgeon

The surgeon is the team Captain in the sense that he or she is responsible for bringing the patient to surgery, choosing the appropriate operation, and managing the patient after surgery. The most effective way to perform this task is to lead with understanding of the components of the team. Each part of the team is working on its portion of the task with its own expertise. One major role of the surgeon is to coordinate the efforts of all team members in the room.

A surgeon should always check-in with the team in the room to make sure they know which operation is being done and if they are ready with the required staff and equipment.[4] For example, in cardiac surgery cases requiring cardiopulmonary

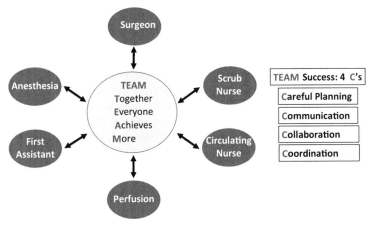

FIGURE 5.1

The components of surgical team success.

bypass, a check-in with perfusion is essential. This is especially true for cases done infrequently. Knowing the expectation for cannulation, myocardial protection strategy, and special equipment needs are key to good outcomes. Miscommunication or lack of communication leads to delays that worsen outcomes. The captain's responsibility is to ensure that everyone involved has a voice and is on the same page.

Anesthesia

Communication with anesthesia is critical. Setting expectations at the beginning of the case includes discussion of comorbid factors such as renal insufficiency, neurologic deficits, and dysrhythmias. Ongoing communication about the management of blood pressure, blood products, and management of air are examples of issues that must be handled as a team.

One author said "An anesthesiologist that looks into the wound is worth his weight in gold"[6] emphasizing the importance of having everyone anticipating and on the same page.

Scrub nurse

The scrub nurse (or scrub technician in many hospitals) is the surgeon's closest ally. Communication with the scrub before, during, and after the case is paramount to success. Preoperative clarification of the operation about to be performed, presence of equipment, and any potential or anticipated deviation from usual practice is necessary to ensure excellent performance.

Collaboration with an experienced scrub nurse can avoid mistakes. The team in the OR needs to have the opportunity to express concerns openly. Ongoing communication is vital. Moments lost with miscommunication end up as costing minutes and then hours. In addition, miscommunication can lead to the wrong instrument passed at the wrong time. It can lead to an incorrect needle or instrument count. A well-trained team can perform an entire operation with few words as each team member anticipates the next step. This level of expertise requires that you intentionally train your team to understand not only the steps of the operation but also the reason for each step. If this is set as the expectation, the team will rise to that level of expectation.

There are times when it is necessary to work with an unfamiliar team. Those include starting a new program or working with new people in an established program. During these times meticulous communication is paramount.

Circulating nurse

The circulating nurse is the surgical team member who is not scrubbed in sterile fashion at the table. They are responsible for assessing the patient immediately before surgery and facilitating a smooth transfer into the OR. Along with the scrub nurse they are responsible for setting up and breaking down the OR. During the procedure they pass supplies up to the table as needed in the order that is planned and expected. Coordination with the surgeon is essential so that the correct instruments and supplies are available at the right time.

Perfusion

The perfusionist controls the cardiopulmonary bypass pump and as such is a critical member of the cardiovascular surgical team. Communication during the open-heart procedure is critical as preparation is made to go on pump and as plans are made to come off pump. This has been described as taking off and landing in an airplane. Like passing a baton in a relay race these critical moments in the case require exact understanding, communication and collaboration among the perfusionist and all of the other team members.

The perfusionist also has a powerful collaborative role and needs to be trained in perioperative management of anticoagulation. In addition to management of heparin on bypass, the perfusionist must have experience with preoperative anticoagulants including Warfarin, Plavix, and novel anticoagulants. It is critical that the perfusion team also has experts in interpreting the thromboelastogram (TEG) preoperatively, intraoperatively, and postoperatively.

This expertise reduces the amount of blood and blood products transfused during cardiac surgery. It also prevents the spiral of complications that come after postoperative bleeding including the need for mediastinal reexploration surgery and massive transfusion.

Surgical first assistant

The surgical first assistant stands opposite the surgeon and provides exposure, follows suture, aids in opening, and often closes the surgical wound. In some operations, they harvest conduit for bypass such as the saphenous vein or radial artery for coronary artery bypass.

This crucial position can be performed by a Registered Nurse First Assistant (RNFA), a Physician Assistant (PA), Surgical Resident, or an Attending Surgeon.

Knowledge of the operation is paramount as the First Assistant is often setting up the next step as the surgeon completes the current step of a precise methodological progression of steps that complete an operation. Like a caddie setting up the professional golfer with the right club at the right time, the First Assistant keeps the flow of the operation moving. They also provide an additional set of eyes and operative experience. This can ensure that steps are not skipped and surgical time is used efficiently.

Traditional approach

Historically surgery was developed with a rigid top-down hierarchy. It was inflexible and did not easily give voice to any but a few team members. The culture was a top-down paramilitary type command structure. It was the culture of the day but had limitations.

Efficiency was limited by the lack of input from the entire team. The discouragement of speaking up led to the cover up of errors. There was a culture of avoiding blame. There was a limited safety net due to a lack of team empowerment.

In clinical practice similar dictates are passed from a senior partner practice who tightly controlled most processes. This was meant to avoid bad outcomes. Yet it at times stifled the talent of the very experienced team.

Today, in general, attempts are made to promote a less hierarchical structure. The surgeon is still the captain, but he or she is more of a team leader than a dictator. They have the responsibility to obtain input from all team members and facilitate collaboration. This requires flexibility and communication. Trust of others and respect are critical. Team members need to be able to speak up, voice concerns, and question. This is the core for safe, reliable, and high-quality performance in the OR.

Careful planning

The dynamic of surgical teamwork begins before the patient enters the OR. In order to complete complex surgical procedures careful preoperative assessment and planning is necessary. The surgeon, the referring cardiologist, and the anesthesiologist must be on the same page about the patient's comorbidities and suitability for surgery.

If the patient has infection, renal insufficiency, or respiratory failure these factors must be identified. A bleeding tendency or the preoperative use of anticoagulants must be carefully assessed by drug type and timing of last dose. OR nursing as well as advanced practice providers are often instrumental in identifying medications that must be stopped days prior to surgery.

A plan must be made to address these factors. Medical treatment is in order until the patient is ready for surgery. There must be a discussion of the risks and benefits. If the patient is at excessive risk the surgery may need to be delayed or canceled. Some smaller centers routinely route higher risk patients to large centers where there are greater resources. A collaboration between centers is beneficial for safe and efficient transfer.

Communication

The ability to perform the many tasks required to complete a complex operation requires precise communication. Once the barriers of hierarchy are broken down there still remains the challenge of performing precisely.

An example of this is preoperative antibiotic administration. The delivery of the preoperative antibiotic 30 min before skin incision reduces the risk of infection and its documentation is required by the Society of Thoracic Surgeons (STS) database. In our experience, the antibiotic administration was not consistent until a question was asked during the preoperative time-out. We would ask "was the preoperative antibiotic given." This was asked before incision was allowed to be made. One institution placed a cover over the scalpel until all preoperative requirements were completed.[4] This increases the ability to achieve a high rate of compliance with nationally endorsed quality measures.

Interestingly despite including this antibiotic administration question in preoperative timeout checklists, there can be lack of evidence in the medical record that the administration of antibiotics had occurred. A discussion with the anesthesiologist revealed that the antibiotic had been given, but documentation was delayed or missed during the busy operation.

In order to get to 100% compliance and ensure best practices were followed, we added an additional phrase to the preoperative antibiotic question. We asked: "was the preoperative antibiotic given and was this recorded in the chart." After we added the additional phrase we soon went to 100% compliance.

Effective communication involves establishing a smooth method of conveying information with accountability and following up that the information has been received and acted upon. Miscommunication has been found to be a major factor in adverse outcomes in cardiac surgery.[3]

Checklists are helpful at the beginning and the end of procedures to ensure that critical components are not overlooked. Yet there is an additional level of communication that is needed. This is the ongoing on the fly communication among team members. Surgery is a step-by-step process from beginning to end. Each step precedes or follows in a logical and technical progression. It's imperative that the OR team is familiar with the steps of the operation, that everyone is thinking and anticipating the next step in a coordinated fashion. In a valve replacement, after exposure of the valve, sutures are placed and sorted, and brought through the new valve in an orderly fashion. After several years, even decades this can be done automatically. The assistant and the scrub each know what the surgeon will do next as they facilitate the next move like a Russian Ballet, an Alvin Ailey troupe performance, or a National Basketball Association (NBA) no look pass on a fast break. My senior partner completed an aortic valve replacement in 90 min skin-to-skin while interviewing me for my first job in Louisville, Kentucky. His team had been together for decades and had nonverbal communication from beginning to end. Teamwork approaching this level of coordination can be achieved by the education of each member. Knowledge of the intricate steps is mandatory. Anticipation and execution comes with practice and experience.

There are regional differences in procedure organization and execution. Some surgical instruments have different names in different places. A Schnidt grasper forceps can be called a Tonsil, or a Vanderbilt depending on where you work. When a new surgeon comes to a practice it is highly recommended for them to scrub as an assistant with one of the established surgeons to see the local method of coordination. New procedures, or new ways of doing the same procedure, can be added later with education and training. A core competency in communication and coordination prevents steps from being missed or sutures from getting tangled. It improves safety through time efficiency and reproducible precision.

Coordination

The organization of activity in the OR is an important part of teamwork. Having the right staff in place at the right time requires coordination among all of the team members. This is particularly important when staffing is in short supply. The development of transcatheter procedures often necessitates two teams: one team from the cardiac catheterization lab and another from the OR. Coordination requires the management of multiple schedules.One solution to this problem is to designate a particular day for transcatheter procedures, e.g., Transcatheter Aortic Valve Replacement (TAVR) Tuesday.

Cardiac surgical teams are highly specialized. Due to the intricacy of the work with multiple complex steps that must be performed under time constraint, having an experienced team is vital. A generic surgical team cannot be substituted. For this reason, cardiac surgical teams often take more on-call responsibility than other types of surgical teams. Cross-training of other teams can help offset the on-call burden for an established cardiac surgery team. Team members from other service lines can learn some of the basic routines of cardiac surgery during normally scheduled cases so that they can give relief during after hours, nights, and weekend cases.

To illustrate the concept of coordination and planning in cardiac surgery, I have had the opportunity to work with a surgical mission training team from Brigham and Women's Hospital in Boston, Massachusetts, and in Kigali, Rwanda, East Africa.

The team comprised of members from multiple hospitals. In this way no single hospital was depleted of a significant part of their team. All were volunteers. All were very experienced. At first the communication began with how do you perform your operations? For example, since we were doing primarily postrheumatic valve replacements the discussions would include types of chest retractor, cannulation sutures and strategy, myocardial protection strategy, valve sutures, aortic or atrial closure sutures, and chest closure technique. Often due to resource limitations there was only one choice available. We had to adapt. After a few cases we no longer needed to talk about most of the fundamentals. We only discussed the patient-specific issues or issues related to equipment availability (e.g., how many valves do we have left in each size). After several operations I was amazed at how well things went. It was like a group of jazz musicians who all knew a standard song. After calling out the key they are able to play in unison. An Olympic sports team is made of members from many schools. They are all elite athletes well trained in fundamentals. Some may be record holders. Yet the team that wins is the one with the best coordination and teamwork.

Actually, a cardiovascular surgical team is more like a 100-meter relay performance. It is a high energy time limited event. There are multiple handoffs and baton exchanges. At any point if the baton is passed slowly, awkwardly, or if it is dropped the race is lost. Careful coordination of all team members is paramount to surgical success.

Collaboration

Having well-defined roles, sharing goals, and creating a culture of mutual trust and respect promote teamwork.[7] This was true in multiple settings including the OR, the emergency department, and in nursing homes. Having accountability for a defined role improved physician well-being.

The aviation industry created a teamwork development model after it recognized the benefit of nontechnical skills in preventing bad outcomes. The "Cockpit Resource Management" programs were developed to improve teamwork.[3] Versions of these principles have been used by emergency departments, medical units, and surgical teams. These programs emphasize nontechnical skills such as communication and leadership make it possible for a team to collaborate effectively. Shared understanding of the task at hand as well as the ability to speak up without penalty leads to an environment that is safe for collaboration. This improves outcomes. It also improves the job satisfaction of the team members.

Training

The National Patient Safety Summit of the American College of Surgeons and the American Academy of Orthopedic Surgeons provided recommendations that surgical OR teamwork training begin in residency.[8] This would include discussion of the benefits of developing nontechnical skills including communication and collaboration. Workshops and didactics would emphasize the development of a culture of collegial respect and the expectation that everyone has a voice in this complex process.

Nontechnical skills are generally developed on the job. Large volume programs of necessity often have streamlined operations. Inefficiencies are weeded out in order to finish a large volume of work in the finite work day. Teamwork has the opportunity to be honed during multiple repetitions in the fire of daily activity. Memory, attention, and thoroughness are enhanced when tasks are performed over and over. There is always room for improvement and it has been said that "'perfect practice' makes perfect" (Vince Lombardi).

Yet smaller programs can perform exceptionally well and many studies have demonstrated this. Often in these cases the small teams are comprised of a dedicated few who have worked together year after year honing their communication and collaboration skills intentionally. At times in larger programs an individual surgeon may have to work with a person with whom they may not have worked with for some time. This level of potential unfamiliarity does not exist in a smaller more intimate program. At Boulder Community Hospital in Colorado I worked with the same partner, surgical assistant, and three scrub nurses for a decade. We had excellent outcomes and great patient satisfaction.

It has been suggested that real-time video recording be used for assessing teamwork in the OR.[9,10] One center used video surveillance during minimally invasive cases to identify opportunities for improvement in teamwork. The legal implications need to be considered but the potential benefit from feedback likely outweighs the risk.

Surgical simulation with an emphasis on teamwork has the potential for significant benefit. Examples of this are advanced cardiac life support (ACLS) and cardiac surgery advanced life support (CALS). In each of these there is opportunity for practice in a simulated environment preparing the team for better performance under pressure in the real-time environment.[11]

Teamwork also creates a better workplace environment. A study of teams that have been coached in the area of nontechnical communication skills demonstrates increased job satisfaction, and better patient outcomes.[7] Improvement in patient safety was also demonstrated.

Critical care handoff

One of the essential parts of the process of cardiac surgery is the safe transfer of the patient to the ICU. The ICU management of the cardiac surgical patient also requires teamwork but is outside of the scope of this discussion.

Upon admission to the ICU the cardiac surgery patient is moving with a ventilator, a transport monitor, multiple IVs, and an arterial line at least. There may be intraaortic balloon pumps, temporary pacemakers, and other devices. It is critical for the transport team to communicate patient's pertinent preoperative history, type of procedure, and any problems that may have been encountered. The type and rate of vasoactive drugs running as well as ventilator settings must be expeditiously communicated.

A "head to toe by systems" approach is often used. A checklist for transfer is very valuable and is used to avoid missing key issues. In one community hospital in Colorado it was common practice for the ICU staff to come into the OR as the operation was concluding to speak with the OR team. They would discuss problems, unusual findings, and get a preliminary assessment of the patient's ventilator settings and vasoactive drips. The communication and collaboration began early and made the subsequent transfer easier.

A checklist kept on the electronic medical record can be used to effectively pass information to the next shift of doctors, nurses, and advanced practice providers. Using an electronic checklist, key data as well as the plan of care can be passed with less risk of losing information in the transfer.

Summary

Teamwork in the OR is essential for safe delivery of care. The creation of well-practiced teams will enhance the delivery of cost-effective care as well. The maintenance of these teams requires practice. High-volume centers have the advantage of daily practice of necessity. Smaller programs have the advantage of close-knit teams with low turnover. They rely upon experienced practitioners with regular collaboration. All teams benefit from the regular review of essential steps and the use of checklists.

The development of simulation laboratories may help in developing surgical teamwork skills in trainees. As efforts are made to improve surgical quality and contain costs, teamwork will be a topic for ongoing study.

References

1. Sevdalis N, Hull L, Birnbach DJ. Improving patient safety in the operating theatre and perioperative care: obstacles, interventions, and priorities for accelerating progress. *Br J Anaesth* 2012;**109**(Suppl 1):i3–16. https://doi.org/10.1093/bja/aes391.
2. Abahuje E, Riviello R. Operation teamwork: improving surgery with non-technical skills training. *Brigham Bulletin* 2019. In this issue, https://bwhbulletin.org/3-15-2019/.
3. Wahr J, et al. Patient safety in the cardiac operating room: human factors and teamwork. *Circulation* 2013;**128**:1139–69.
4. Gavin K. *The more doctors interact, the better their patients do.* The Univ of Maryland Rounds; November 08, 2016.

5. Gawande A. *The checklist manifesto: how to get things right*. New York: Metropolitan Books; 2010.
6. Waters DJ. *A surgeon's little instruction book*. Cleveland: Taylor and Francis; 1998.
7. Smith CD, Balatbat C, Corbridge S, Dopp AL, Fried J, Harter R, et al. *Implementing optimal team-based care to reduce clinician burnout. NAM Perspectives*. Discussion Paper. Washington, DC: National Academy of Medicine; 2018. https://doi.org/10.31478/201809c.
8. Teamwork and communication training for surgical safety. August 9, 2016. https://healthmanagement.org/c/hospital/news/teamwork-and-communication-training-for-surgical-safety.
9. Warnock GL. Building the high-reliability surgical team. *Can J Surg* 2006;**49**(1):6−9. PMID: 16524135; PMCID: PMC3207520.
10. Boet S. *Could better teamwork and communications in the operating room make surgery safer for patients?* The Ottawa Hospital Copyright; 2018.
11. Fleming M, Smith S, Slaunwhite J, et al. Investigating interpersonal competencies of cardiac surgery teams. *Can J Surg* 2006;**49**(1):22−30.

Structured perioperative team communication

Katherine G. Verdi, MD [1], Hadley K. Wesson, MD MPH [2],
Robert Higgins, MD MSHA [3]

[1]*Resident, Department of Surgery, Johns Hopkins School of Medicine, Baltimore, MD, United States;* [2]*Assistant Professor, Department of Surgery, Johns Hopkins School of Medicine, Baltimore, MD, United States;* [3]*President, Brigham and Women's Hospital, Executive Vice President, Mass General Brigham, Brigham and Women's Hospital, Boston, MA, United States*

Structured and effective communication is critical to a successful operation and perioperative care. It plays an essential role in facilitating teamwork. We define communication as the transfer of information from one person to another or to a group of individuals, either via verbal language, gestures or cues, or written messages.[1] Effective communication allows a message or concern to be efficiently and clearly delivered to and understood by the intended recipient. Structured communication describes frameworks in which systems are put in place to allow for the delivery of this message or concern.

In the operating room and perioperative setting, the surgical care team must be able to clearly convey the plan of care, discuss obstacles, and debrief. The operating room, however, presents unique challenges to accomplish this, such as the physical barriers of surgical masks and sterile drapes, handoffs of care between team members, the potential for unexpected adversity or stress, and the traditional hierarchical structure of the medical team. Ultimately poor communication can result in the most dreaded complications: wrong procedure, wrong site surgery, use of incorrect or expired implants, increased morbidity, and even mortality.[2–5]

This chapter will examine the importance of perioperative team communication. We will summarize the history behind formalizing and mandating surgical time-outs. We will also present evidence to support other interventions that enhance structured communication, including preoperative briefings, surgical checklists, postoperative debriefings, and handoffs. We will review the benefits and perceived limitations in implementing these interventions. Finally, we will outline strategies to help you achieve structured and effective communication in your operating room.

The need for structured and effective perioperative team communication

The perioperative surgical team consists of surgical members in three different locations: the preoperative, intraoperative, and postoperative areas. Team members include preoperative nurses and clinical technicians, the anesthesia care team, the operating room nurse, the scrub technician, the surgeon and their assistants, postoperative nurses, and the postoperative care team in the intensive care unit or the inpatient ward. Each team member provides a different skill set, all of which are crucial to patient care. Not only are multiple team members involved, but there are also multiple transitions of care inherent in the operative care of a patient. Effective teamwork entails cooperation and communication among the various care providers with the common goal of providing the best possible patient care. Its value is highlighted by evidence showing that poor teamwork results in errors, adverse events, and poor patient outcomes.[6–8]

Despite a team's best intentions, the operating room presents several distinct challenges that can potentially limit effective communication. Many of the visual and auditory cues inherent to communication are precluded or dampened by the very nature of the operating room. For instance, the operating surgeon may not be able to look up from the patient for any visual cues while communicating with the first assistant, the scrub technician, the circulating nurse, or the anesthesiologist, who is additionally behind the curtain of the sterile drapes. Facemasks further cover nonverbal facial expressions and muffle verbal speech. The environment can be chaotic, such as during an unplanned, emergent operation in an unstable patient or an unexpected adverse event during the course of a planned operation. Such high stress, high stakes environments are associated with cognitive overload and breakdown of communication.[9] This only helps to fuel a traditionally hierarchical team structure, both between the various health professionals and within the same category of healthcare professional based on level of experience. This hierarchy can breed an unsafe environment where team members might not speak up regarding a safety concern or question out of fear or formality.[2,10]

Poor communication has been linked to many adverse outcomes, including wrong procedure, wrong site surgery, retained foreign objects, and use of incorrect or expired implants.[2–4] Beyond individual adverse events, the evidence suggests that ineffective communication is independently associated with poorer overall outcomes for patients. For instance, Mazzocco et al. observed surgical teams in the operating room and found when teamwork behavior was infrequently observed, patients were statistically significantly more likely to experience a complication within 30 days of surgery, with an adjusted odds ratio of 4.82. Complications included in this analysis included death, intraoperative complications such as surgical burn, adverse drug reaction, wrong laterality or procedure, and retained foreign objects, and postoperative complications including respiratory failure, wound dehiscence, myocardial infarction, and cerebrovascular accident.[5] As such, the need for effective and structured perioperative team communication is ever present.

The Joint Commission's surgical time-out

In 2004, The Joint Commission introduced the universal protocol to prevent wrong site, wrong procedure, and wrong person surgery as a mandatory quality standard.

This is arguably the first time a structure was put in place to mandate a perioperative team communication initiative. The protocol includes a preprocedure verification process, surgical site marking, and a surgical time-out prior to starting the procedure.[11] The time-out component of the universal protocol was initially defined as a designated time during which all members of the team pause to confirm the correct patient, operation, and laterality (Table 6.1). All members of the operative team, including the anesthesiologist, surgeon, circulating nurse, and technician, must be present and engaged during the time-out.

Since it was first implemented, The Joint Commission's surgical time-out has expanded to include verification of patient positioning, availability of equipment, patient allergies, and the need for essential medications including antibiotics, beta-blockers, and venous thromboembolism prophylaxis.[12] The expanded time-out also includes the introduction of all team members by both name and role.[13] The Joint Commission mandates that this is not only implemented before every invasive procedure, but that the procedure does not start until all questions and concerns are addressed. Failure to comply may result in the loss of accreditation of the medical center.

Unfortunately, despite The Joint Commission's universal protocol, operative errors still occur. Between 2005, when the time-out was first mandated, and 2016, 1281 wrong patient, wrong site, or wrong procedure sentinel events were reported to The Joint Commission.[14] In 2018 alone, 94 wrong site surgeries were reported.[15] This highlights that The Joint Commission's surgical time-out is a starting point, and not end point, to achieve structured and effective perioperative communication. The remainder of this chapter will focus on initiatives put forth by the World Health Organization (WHO) and other researchers that support preoperative briefings, surgical checklists, postoperative debriefings, and handoffs (Fig. 6.1).

Table 6.1 Components of The Joint Commission's surgical time-out.[a]

- Conduct a time-out immediately before starting the invasive procedure or making the incision
- A designated member of the team starts the time-out
- The time-out is standardized
- The time-out involves the immediate members of the procedure team
- All relevant members of the procedure team actively communicate during the time-out
- During the time-out, the team members agree, at a minimum, on the following:
  1. Correct patient identity
  2. Correct site
  3. Procedure to be done
- If the same patient has two or more procedures: If the person performing the procedure changes, another time-out needs to be performed before starting each procedure
- Document the completion of the time-out

---

[a] *Source: The Joint Commission. "The Universal Protocol for Preventing Wrong Site, Wrong Procedure, and Wrong Person Surgery: Guidance for health care professionals." https://www.jointcommission.org/assets/1/18/UP_Poster1.PDF. Accessed: July 5, 2019.*

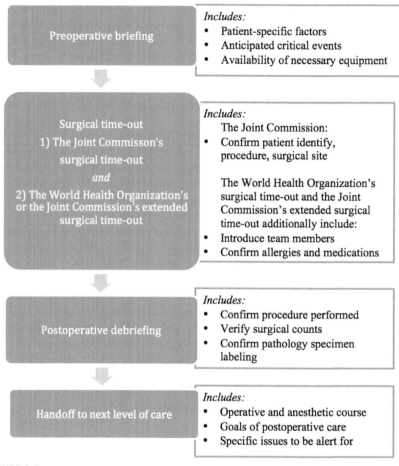

Preoperative briefing

Includes:
- Patient-specific factors
- Anticipated critical events
- Availability of necessary equipment

Surgical time-out
1) The Joint Commisson's surgical time-out
and
2) The World Health Organization's or the Joint Commission's extended surgical time-out

Includes:
The Joint Commission:
- Confirm patient identify, procedure, surgical site

The World Health Organization's surgical time-out and the Joint Commission's extended surgical time-out additionally include:
- Introduce team members
- Confirm allergies and medications

Postoperative debriefing

Includes:
- Confirm procedure performed
- Verify surgical counts
- Confirm pathology specimen labeling

Handoff to next level of care

Includes:
- Operative and anesthetic course
- Goals of postoperative care
- Specific issues to be alert for

FIGURE 6.1

Structured communication at each stage of the patient's operative care.

The World Health Organization's surgical checklists

In 2009, the WHO officially recommended the universal use of its Surgical Safety Checklist, developed in 2007.[16] The checklist formalizes three designated times for the surgical team to pause and communicate: (1) before the induction of anesthesia, (2) before skin incision (i.e., the "time-out"), and (3) after skin closure. The time-out before skin incision is similar to the Joint Commission's extended time-out in that it consists of all team members introducing themselves by name and role, confirming the patient's name, procedure, where the incision will be made, that antibiotic prophylaxis has been given within the last hour, that essential imaging is displayed, but also includes discussing anticipated critical events such as duration of the operation, anticipated blood loss, equipment issues, and any patient-specific concerns.[16] The WHO's recommendation resulted from a 2009 study that assessed 30-day postoperative outcomes in eight hospitals before and after the introduction of the checklist. After the implementation of the checklist, mortality significantly decreased by 47% and morbidity significantly decreased by 36%.[17]

The benefit of the WHO Surgical Safety Checklist was further established by a 2012 retrospective study of over 25,000 patients. Adjusted mortality significantly decreased after the checklist implementation, with an odds ratio of 0.85 for the primary outcome of in-hospital mortality within 30 days of surgery.[18] The study found the mortality benefit was strongly related to checklist compliance, with the largest mortality benefit observed in cases where the full checklist was completed (odds ratio of 0.44). This led the WHO to explicitly define the importance of team communication in promoting patient safety and to prioritize effective communication as a top 10 objective for safe surgery.[19]

Moreover, the use of the WHO Surgical Safety Checklist has been demonstrated to improve knowledge of the names and roles of team members, increase the preemptive discussion of anticipated critical events between anesthesiologists and surgeons, and reduce communication failures.[20,21] The structured surgical time-out has significantly decreased uncertainty regarding surgical site location among surgical team members and enhanced teamwork among the surgery and anesthesia providers.[2,22] Specifically, implementing a checklist that outlines the components of the WHO's surgical time-out has shown significant reductions in 30-day morbidity, increased rates of properly timed and administered prophylactic antibiotics, and improvements in the sense of teamwork.[23–25]

Preoperative briefings

Structured preoperative briefings that occur before the patient arrives in the operating room build on The Joint Commission's mandated surgical time-out to provide an additional formalized time to enhance communication between members of the surgical care team.[26] Such briefings include three key components: (1) the traditional Joint Commission time-out, (2) team member introductions, and (3) a review of the proposed operative plan by the surgical, anesthesia, and nursing teams.[26] Studies show preoperative briefings can be accomplished in less than 2 min, leading to improved operating room efficiency and increased first case start times.[27]

Data suggest that engaging in regular surgical briefings correlate with staff perceptions of a positive safety culture.[22] Hicks et al.'s review of the literature found that in addition to improving the perception of better safety climate, preoperative briefings resulted in a significant decrease in communication failures, an increase in the appropriate administration of perioperative antibiotics and deep venous thrombosis prophylaxis, and a reduction in both surgical morbidity and mortality.[5,22,25–33]

Despite the evidence that preoperative briefings enhance safety culture and improve patient outcomes, we recognize there are several barriers to implementation.

The first barrier is the infrastructure required to create a protocol to implement preoperative briefings. A second concern is the perception that preoperative briefings take time and thus have the potential to delay case start.[22] To address the validity of these concerns, a 2011 study assessed how a surgical debriefing affects the average operating room start times.[31] Their preoperative safety briefing occurred between the anesthesia staff, surgeons, operating room nurses, and operating department practitioners. Included in the briefing were team member introductions, statement of the planned procedures and patient position, verification of equipment sterility and the availability of required imaging, and patient-specific issues such as airway, monitoring requirements, allergies, and anticipated blood loss during the surgery. These meetings took approximately 5−10 min and occurred before the arrival of the first patient. After implementation of this debriefing, there was no significant difference in the operating room start time.[31] Furthermore, staff members reported that the briefings were positively received; specifically, 89% of staff members found the briefings made them more aware of the cases and were an effective tool to improve communication; 97% of staff members felt the briefings highlighted potential patient problems and wanted them to continue.[31] Leong et al. similarly demonstrated that the introduction of a preoperative briefing positively enhanced the perception of the team climate among operative staff members.[34]

Postoperative debriefings

A postoperative debriefing, which occurs after the critical portions of the operation are complete, is a time when the team can review the procedure performed and address any concerns or deficits that occurred during the case.[6,35] Berenholtz et al. implemented a standardized debriefing process that was initiated by the operating room nurse after the first counts were conducted.[35] The attending surgeon was required to be present for the debriefing. On average, the debriefing took 2.5 min to complete. Seventy-two percent of surveyed participants felt that the debriefing was an effective strategy to improve teamwork, and 70% felt it was feasible given current workload.[35]

The WHO's surgical safety checklist includes a sign-out to be completed before the patient leaves the operating room. In it, the nurse verbally confirms the name of the procedure, completion of instrument, sponge, and needle counts, specimen labeling, and whether there are any equipment problems to be addressed.[16] There is also an opportunity for the surgeon, anesthesiologist, and operating room nurse to state any key concerns regarding the recovery and management of the patient. Completing this debriefing has been shown to significantly decrease the number of surgical specimen labeling errors.[36]

Handoffs to next level of care

After the operation is complete, the care of the patient transitions either to an intensive care unit (ICU) team or to a postanesthesia care unit (PACU) care team, followed by either discharge from the hospital or admission to an inpatient ward.

This transition of care represents another period in which communication is critical, so that those caring for the patient understand what occurred in the operating room, what complications to specifically look out for, and what care the patient will require. This handoff of care is particularly well studied in the cardiac surgery patient population, where nearly all patients transition to care in an ICU postoperatively. For example, Hall et al. developed and implemented a multidisciplinary formalized transfer of care process for postoperative cardiac surgery patients in an academic tertiary care center. They found that implementing this process significantly decreased preventable complications, including cardiac arrest, postoperative hypotension, line complications, anaphylaxis and allergic reactions, drug/dosage errors, and iatrogenic pneumothoraces.[37] Specifically, after adjusting for age and sex, the odds ratio for having a preventable complication was significantly less at 0.35 for postintervention patients compared to preintervention patients. Furthermore, the authors found that using the structured handoff template did not significantly increase the time the sign-out process took.[37]

In the Handoffs and Transitions in Critical Care (HATRICC) Prospective Cohort Study, a standardized operating room to ICU handoff process was implemented in two mixed surgical ICUs at two hospitals within an academic tertiary care health system.[38] The process began with a pre-handoff telephone call, during which the operating room nurse communicated with the ICU staff prior to the patient leaving the operating room. In the ICU, the handoff included introduction of the clinicians, stabilization of the patient, and transfer of monitors by the nursing staff, followed by a report given by the surgeon and then the anesthesiologist. As a final step, the ICU provider provides a synopsis of the immediate postoperative concerns. The authors found that the duration of the handoff process significantly increased, from an average of 4.1 to 8.0 min.[38] However, the number of information omissions per handoff decreased significantly by 21% and the percentage of handoffs rated as unsatisfactory also significantly decreased by 59%. The literature similarly demonstrates a structured postoperative handover between the operating room team and the PACU nurse receiving the patient reduces information omissions and increases teamwork and nurse satisfaction.[39–41]

Tools to implement structured and effective communication

So far we have outlined the benefits and addressed the perceived limitations of structured perioperative communication processes (Table 6.2). But how do you implement these interventions in your practice? Recognizing the importance of teamwork and communication in the perioperative period, several organizations have developed formalized team training to address this very question. The Agency for Healthcare Research and Quality and the Department of Defense jointly developed Team Strategies and Tools to Enhance Performance and Patient Safety (TeamSTEPPS), an evidence-based toolkit intended to improve patient safety through enhanced communication and teamwork skills in the perioperative

Table 6.2 Outcomes from initiatives to enhance perioperative communication.

Initiative	Improves mortality	Improves morbidity	Improves staff satisfaction	Time to implement (minutes)	Limitations
Preoperative briefing	✓5, 33	✓5, 25, 32, 33	✓22, 31, 34	5–10 min	• Requires organizational and team dedication to implement
WHO's surgical checklist	✓17	✓17	✓5, 22	Not studied	• Requires organizational and team dedication to implement
Postoperative debriefing	Not studied	✓36	✓35	2.5 min	• Requires team dedication to implement this before members of the surgical team leave the operating room
Postoperative handoffs	Not studied	✓39–41	✓39–41	4–8 min	• Requires organizational and team dedication to implement

setting.[42] At the San Antonio Military Medical Center, all operating room health care personnel participated in TeamSTEPPS training, which included didactic-based modules on leadership, situation monitoring, mutual support, and communication.[43] A standardized preoperative briefing and postoperative debriefing was also implemented. With the use of TeamSTEPPS, the incidence of patient safety issues significantly decreased. Furthermore, the mean case time decreased and the on-time first-start rate was significantly higher.[43] Using tools such as TeamSTEPPS, we would encourage you to work with your operative team and administration to implement structured communication initiatives such as those described in this chapter.

Future directions

Structured and effective perioperative team communication has consistently shown to improve surgical patient outcomes and enhance the perceived sense of teamwork between members of the operative care team. The Joint Commission's surgical time-out, performed with the surgeon, anesthesiologist, and operating room nurse prior to incision, has become a mandated component of the operating room practice and has led to a decrease in wrong person, wrong site, and wrong procedure operations. An abundance of data also suggests that increasing and formalizing structured perioperative communication in the forms of checklists, preoperative briefings, postoperative debriefings, and standardized handoffs to the next level of care improves outcomes for patients. A perceived limitation to implementing these initiatives is the amount of work it would take to establish these systems. But as healthcare providers, our entire purpose is to do no harm. We can do this by promoting a culture of safety, as supported by The Joint Commission. It requires buy-in from all parties of the surgical team and an organization's administration. Through dedication and commitment to invest in enhanced perioperative communication, we have the potential to decrease the rate of morbidity and mortality for our patients.

References

1. Pierre St M, ProQuest (Firm). *Crisis management in acute care settings human factors, team psychology, and patient safety in a high stakes environment*. New York: Springer; 2011.
2. Makary MA, Mukherjee A, Sexton JB, Syin D, Goodrich E, Hartmann E, Rowen L, Behrens DC, Marohn M, Pronovost PJ. Operating room briefings and wrong-site surgery. *J Am Coll Surg* 2007;**204**:236—43.
3. Gawande AA, Studdert DM, Orav EJ, Brennan TA, Zinner MJ. Risk factors for retained instruments and sponges after surgery. *N Engl J Med* 2003;**348**:229—35.
4. Saufl NM. Universal protocol for preventing wrong site, wrong procedure, wrong person surgery. *J Perianesth Nurs* 2004;**19**:348—51.

5. Mazzocco K, Petitti DB, Fong KT, Bonacum D, Brookey J, Graham S, Lasky RE, Sexton JB, Thomas EJ. Surgical team behaviors and patient outcomes. *Am J Surg* 2009;**197**:678−85.

6. Gluyas H. Effective communication and teamwork promotes patient safety. *Nurs Stand* 2015;**29**:50−7.

7. Lyons VE, Popejoy LL. Meta-analysis of surgical safety checklist effects on teamwork, communication, morbidity, mortality, and safety. *West J Nurs Res* 2014;**36**:245−61.

8. Treadwell JR, Lucas S, Tsou AY. Surgical checklists: a systematic review of impacts and implementation. *BMJ Qual Saf* 2014;**23**:299−318.

9. Salvendy G, editor. *Handbook of human factors and ergonomics*. 4th ed. Hoboken, NJ: Wiley; 2012.

10. Nugus P, Greenfield D, Travaglia J, Westbrook J, Braithwaite J. How and where clinicians exercise power: interprofessional relations in health care. *Soc Sci Med* 2010;**71**: 898−909.

11. JOINT COMMISSION ACCREDITATION. *Comprehensive accreditation manual: camh for hospitals effective january 1, 2019*. JT COMM OF ACCRED HEALTH; 2018 [Place of publication not identified].

12. Hunter JG. Extend the universal protocol, not just the surgical time out. *J Am Coll Surg* 2007;**205**:e4−5.

13. Stahel PF, Mehler PS, Clarke TJ, Varnell J. The 5th anniversary of the "Universal Protocol": pitfalls and pearls revisited. *Patient Saf Surg* 2009;**3**:14.

14. Summary data of sentinel events reviewed by The Joint Commision.

15. Summary data of events reviewed by The Joint Commission.

16. WHO's patient-safety checklist for surgery. *Lancet* 2008;**372**:1.

17. Haynes AB, Weiser TG, Berry WR, et al. A surgical safety checklist to reduce morbidity and mortality in a global population. *N Engl J Med* 2009;**360**:491−9.

18. van Klei WA, Hoff RG, van Aarnhem EEHL, Simmermacher RKJ, Regli LPE, Kappen TH, van Wolfswinkel L, Kalkman CJ, Buhre WF, Peelen LM. Effects of the introduction of the WHO "Surgical Safety Checklist" on in-hospital mortality: a cohort study. *Ann Surg* 2012;**255**:44−9.

19. World Health Organization, Patient Safety. *WHO guidelines for safe surgery 2009: safe surgery saves lives*. 2009.

20. Takala RSK, Pauniaho S-L, Kotkansalo A, et al. A pilot study of the implementation of WHO surgical checklist in Finland: improvements in activities and communication. *Acta Anaesthesiol Scand* 2011;**55**:1206−14.

21. Fudickar A, Hörle K, Wiltfang J, Bein B. The effect of the WHO Surgical Safety Checklist on complication rate and communication. *Dtsch Arztebl Int* 2012;**109**:695−701.

22. Allard J, Bleakley A, Hobbs A, Coombes L. Pre-surgery briefings and safety climate in the operating theatre. *BMJ Qual Saf* 2011;**20**:711−7.

23. Bliss LA, Ross-Richardson CB, Sanzari LJ, Shapiro DS, Lukianoff AE, Bernstein BA, Ellner SJ. Thirty-day outcomes support implementation of a surgical safety checklist. *J Am Coll Surg* 2012;**215**:766−76.

24. Johnston FM, Tergas AI, Bennett JL, Valero V, Morrissey CK, Fader AN, Hobson DB, Weaver SJ, Rosen MA, Wick EC. Measuring briefing and checklist compliance in surgery: a tool for quality improvement. *Am J Med Qual* 2014;**29**:491−8.

25. Lingard L, Regehr G, Cartmill C, Orser B, Espin S, Bohnen J, Reznick R, Baker R, Rotstein L, Doran D. Evaluation of a preoperative team briefing: a new communication routine results in improved clinical practice. *BMJ Qual Saf* 2011;**20**:475−82.

26. Hicks CW, Rosen M, Hobson DB, Ko C, Wick EC. Improving safety and quality of care with enhanced teamwork through operating room briefings. *JAMA Surg* 2014;**149**: 863−8.

27. Henrickson SE, Wadhera RK, Elbardissi AW, Wiegmann DA, Sundt TM. Development and pilot evaluation of a preoperative briefing protocol for cardiovascular surgery. *J Am Coll Surg* 2009;**208**:1115−23.

28. Lingard L, Regehr G, Orser B, Reznick R, Baker GR, Doran D, Espin S, Bohnen J, Whyte S. Evaluation of a preoperative checklist and team briefing among surgeons, nurses, and anesthesiologists to reduce failures in communication. *Arch Surg* 2008; **143**:12−7. discussion 18.

29. Nundy S, Mukherjee A, Sexton JB, Pronovost PJ, Knight A, Rowen LC, Duncan M, Syin D, Makary MA. Impact of preoperative briefings on operating room delays: a preliminary report. *Arch Surg* 2008;**143**:1068−72.

30. Bandari J, Schumacher K, Simon M, Cameron D, Goeschel CA, Holzmueller CG, Makary MA, Welsh RJ, Berenholtz SM. Surfacing safety hazards using standardized operating room briefings and debriefings at a large regional medical center. *Joint Comm J Qual Patient Saf* 2012;**38**:154−60.

31. Ali M, Osborne A, Bethune R, Pullyblank A. Preoperative surgical briefings do not delay operating room start times and are popular with surgical team members. *J Patient Saf* 2011;**7**:139−43.

32. Paull DE, Mazzia LM, Wood SD, Theis MS, Robinson LD, Carney B, Neily J, Mills PD, Bagian JP. Briefing guide study: preoperative briefing and postoperative debriefing checklists in the Veterans Health Administration medical team training program. *Am J Surg* 2010;**200**:620−3.

33. Neily J, Mills PD, Eldridge N, Carney BT, Pfeffer D, Turner JR, Young-Xu Y, Gunnar W, Bagian JP. Incorrect surgical procedures within and outside of the operating room: a follow-up report. *Arch Surg* 2011;**146**:1235−9.

34. Leong KBMSL, Hanskamp-Sebregts M, van der Wal RA, Wolff AP. Effects of perioperative briefing and debriefing on patient safety: a prospective intervention study. *BMJ Open* 2017;**7**:e018367.

35. Berenholtz SM, Schumacher K, Hayanga AJ, Simon M, Goeschel C, Pronovost PJ, Shanley CJ, Welsh RJ. Implementing standardized operating room briefings and debriefings at a large regional medical center. *Joint Comm J Qual Patient Saf* 2009;**35**:391−7.

36. Martis WR, Hannam JA, Lee T, Merry AF, Mitchell SJ. Improved compliance with the World Health Organization Surgical Safety Checklist is associated with reduced surgical specimen labelling errors. *N Z Med J* 2016;**129**:63−7.

37. Hall M, Robertson J, Merkel M, Aziz M, Hutchens M. A structured transfer of care process reduces perioperative complications in cardiac surgery patients. *Anesth Analg* 2017; **125**:477−82.

38. Lane-Fall MB, Pascual JL, Peifer HG, et al. A partially structured postoperative handoff protocol improves communication in 2 mixed surgical intensive care units: findings from the handoffs and transitions in critical care (HATRICC) prospective cohort study. *Ann Surg* 2018. https://doi.org/10.1097/SLA.0000000000003137.

39. Nagpal K, Abboudi M, Manchanda C, Vats A, Sevdalis N, Bicknell C, Vincent C, Moorthy K. Improving postoperative handover: a prospective observational study. *Am J Surg* 2013;**206**:494−501.

40. Barbeito A, Agarwala AV, Lorinc A. Handovers in perioperative care. *Anesthesiol Clin* 2018;**36**:87−98.

41. Robinson NL. Promoting patient safety with perioperative hand-off communication. *J Perianesth Nurs* 2016;**31**:245−53.
42. Clancy CM. TeamSTEPPS: optimizing teamwork in the perioperative setting. *AORN J* 2007;**86**:18−22.
43. Weld LR, Stringer MT, Ebertowski JS, Baumgartner TS, Kasprenski MC, Kelley JC, Cho DS, Tieva EA, Novak TE. TeamSTEPPS improves operating room efficiency and patient safety. *Am J Med Qual* 2016;**31**:408−14.

Human factors and ergonomics in the operating room

Kristen L.W. Webster, PhD[1], Elliott R. Haut, MD, PhD, FACS[2,3,4]

[1]Department of Patient Safety, Regulatory, and Accreditation, Cincinnati Children's Hospital Medical Center, Cincinnati, OH, United States; [2]Department of Surgery, Department of Anesthesiology and Critical Care Medicine, Department of Emergency Medicine, The Johns Hopkins University School of Medicine, Baltimore, MD, United States; [3]The Armstrong Institute for Patient Safety and Quality, Johns Hopkins Medicine, Baltimore, MD, United States; [4]Department of Health Policy and Management, The Johns Hopkins Bloomberg School of Public Health, Baltimore, MD, United States

Defining human factors and ergonomics

Human Factors/Ergonomics is the application of psychology and physiology for the purpose of designing products, processes, and systems with the purpose of increasing safety and comfort for the human that interacts within the product, process, or system[1] and is divided into physical, cognitive, and organizational ergonomics.[2] While "ergonomics" is the term commonly used throughout the rest of the world, North America differentiates the terms "human factors" and "ergonomics" to cover the cognitive/organizational and physical ergonomics. The term "human factors" tends to include cognitive and organizational ergonomics while "ergonomics" refers to physical ergonomics.[3] Cognitive ergonomics includes the psychosocial attributes of the work system including workload, reliability, stress, communication, etc. Organizational ergonomics includes the optimization of the work system within the organization's mandatory structures, policies, and processes. Physical ergonomics is concerned with the biomechanical attributes within a work system and the effects of that work system on the human body.

Because much of this book focuses on cognitive and organizational ergonomics (human factors) as it applies to safety in the operating room (OR), this chapter will focus on the physical and biomechanical ergonomics, with only small sections on human factors to compliment the other chapters.

Ergonomics is concerned with the optimization of performance. Optimization occurs through examination of the biomechanical and physiological capabilities of the worker, their limitations, and the development of an environment or work system that supports performance while decreasing injury as much as possible. The goal of ergonomics is to achieve the optimal compatibility between human, system, and environment.[4,5]

The goal of ergonomics suggests that rather than forcing an employee to conform to a limited or compromising work environment, that the employee either be selected for a job which is tailored to his/her individual skills and abilities or the work environment be tailored to the employee's physical abilities.[6] Simply said, the goal is to "fit the task to the individual, not the individual to the task."[3] In this way ergonomics places emphasis on the work system, the job design, and the adaption ability of the worker.[6] Ergonomics carefully balances employee safety and employee capability, while advancing the company's productivity.[6] Understanding this principle, healthcare has transitioned from the triple aim including population health, patient experience, and cost to a quadruple aim which adds staff satisfaction, wellness, and/or safety as one of the four aims.[7] In this manner, the healthcare industry commits to protecting their staff mentally, physically, and emotionally by creating systems and environments that support well-being.

Human factors and ergonomics in healthcare

Many high-risk industries, such as aviation and nuclear power, have relied upon human factors principles to reduce human error and react quickly to errors within the system to prevent failure. With the publishing of the Institute of Medicine's report, *To Err is Human: Building a Safer Health System,*[8] it was demonstrated that preventable errors within healthcare were no the result of poor performance but were instead insidious systematic failures that had gone unaddressed.[9] Since the publication, the healthcare industry and human factors field have begun integrating. Some well recognized areas of application of human factors principles include improving the human and computer interface within electronic health records, usability designing and testing for medical equipment, implementation of checklists and memory aids, analysis of task saturation and over loading on providers, process analysis to improve efficiency and decrease risk, improved communication, and root cause analysis investigation, team skills and training, team and organizational culture change, and more.

Addition of a human factors practitioner within the hospital's quality and safety department can provide the facility with a new lens to improve patient care, patient satisfaction, and providers' safety and well-being. Practitioners and researchers in the field have varied backgrounds and education levels ranging from the certificate level through doctorate degree. All healthcare workers can benefit from having a basic understanding of how human factors influences their daily tasks[10] and as such, some nursing and residency programs have begun including human factors as part of the curriculum.[9,11–13] However, having an embedded human factors practitioner or team within a hospital provides the opportunity to build trust, promotes the use of multidisciplinary teams, creates transparency, and supports continuous outcomes measurement and planning.[14]

The effects of poor physical ergonomics
Physical pain and discomfort

The results of poor physical ergonomics can vary based upon the biomechanical exposures, psychosocial stressors, and individual risk factors for each employee performing a specific job task.[15] Most commonly, poor physical ergonomics results in biomechanical stresses that contribute to work-related musculoskeletal disorders (WRMSDs) resulting from tasks such as repetitive, continuous, or high force motions and deviation from neutral body alignments.[16] Influencing the employee's muscles, nerves, and connective tissues like tendons and ligaments, these disorders can cause muscle fatigue, pain, injury, illness, and loss of work time/ability. Musculoskeletal disorders (MSDs) manifest in different ways dependent upon the employee's role (surgeon, nurse, anesthesiologist, perfusionist, or others) when as a part of that role they may be required to maintain static positions, sustain continuous use, or bear strain.

Surgeons are more likely to report pain in the neck, erector muscles, and deltoids.[15] In a systematic review of 21 articles, with over 5000 surgeons and interventionalists, the most common MSDs were cervical spine disease (17%), rotator cuff pathology (18%), lumbar spine disease (19%), and carpal tunnel syndrome (9%).[17] OR nurses most commonly report lower back pain followed by pain in the rest of the joints.[7] Of these wrists and shoulders were cited as giving discomfort most frequently. Furthermore, MSDs manifest differently within roles. For example, reports of WRMSDs varied based upon nurses' roles and specialties. Assistant nurses were more likely to report discomfort in the hands and elbows when compared with OR nurses who reported pain in the neck and shoulders.[18] Furthermore, orthopedics and neurosurgery OR nurses were more likely to report knee pain when compared to cardiac or other general surgery OR nurses.[19] WRMSD pain and injury results in pain, injury, and necessary absenteeism sometimes requiring workman's compensation. This can lessen the provider's ability to work in the OR, or prompt them to change roles/occupations. In extreme cases, WRMSDs can cause providers to lose their jobs, or retire early.[19,20] Literature supports that nearly 70% of nurses leave the profession due to reasons related to WRMSDs.[19–22] Anesthesiologists reported discomfort when providing spinal anesthesia due to low operating table heights. Researchers noted that anesthesiologists compensated for lower table heights by unduly flexing their necks, lower backs, and knees.[23] More insight and study of the ergonomic implications of equipment and tools are needed before implementation. Emphatically, more research is needed to investigate the ergonomic risk factors for all roles within the OR setting as the most prevalently studied roles include surgeons, anesthetists, and nurses. At publication of this book, not a single article reviewing perfusionist ergonomic risk could be found.

Job dissatisfaction and performance

With the reported amount of discomfort and pain, it's easy to understand the connection between ergonomics and job satisfaction. Proper ergonomics in the workplace can stimulate employee morale, performance, and job satisfaction.[24,25] For those who spend long hours stationed in front of computer screens or locked into stances necessary to surgical proficiency proper ergonomics can significantly improve job satisfaction.[26,27] Organizations have a history of addressing stress through interventions focused on the individual, i.e., employee assistance programs. These programs often rely on offering the employee relaxation techniques, medications, and supportive exercise routines and even extend psychological resources.[17] However, these individual interventions do little to address the cause of the stress itself.[16] The effectiveness of individual interventions is weakened since the employee must return to the same unchanged stress inducing environment.[28] A comfortable workspace with as little physical discomfort as possible aids in eliminating stress, thus increasing job satisfaction. Considering the high rates of burnout in surgeons, it is critical to include approaches to address ergonomic fatigue and injury rather than placing the weight of the issue directly onto the clinicians' shoulders.

Physical ergonomic considerations and recommendations

Due to the risk factors associated with poor physical ergonomic conditions, improvement is necessary to reduce the risk of WRMSDs in healthcare providers. This section will provide an overview of some of the most commonly cited ergonomic risk factors in the OR and potential suggestions for improvement which can be made to decrease risk for providers.

The overriding ergonomic concern is to reduce strain and stress on the musculoskeletal structure. Inappropriate placement of equipment, visual constraints, and poor equipment design can increase force and pressure on the spine and other joints causing discomfort, pain, and damage. Poor physical ergonomics requires the providers to compensate by manipulating their own posture, deviating from neutral positions repetitively, and in doing so, sacrificing their own well-being. Evidence has demonstrated that improved ergonomic performance and well-being result from training as *a part of* ergonomic system implementation, thereby reducing the full weight of responsibility on the person as training cannot stand alone to reduce poor physical ergonomic outcomes.[29] Those who have presented training in correct ergonomic body posture, including video feedback to providers, still maintain that work system design is the foundation for gaining healthy and pain-free surgery.

Training can be used to address some risk factors that influence physical ergonomics but is recommended as a last resort when no other options are available or feasible. This is because human factors focus on the adaption of the environment rather than the adaption of the human. When placing liquid in a square container, we cannot reasonably expect or demand that the liquid maintain a cylindrical shape.

Likewise, we cannot expect our employees and providers to maintain perfect posture in a system that does not support correct anatomical posture.

Recommendations to improve posture: Sit whenever possible. When sitting, keep the body as symmetrical as possible. Have both feet resting on the floor. If a foot pump is needed while standing do not leave the controlling foot on the pedal continuously. Instead return it to neutral ground when not exerting foot control to the pump. If using a foot pump while sitting, place a block or riser under your other foot so that the feet are at the same height. When tasks require sitting, use lower lumbar support to maintain a lordotic position in the lower back. When tasks require standing for long periods of time, keep your knees slightly bent and transfer your body weight from one side to the other every couple of minutes. Providers should conduct treatments/therapies at a proper table height to avoid bending. When necessary, provide safe and sturdy stools for other involved/assisting providers to stand on if the table height is too tall for them. Take breaks to stretch when possible, both inside and outside the OR.[30] Targeted stretching microbreaks may improve surgeon pain scores, without significantly lengthening procedural times.[31]

Equipment positioning

While every hospital has different structural parameters within their ORs, regardless of size of the OR, layout and use of space can become an issue. Layout of the OR can be difficult as multiple machines must coexist with the providers in the same space. Because the flow of work surrounds the patient, equipment is circled around the patient. Further, certain machines like the cardiopulmonary bypass pump must be maintained within a certain distance from the patient, with closer being optimal. Adjusting table heights or providing stools (for standing or sitting) when appropriate has been recommend to combat ergonomic problems.[32]

Commonly, endoscopic or laparoscopic monitors are placed on top of other pieces of equipment above eye level. Confounding the low resolution and instability of endoscopic images is the placement of the technology responsible for displaying the image. Preferred viewing angles of this type of technology are between 10 and 25 degrees below the line of sight.[33] In the future, new advancements such as head mounted displays (such as a pair of glasses) will eliminate some of these current issues while creating others. As discussed earlier, posture and neutral anatomical positioning is vital to the prevention of WRMSDs. When equipment is placed out of arms reach or treatment requires providers to lean, proper posture cannot be maintained. Further, poor equipment positioning can lead to inadequate spaces for providers to move through and require providers to step over wires, tubing, and electrical connections. While layout issues can cause problems for any role in the OR, the perfusionists experience greater deviations from their workflow.[34]

Ideally, teams should arrange monitors and other tools optimally by installing flexible ceiling mounted booms rather than placing them on the tops of other equipment. This allows providers a range of usage for that equipment and can more easily accommodate musculoskeletal function regardless of provider heights or provider positioning.[35,36]

For more information about redesigning the OR workspace, see Chapter 12: Redesigning the Operating Room for Safety.

Visual considerations

From lighting to the positioning of the patient and equipment, visualization is of utmost importance during surgery. Providers must be able to see the surgical field, (aided or unaided by technology), the read out of monitors, and their surroundings including equipment and personnel.

Within the hospital, the OR is one of the few areas that require specialized lighting. A combination of general ambient light precision light and high light levels is needed depending on the task or precision required.[37] Surgical lights are unique as they are constantly manipulated by their users. However, the lights are often described as hard to move, moving of their own volition, or difficult to grasp firmly due to small handles or general weightiness. Further, depending on their placement, they can cast shadows over the surgical field. With the use of a monoscopic camera, advances in endoscopic surgery have shifted the view of the operating field. The low resolution of the image and other factors such as inability to maintain a still image and lack of light inside a body cavity create difficult visualization. Evidence suggests that these conditions delay the completion of surgical tasks when compared to direct observation.[38]

Other sightlines are compromised using certain materials. For example, clear drapes are not the norm, but may be preferred as they enable anesthesiologists to see what is happening in the operating field allowing them to maintain situation awareness of the case.[39]

Recommendations: An increase in lighting in the OR may alleviate the need to constantly reposition the surgical lights and decrease shadows.[40] Additionally, regular maintenance of the OR light hinges/joints and replacement/extension of small handles would make them easier to manipulate and place as needed.

Equipment design

Personal equipment used during surgery ranges from stools and headlamps to surgical instruments like scissors, scalpels, forceps, clamps, and retractors. The design of standardized surgical equipment has focused on the ability to be mass produced and rapidly sterilized rather than for ergonomic sustainability of the user. Dental Loupes corrected the posture of dental students' trunks, heads, and necks when used during cavity preparation.[41] Other studies have demonstrated the opposite that loupes and headlamps contribute to neck pain, thus demonstrating that the solution is not one size fits all. Depending on the role, job requirements, and individual factors associated with a person, solutions to maintain proper posture may be difficult. This difference could potentially be explained by the common seated versus standing positions of dental providers compared with surgical providers.[42]

Further, the nature of surgery requires providers to maintain static positions, even for maintenance tasks such as holding an instrument for a long period of time. New technologies and devices allow for relief of these obligations during surgery sparing the provider physical strain and free him or her up for other tasks. Self-retaining retractors for abdominal surgery (i.e., Bookwalter, Thompson, Omni-Tract), cardiothoracic surgery (i.e., Finochietto), or musculoskeletal surgery (i.e., Weitlaner) allow ideal exposure with limited human capital needs. For example, residents and nurses who would traditionally be responsible for holding pannus steadily over a long period of time can be relieved of this task by implementing a device which maintains the retraction without inducing physical stress or fatigue in the provider.[31] While some tasks require certain positions and can be alleviated by introduction of a new supportive device, other current devices cause pain and discomfort. These devices are unavoidable. For instance, minimally invasive surgery requires providers to deviate their hands and wrists from the neutral anatomical position. Redesigning these tools can provide relief by redirecting force away from pressure points and distributing it to maximal surface area.[43] Similarly, a redesign of needle drivers decreased muscle fatigue and the necessary muscle power to complete endoscopic suturing.[44] Rather than the traditional design, pistol-shaped forceps and scissors have been demonstrated to reduce muscle strain, pressure areas, and pain without decreasing effectiveness or efficiency.[45]

The following recommendations may help when planning OR design. Provider workload and necessity to maintain static positions can be reduced or avoided by adopting ergonomic supportive devices. Handheld equipment should accommodate multiple hand sizes[46–48] and wrist positions, especially as the gender gap within the OR continues to close.[49,50] Adjust loupes so that the head, neck, and trunk remain in a neutral position if possible. Use ergonomically designed surgical instruments. Try to maintain correct body posture while using these tools by keeping your extremities as close to your core as possible. For instance, providers should maintain elbows as close to a 90-degree bend as possible while keeping them tucked close into their sides.

Posture analysis tools

Now that we have presented some of the most common physical ergonomic risk factors, we will briefly present the methods by which you can analyze posture in your OR to identify and potentially improve the safety of the providers.

Analysis of posture can be conducted using multiple methods including the Rapid Entire Body Assessment (REBA) method,[51] Rapid Upper Limb Assessment (RULA) method,[52] the Quick Exposure Check (QEC) method,[53] the Nordic Questionnaire,[54] Postural Ergonomic Risk Assessment (PERA) method,[55] the Body Part Discomfort (BPD) scale,[48] the Lifting Fatigue Failure Tool (LiFFT), and the National Aeronautics and Space Administration Task Load index (NASA-TLX).[56]

Even more methods exist to evaluate risk factors which contribute to musculoskeletal disorders, and as Chiasson et al. demonstrate, no two are alike.[57] For this reason, great care must be taken when selecting a method for analysis. For example, the LiFFT method focuses explicitly on the cumulative loading and fatigue failure associated with the lower back.[58] Additionally, as we learn more about ergonomic risk factors and the musculoskeletal system, the methods are revised and updated. As an example, the NIOSH lifting equation is now known as the Revised NIOSH Lifting Equation.[59]

In conclusion, physical ergonomic improvement begins with the environment and the work system. The goal of a properly designed ergonomic work system is to support the health and well-being of the people within that system, adapting to the user rather than constraining the user. Studies have demonstrated that ergonomic improvement can lead to injury reduction, cost reduction, and reduction of absenteeism and that these outcomes can be achieved by implementing low-cost solutions.[25,60]

For more information or to reach out to a Human Factors Engineer/Researcher/Practitioner, please use the following resources:

The Human Factors and Ergonomics Society: www.hfes.org.

Human Factors Transforming Healthcare: www.hfthnetwork.org.

Agency for Healthcare Research and Quality: https://psnet.ahrq.gov/primer/human-factors-engineering.

Institute for Healthcare improvement: http://www.ihi.org/education/IHIOpenSchool/resources/Pages/Activities/ExerciseHumanFactors.aspx.

MedStar Health's National Center for Human Factors in Healthcare: www.medicalhumanfactors.net.

The Johns Hopkins' Armstrong Institute Center for Health Care Human Factors: https://www.hopkinsmedicine.org/armstrong_institute/centers/human_factors_engineering.

Other overarching articles of interest:

From discovery to design: The evolution of human factors in healthcare.[61]

Human factors in healthcare: Welcome progress, but still scratching the surface.[62]

The science of human factors: Separating fact from fiction.[63]

SEIPS 2.0: A human factors framework for studying and improving the work of healthcare professionals and patients.[64]

References

1. Wickens CD, editor. *An introduction to human factors engineering*, vol. 2. Upper Saddle River, NJ: Pearson/Prentice Hall; 2004.
2. Hagberg M, Silverstein B, Smith M, Hendrick H, Carayon P. *Work related musculoskeletal disorders (WMSDs): a reference book for prevention*. London: Taylor & Francis; 1995.

3. Human-factors engineering | definition, ergonomics, & examples. Encyclopedia Britannica. https://www.britannica.com/topic/human-factors-engineering. Accessed February 18, 2020.

4. Tayyari F, Smith J. *Occupational ergonomics: principles and applications.* 1st ed. London: Chapman & Hall; 1997.

5. Lee KS. Ergonomics in total quality management: how can we sell ergonomics to management? *Ergonomics* 2005;**48**(5):547−58. https://doi.org/10.1080/001401304000 29282.

6. Jaffar N, Jaffar A, Mohd-Kamar I, Lop N. A literature review of ergonomics risk factors in construction industry. *Procedia Eng* 2011;**20**:89−97.

7. Bodenheimer T, Sinsky C. From triple to quadruple aim: care of the patient requires care of the provider. *Ann Fam Med* 2014;**12**(6):573−6. https://doi.org/10.1370/afm.1713.

8. Institute of Medicine (US) Committee on Quality of Health Care in America. To err is human: building a safer health system. In: Kohn LT, Corrigan JM, Donaldson MS, editors. Washington, DC: National Academies Press (US); 2000. http://www.ncbi.nlm.nih.gov/books/NBK225182/. [Accessed 18 February 2020].

9. Henriksen K, Dayton E, Keyes MA, Carayon P, Hughes R. Understanding adverse events: a human factors framework. In: Hughes RG, editor. *Patient safety and quality: an evidence-based handbook for nurses. Advances in patient safety.* Rockville, MD: Agency for Healthcare Research and Quality (US); 2008. http://www.ncbi.nlm.nih.gov/books/NBK2666/. [Accessed 18 February 2020].

10. World Health Organization. What is human factors and why is it important to patient safety? https://www.who.int/patientsafety/education/curriculum/who_mc_topic-2.pdf. Accessed September 24, 2019.

11. Sachdeva AK, Philibert I, Leach DC, et al. Patient safety curriculum for surgical residency programs: results of a national consensus conference. *Surgery* 2007;**141**(4):427−41. https://doi.org/10.1016/j.surg.2006.12.009.

12. Yeung A, Greenwalt J. A framework for quality improvement and patient safety education in radiation oncology residency programs. *Practic Radiat Oncol* 2015;**5**(6):423−6. https://doi.org/10.1016/j.prro.2015.07.008.

13. Beyea SC, Slattery MJ, von Reyn LJ. Outcomes of a simulation-based nurse residency program. *Clin Simul Nurs* 2010;**6**(5):e169−75. https://doi.org/10.1016/j.ecns.2010.01.005.

14. Kennedy BP. Human factors science being used to improve health care systems, patient care. *AAP News* February 2020. https://www.aappublications.org/news/2019/10/11/hit101119. [Accessed 18 February 2020].

15. Bongers PM, Kremer AM, ter Laak J. Are psychosocial factors, risk factors for symptoms and signs of the shoulder, elbow, or hand/wrist? A review of the epidemiological literature. *Am J Ind Med* 2002;**41**(5):315−42. https://doi.org/10.1002/ajim.10050.

16. National Research Council and The Institute of Medicine. *Musculoskeletal disorders and the workplace: low back and upper extremities. Panel on musculoskeletal disorders and the workplace.* Washington, DC: National Academy Press; 2001.

17. Epstein S, Sparer EH, Tran BN, et al. Prevalence of work-related musculoskeletal disorders among surgeons and Interventionalists: a systematic review and meta-analysis. *JAMA Surg* 2018;**153**(2). https://doi.org/10.1001/jamasurg.2017.4947. e174947-e174947.

18. Simonsen JG, Arvidsson I, Nordander C. Ergonomics in the operating room. *Work* 2012;**41**(Suppl. 1):5644−6. https://doi.org/10.3233/WOR-2012-0905-5644.

19. Choobineh A, Movahed M, Tabatabaie SH, Kumashiro M. Perceived demands and musculoskeletal disorders in operating room nurses of Shiraz city hospitals. *Ind Health* 2010;**48**(1):74−84. https://doi.org/10.2486/indhealth.48.74.

20. Sheikhzadeh A, Gore C, Zuckerman JD, Nordin M. Perioperating nurses and technicians' perceptions of ergonomic risk factors in the surgical environment. *Appl Ergon* 2009;**40**(5):833−9. https://doi.org/10.1016/j.apergo.2008.09.012.

21. Long MH, Johnston V, Bogossian F. Work-related upper quadrant musculoskeletal disorders in midwives, nurses and physicians: a systematic review of risk factors and functional consequences. *Appl Ergon* 2012;**43**(3):455−67. https://doi.org/10.1016/j.apergo.2011.07.002.

22. Schlossmacher R, Amaral FG. Low back injuries related to nursing professionals working conditions: a systematic review. *Work* 2012;**41**(Suppl. 1):5737−8. https://doi.org/10.3233/WOR-2012-0935-5737.

23. Sohn H-M, Kim H, Hong J-P, Lee KM, Kim J. Higher operating table for optimal needle-entry angle and less discomfort during spinal anesthesia. *Anesth Analg* 2018;**126**(4):1349. https://doi.org/10.1213/ANE.0000000000002534.

24. Leblebici D. Impact of workplace quality on employee's productivity: case study of a bank in Turkey. *J Bus Econ Finan* 2012;**1**(1):38−49. http://agris.fao.org/agris-search/search.do?recordID=TR2016013061. [Accessed 18 February 2020].

25. Evanoff BA, Bohr PC, Wolf LD. Effects of a participatory ergonomics team among hospital orderlies. *Am J Ind Med* 1999;**35**(4):358−65. https://doi.org/10.1002/(SICI)1097-0274(199904)35:4<358::AID-AJIM6>3.0.CO;2-R.

26. Ikonne CN, Onuoha UD. Factors influencing job satisfaction of librarians in Federal and State University Libraries in Southern Nigeria. *Open Access Libr J* 2015;**2**(2):1−9. https://doi.org/10.4236/oalib.1101337.

27. Miles AK, Perrewé PL. The relationship between person−environment fit, control, and strain: the role of ergonomic work design and training. *J Appl Soc Psychol* 2011;**41**(4):729−72. https://doi.org/10.1111/j.1559-1816.2011.00734.x.

28. Cartwright S, Cooper C, Murphy L. Diagnosing a health organization: a proactive approach to stress in the workplace. In: *Job stress interventions*. Washington, DC: American Psychological Association; 1995. p. 217−33.

29. Robertson MM, Maynard WS. Office ergonomics training: an instructional systems model for developing an effective program. *Prof Saf*:22-30.

30. Rohrich RJ. Why I hate the headlight and other ways to protect your cervical spine. *Plast Reconstr Surg* 2001;**107**(4):1037−8. https://doi.org/10.1097/00006534-200104010-00021.

31. Park AE, Zahiri HR, Hallbeck MS, et al. Intraoperative "micro breaks" with targeted stretching enhance surgeon physical function and mental focus: a multicenter cohort study. *Ann Surg* 2017;**265**(2):340−6. https://doi.org/10.1097/SLA.0000000000001665.

32. Matern U, Koneczny S. Safety, hazards and ergonomics in the operating room. *Surg Endosc* 2007;**21**:1965−9. https://doi.org/10.1007/s00464-007-9396-4.

33. Menozzi M., von Buol A, Krueger H, Miège C. Direction of gaze and comfort: discovering the relation for the ergonomic optimization of visual tasks. *Ophthalmic Physiol Opt: the Journal of the British College of Ophthalmic Opticians (Optometrists)* 1994 Oct;**14**(4):393-399. https://doi.org/10.1111/j.1475-1313.1994.tb00131.x. PMID: 7845698.

34. Cohen TN, Cabrera JS, Sisk OD, et al. Identifying workflow disruptions in the cardiovascular operating room. *Anaesthesia* 2016;**71**(8):948−54. https://doi.org/10.1111/anae.13521.

35. Kelts GI, McMains KC, Chen PG, Weitzel EK. Monitor height ergonomics: a comparison of operating room video display terminals. *Allergy Rhinol (Providence)* 2015;**6**(1): 28−32. https://doi.org/10.2500/ar.2015.6.0119.

36. Sugita S, Sugita K. Modified ceiling-mounted zoom operating microscope. *Am J Ophthalmol* 1971;**72**(5):972−4. https://doi.org/10.1016/0002-9394(71)91700-4.

37. Rostenberg B, Barach PR. Design of cardiovascular operating rooms for tomorrow's technology and clinical practice—Part 2. *Prog Pediatr Cardiol* 2012;**33**(1):57−65. https://doi.org/10.1016/j.ppedcard.2011.12.010.

38. Tendick F, Jennings RW, Tharp G, Stark L. Sensing and manipulation problems in endoscopic surgery: experiment, analysis, and observation. *Presence Teleoperators Virtual Environ* 1993;**2**(1):66−81. https://doi.org/10.1162/pres.1993.2.1.66.

39. Guttman O, Lazzara E, Keebler J, Webster KL, Gisick L, Baker A. Dissecting communication barriers in healthcare: a path to enhancing communication resiliency, reliability, and patient safety. *J Patient Saf* 2018. https://doi.org/10.1097/PTS.0000000000000541. Publish Ahead of Print.

40. Joseph A, Bayramzadeh S, Zamani Z, Rostenberg B. Safety, performance, and satisfaction outcomes in the operating room: a literature review. *HERD* 2018;**11**(2):137−50. https://doi.org/10.1177/1937586717705107.

41. Carpentier M, Aubeux D, Armengol V, Pérez F, Prud'homme T, Gaudin A. The effect of magnification loupes on spontaneous posture change of dental students during preclinical restorative training. *J Dent Educ* 2019;**83**(4):407−15. https://doi.org/10.21815/JDE.019.044.

42. Neck postures and cervical spine loading among microsurgeons operating with loupes and headlamp: IIE Transactions on Occupational Ergonomics and Human Factors: Vol 1, No 4. https://www.tandfonline.com/doi/abs/10.1080/21577323.2013.840342. Accessed February 18, 2020.

43. Sancibrian R, Gutierrez-Diez MC, Torre-Ferrero C, Benito-Gonzalez MA, Redondo-Figuero C, Manuel-Palazuelos JC. Design and evaluation of a new ergonomic handle for instruments in minimally invasive surgery. *J Surg Res* 2014;**188**(1):88−99. https://doi.org/10.1016/j.jss.2013.12.021.

44. Emam TA, Frank TG, Hanna GB, Cuschieri A. Influence of handle design on the surgeon's upper limb movements, muscle recruitment, and fatigue during endoscopic suturing. *Surg Endosc* 2001;**15**(7):667−72. https://doi.org/10.1007/s004640080141.

45. Büchel D, Mårvik R, Hallabrin B, Matern U. Ergonomics of disposable handles for minimally invasive surgery. *Surg Endosc* 2010;**24**(5):992−1004. https://doi.org/10.1007/s00464-009-0714-x.

46. Berguer R, Hreljac A. The relationship between hand size and difficulty using surgical instruments: a survey of 726 laparoscopic surgeons. *Surg Endosc* 2004;**18**(3):508−12. https://doi.org/10.1007/s00464-003-8824-3.

47. Hands of a Woman…Surgeon…. The Academic Surgeon. https://www.aasurg.org/blog/hands-of-a-womansurgeon/. Published July 20, 2015. Accessed February 18, 2020.

48. Sutton E, Irvin M, Zeigler C, Lee G, Park A. The ergonomics of women in surgery. *Surg Endosc* 2014;**28**(4):1051−5. https://doi.org/10.1007/s00464-013-3281-0.

49. Wolfe L. How many women surgeons are there in the United States? The balance careers. https://www.thebalancecareers.com/number-of-women-surgeons-in-the-us-3972900. Accessed February 18, 2020.

50. Mueller C, Wright R, Girod S. The publication gender gap in US academic surgery. *BMC Surg* 2017;**17**(1):16. https://doi.org/10.1186/s12893-017-0211-4.

51. Hignett S, McAtamney L. Rapid entire body assessment (REBA). *Appl Ergon* 2000; **31**(2):201−5. https://doi.org/10.1016/s0003-6870(99)00039-3.
52. McAtamney L, Nigel Corlett E. RULA: a survey method for the investigation of work-related upper limb disorders. *Appl Ergon* 1993;**24**(2):91−9. https://doi.org/10.1016/0003-6870(93)90080-s.
53. David G, Woods V, Li G, Buckle P. The development of the quick exposure check (QEC) for assessing exposure to risk factors for work-related musculoskeletal disorders. *Appl Ergon* 2008;**39**(1):57−69. https://doi.org/10.1016/j.apergo.2007.03.002.
54. Bernal D, Campos-Serna J, Tobias A, Vargas-Prada S, Benavides FG, Serra C. Work-related psychosocial risk factors and musculoskeletal disorders in hospital nurses and nursing aides: a systematic review and meta-analysis. *Int J Nurs Stud* 2015;**52**(2): 635−48. https://doi.org/10.1016/j.ijnurstu.2014.11.003.
55. An observational method for Postural Ergonomic Risk Assessment (PERA) - ScienceDirect. https://www.sciencedirect.com/science/article/pii/S0169814116302657. Accessed February 18, 2020.
56. Hart SG. *NASA task load index (TLX). Volume 1.0;* Paper and pencil package. Moffett Field, CA United States: NASA Ames Research Center; 1986. p. 1−26. https://ntrs.nasa.gov/archive/nasa/casi.ntrs.nasa.gov/20000021488.pdf. [Accessed 20 February 2020].
57. Chiasson M-È, Imbeau D, Aubry K, Delisle A. Comparing the results of eight methods used to evaluate risk factors associated with musculoskeletal disorders. *Int J Ind Ergon* 2012;**42**(5):478−88.
58. Gallagher S, Sesek RF, Schall MC, Huangfu R. Development and validation of an easy-to-use risk assessment tool for cumulative low back loading: the lifting fatigue failure tool (LiFFT). *Appl Ergon* 2017;**63**:142−50. https://doi.org/10.1016/j.apergo.2017.04.016.
59. Barim MS, Sesek RF, Capanoglu MF, et al. Improving the risk assessment capability of the revised NIOSH lifting equation by incorporating personal characteristics. *Appl Ergon* 2019;**74**:67−73. https://doi.org/10.1016/j.apergo.2018.08.007.
60. Juul-Kristensen B, Jensen C. Self-reported workplace related ergonomic conditions as prognostic factors for musculoskeletal symptoms: the "BIT" follow up study on office workers. *Occup Environ Med* 2005;**62**(3):188−94. https://doi.org/10.1136/oem.2004.013920.
61. Cafazzo J, St-Cyr O. From discovery to design: the evolution of human factors in healthcare. *Hcq* 2012;**15**(sp):24−9. https://doi.org/10.12927/hcq.2012.22845.
62. Waterson P, Catchpole K. Human factors in healthcare: welcome progress, but still scratching the surface. *BMJ Qual Saf* 2016;**25**(7):480−4. https://doi.org/10.1136/bmjqs-2015-005074.
63. Russ AL, Fairbanks RJ, Karsh B-T, Militello LG, Saleem JJ, Wears RL. The science of human factors: separating fact from fiction. *BMJ Qual Saf* 2013;**22**(10):802−8. https://doi.org/10.1136/bmjqs-2012-001450.
64. Holden RJ, Carayon P, Gurses AP, et al. SEIPS 2.0: a human factors framework for studying and improving the work of healthcare professionals and patients. *Ergonomics* 2013;**56**(11):1669−86. https://doi.org/10.1080/00140139.2013.838643.

Prehabilitation and enhanced recovery after surgery

Artem Shmelev, MD [1], Steven C. Cunningham, MD, FACS [2]

[1]*Department of Surgery, Columbia University Medical Center, New York, NY, United States;*
[2]*Division of Pancreatic and Hepatobiliary Surgery, Ascension Saint Agnes Hospital Center and Cancer Institute, Baltimore, MD, United States*

Introduction

Background and history

Enhancing recovery after surgery has, of course, been the goal of surgeons since the beginning of surgery. It was not until the 1990s, however, that what we now refer to as "enhanced recovery after surgery" (ERAS) began to take its more formalized, programmatic shape, initially under the name "Fast Track" surgery in a publication on coronary bypass patients showing shorter intensive care unit and overall postoperative lengths of stay in the "fast track" group managed with a bundle of pre-, intra-, and postoperative principles.[1] Shortly later, similar reports followed, describing bundle-enhanced recovery after colonic resections.[2,3] Then, in 2001, the ERAS Study Group formed, gathered in London to optimize a protocol based on published evidence, met again in 2003 in Stockholm as the 1st ERAS Symposium, and in 2005 produced a consensus paper[4] describing approximately 20 pre-, intra-, and postoperative interventions that now form the backbone of 17 specialty-specific ERAS guidelines,[5] most with a high level of evidence, that are currently (and freely) available via The ERAS Society (erassociety.org), which was founded and registered as a nonprofit in 2010.[6] Even from the earliest designs, the perioperative interventions have covered the gamut of perioperative care, from the earliest stages of patient education and prehabilitation, to beyond the end of the postoperative care of any one patient, to include—and this is essential—an audit of the ERAS process for future patients, as shown in the ERAS protocol in Table 8.1.

Why ERAS works

If one had to identify a single source of value in ERAS, it would likely be multimodality. However, this refers not merely to the multiplicity of the modal elements in the bundle (no single modality would be expected to yield drastic results,[7] but instead it is the combination of interventions that produces a larger benefit). Rather, a broader multimodality helps explain why the larger benefit that comes with the

Handbook of Perioperative and Procedural Patient Safety. https://doi.org/10.1016/B978-0-323-66179-9.00017-8

Table 8.1 Elements of a typical ERAS protocol (e.g., for gastrointestinal surgery, hernia surgery, etc.).

Element	Goal
Preoperative (months to weeks)	
Medical optimization of chronic diseases; BMI reduction; diabetes control	Reduce SSI, cardiopulmonary complications, hernia recurrence, etc.
Prehabilitation and exercise	Improve functional status; engage patients in their care; reduce deconditioning postoperatively
Nutritional screening and supplementation	Reduce wound and other complications
Cessation of smoking and excessive alcohol use	Reduce wound and other complications
Counseling of patients and their supporters	Reduce anxiety; strengthen rapport and compliance
Preoperative (days to hours)	
Skin preparation; MRSA decolonization; antibiotics	Reduce SSI
Avoidance of bowel preparation	Reduce dehydration, electrolytes imbalances; preserve protective GI flora
DR and/or carbohydrate loading[a]	Reduce insulin resistance; improve well-being
Avoiding sedative premedication	Hasten recovery from anesthesia
VTE prophylaxis (based on Caprini or other scale)	Reduce VTE
Multimodal anesthesia	Reduce pain, PONV, and ileus
Intraoperative	
Balanced fluid management	Avoid edema; reduce ileus and other complications
Maintenance of normothermia	Reduce various complications including SSI
Epidural or regional anesthesia for open surgery	Reduce stress response and insulin resistance; minimize opioid use
Minimally invasive surgical approach	Hasten recovery; reduce pain and opioid use
Multimodal anesthesia; avoiding long-acting opioids and excessively deep anesthesia	Reduce pain and PONV; hasten recovery from anesthesia; reduce stress and ileus
Restrictive use of surgical drains	Facilitate mobilization; reduce discomfort
Removal of NGT before reversal of anesthesia	Reduce pulmonary complications; hasten PO intake

Table 8.1 Elements of a typical ERAS protocol (e.g., for gastrointestinal surgery, hernia surgery, etc.).—*cont'd*

Element	Goal
Postoperative	
Early mobilization (beginning the day of surgery)	Hasten recovery and return of bowel function; reduce VTE and respiratory complications
Multimodal, opioid-sparing analgesia	Reduce pain, PONV, and ileus; hasten overall recovery
Multimodal approach to PONV	Minimize PONV and enhance PO intake
Avoidance or early removal of urinary catheters	Reduce UTI
Use of chewing gum, laxatives, prokinetics, and/or (when using opioids) peripheral opioid antagonists	Hasten return of bowel function
Early oral intake with nutrient-rich supplements	Enhanced nutritional support of healing; reduce insulin resistance
Restrictive postoperative fluid management	Reduce edema- and hypervolemia-related complications; hasten return of bowel function
Postoperative glucose control	Reduce risk of SSI
Continued mechanical and/or chemical VTE prophylaxis; early mobilization	Reduce VTE
Planned early discharge	Avoid delays in discharge; reduce healthcare-associated complications
Audit of outcomes and process in a multidisciplinary team on a regular basis	Control adherence to ERAS protocols and improve outcomes

Abbreviations: DR, dietary restriction; GI, gastrointestinal; MRSA, methicillin-resistant Staphylococcus aureus; NGT, nasogastric tube; NSAID, nonsteroidal, antiinflammatory drug; PONV, postoperative nausea and vomiting; SSI, surgical-site infection; UTI, urinary-tract infection; VTE, venous thromboembolism.
[a] *See text for details.*

bundle of interventions is not merely additive, but rather is likely synergistic (meaning that, for example, 10 interventions each with a benefit of 1 hypothetical unit "add up" to >10 units of benefit). When one considers the surgical truism that "complications beget complications," it becomes intuitive that an inverse process explains the synergy of ERAS bundles: each intervention in the bundle serves to set up all others for success. However, when one further considers the even less tangible effects of all the coordination, communication, and teamwork—among different types of care providers, different departments, the patients themselves and their families, etc.—that are required to build and run a robust ERAS program, it becomes increasingly clear that there is a further synergy that occurs as a result of "the coordinated team effort," of the breaking down of silos to achieve a unified collaboration, of the resultant culture change that invariably accompanies the extensive process of developing an ERAS program. Of course, the degree to which this additional synergy occurs is directly proportional to the degree to which the ERAS process is developed in a substantive, deeply rooted manner, as opposed to nominally going through the motions.

The essential inclusion in the process of a way to audit the process using various metrics invokes the adage that "you can't manage what you can't measure." While there is much useful truth here, it is important not to confuse measurability with value; indeed, many things with little to no value are highly measurable—and manageable—and countless things are intangible and largely unmeasurable but yet have tremendous value, such as culture. The ethos that develops in a multidisciplinary ERAS team coming together to break down interdepartmental silos and to build and run ERAS program is infectious throughout the institution. And the self-critical preoccupation with failure that accompanies a good audit process is a mark of a high-reliability organization.

Enhanced recovery before surgery

One of the most important aspects of ERAS is that it starts *before* surgery, with preoperative interventions such as prehabilitation. Rehabilitation will always be required postoperatively, of course, in the sense that any major surgical intervention will require a rehabilitation during recovery and convalescence of the patient back toward their preoperative baseline. But the shift in emphasis in the ERAS era, from *re*habilitation alone to *pre*habilitation, is essential.

It is not that prehabilitation, per se, is so important. Indeed, the evidence supporting the effectiveness of physical prehabilitation, as discussed below, is conflicting. Prehabilitation is, in fact, just another, single element in an ERAS bundle, and not an overwhelmingly effective one in isolation. What is essential about it, however, is that it is one of the *first* elements, and as such it *sets the tone and the cadence* of the entire perioperative experience. Having an operation is a significantly stressful trauma to the body, not unlike running a marathon, and just like attempting a marathon without training would be foolish, so too would having an elective major operation be, without first "training." Indeed, all the components of an ERAS protocol share the common focus of stress: minimizing it, and maximizing the patient's ability to respond to it.

Prehabilitation: preoperative ERAS elements

Although prehabilitation generally refers to a program of physical conditioning, here it may refer more broadly to the entire, preoperative, "training" period, including not only increasing physical conditioning, but also preparing psychologically and socially. Specific components of this preoperative phase, as shown in Table 8.1, include counseling of the patient and family, including assessing and shoring up social support; cessation of smoking, excessive alcohol use, and over-the-counter dietary supplements; assessing frailty; nutritional care; standard cardiac and medical risk stratification and optimization of comorbidities, including in particular controlling diabetes and addressing preoperative anemia; and, of course, the actual physical exercise generally associated with the term "prehabilitation."

Counseling

The first and most important step in counseling is establishing rapport; nothing good can be expected to result from a surgeon-patient relationship that lacks good rapport, especially in the elective setting. Facing a life-threatening situation such as a major operation is a highly meaningful experience for patients, one that profoundly impacts their humanity and spirituality, and therefore the meaning that patients attribute to their disease and the proposed operation is eminently relevant, as evidenced by studies showing that this *meaning*, per se, contributes to a patient's psychological and physiologic response.[8,9] And the way that surgeons impact this meaning is through their communication—their rapport—with patients. Indeed, an abundance of experience and data, including randomized data, has established the benefit of good communication on patient outcomes,[10,11] and optimal communication is patient-centered and value-sensitive regarding patients' religion/spirituality.[12,13] Although many providers may not have a sufficient degree of comfort to meet the spiritual and religious needs of their patients,[13] several good resources are available.[12,14]

Once rapport is established, patients will generally be more receptive to all subsequent counseling, and that counseling should include high-quality informed consent, estate planning (in particular, establishing medical power of attorney and healthcare directives), and optimizing and enlisting the collaboration of the patient's social support. A trusting relationship grows rapidly out of good rapport and will also facilitate successful counseling regarding the need to cease smoking[15] and excessive alcohol,[16] both ideally 4—8 weeks prior to operation, and dietary supplements,[17] 2—3 weeks prior, all of which is associated with a reduction in postoperative complications.

Assessing frailty

An increasingly recognized opportunity to further improve ERAS protocols is the assessment of frailty,[18] a syndrome of decreased physiologic reserve and resistance to stressors (viz, operations), which leaves patients vulnerable to worse postoperative outcomes.[19] The American College of Surgeons National Surgical Quality Improvement Program (ACS NSQIP)/American Geriatrics Society (AGS) Best Practices Guidelines list 5 criteria for frailty: weight loss, weakness, exhaustion, low physical activity, and slowness.[19] As shown in Table 8.2, these five criteria have definitions and cutoffs, whereby each criterion scores 1 point if positive, for

Table 8.2 ACS NSQIP/AGS best practice guidelines for frailty assessment.

Pts	Criteria	ACS definition	Positive (1 point scored) if ...
1	Weight loss	Lb lost in past year	>10 lb
1	Weakness	Grip strength	Lowest 20th percentile by gender and BMI
1	Exhaustion	Self-reported (Fried's Frailty[20])	Any answer of "moderate amount" or "most of the time"
1	Low physical activity	Weekly energy expenditure	Lowest 20th percentile by gender: Men: <383 kcal/week; Women: <270 kcal/week
1	Slowness	Walking	Lowest 20th percentile by gender and height

Legend: 0–1 = not frail; 2–3 = intermediate frail (pre-frail); 4–5 = frail (see text and Ref.[19] for details).

a total score of 0 (least frail) to 5 (most frail). In brief, the cutoff for weight loss is 10 lb; for exhaustion it is any positive answer to either of the two questions in Fried's Frailty test[20] (see below); and for the other three, it is being in the lowest 20th percentile. Based on this simple, 5-point scale, frail patients score 0–1, intermediate-frail patients 2–3, and frankly frail patients score 4–5. Increasing frailty is directly associated with increasing risk of poor outcomes: Intermediate-frail patients have a substantially elevated risk (but less than frankly frail patients) and further face a two-fold risk of *becoming* frankly frail over the next three years. Accordingly, frankly frail patients are at an even higher risk of poor postoperative outcomes,[19] and accordingly warrant a particularly assiduous risk–benefit analysis prior to operation, and strict adherence to ERAS protocols if operation is pursued.

In our practice, we assess frailty in any patient who is not obviously young and healthy and is being considered for a major operation. Many good tools for assessing frailty in addition to those in Table 8.2 are available and easy to administer and to score. We have found three instruments to be particularly useful and user-friendly: One is the Fried's Frailty tool recommended by the ACS/NSQIP/AGS Guidelines, which is a simple, 2-question survey that asks patients, regarding the last week, (1) how often they feel like "everything I did is an effort," and (2) how often "I could not get going"; the second is the G-8 test,[21] a simple, 8-question survey with a maximum score of 17, whereby a score of ≤14 identifies at-risk individuals; and the third is the vulnerable-elders survey (VES)-13,[22] which is a 13-question survey with a maximum score of 10 points, whereby a score of ≥3 identifies individuals with four times the risk of death or functional decline compared to individuals scoring <3. The beauty of these three survey instruments is that patients can work on them in the waiting room, after which it is easy to review and score them in the exam room.

Nutritional care

Because surgical stress is known to cause insulin resistance,[23] which increases the risk of postoperative nausea and vomiting (PONV)[24] and complications,[25,26] and because traditional, after-midnight fasting causes insulin resistance, which is mitigated by preoperative carbohydrate loading,[27] the omission of overnight fasting and the addition of carbohydrate loading have become a standard part of ERAS protocols, for both well- and malnourished patients. Fasts are now only 2–4 h prior to operation, with no increases in aspiration events in multiple studies.

The first step, however, in nutritional care is simply assessment, which can be done adequately and easily using the preoperative nutritional screen (PONS) score, which was designed by the Perioperative Quality Initiative 2 Workgroup[28] to be quickly (<5 min) administered by nursing staff in preoperative clinics/offices. Per the PONS score, patients with a low BMI (<18.5 [or <20 if age >65]), or unintentional weight loss (8–10 pounds in prior 6 mo), or eating <50% of their normal diet in past week, or a serum albumin <3 g/dL are considered at high risk for malnutrition-associated postoperative complications and should receive focused nutritional care, ideally with a nutrition consult if available. Preoperative nutritional supplementation for at-risk patients, ideally enterally and with immune-modulating formulae (e.g., containing arginine, omega-3 fatty acids, and ribonucleotides), has been shown in many meta-analyses of trials to associate with decreased postoperative complications and shorter length of stay.[29]

Because malnutrition is common, especially in older surgical patients,[30] and because it correlates reliably with complications,[31] providing preoperative nutritional supplementation to *malnourished* patients is uncontroversial. Given this knowledge, and given the above considerations on carbohydrate loading, most or all ERAS protocols eliminate the traditional overnight fast because it is *too much* fasting. However, for *well-nourished* patients, some have asked if overnight fasting is perhaps *not enough* fasting.[32] Indeed, dietary restriction (DR) has received increasing attention in recent decades for its health benefits. DR is best known for being the only intervention to extend both life span and health span, across species.[33,34] In addition to this well-known effect of DR, however, emerging data support a role for reducing postoperative complications[35]: Animal models of short-term, preoperative DR, followed by normal feeding postoperatively, show protection against ischemia reperfusion injury and vascular restenosis (intimal hyperplasia), with improved postoperative outcomes.[32] And in humans, supportive data are accruing. For example, short-term fasts (24- to 36-h) prior to chemotherapy attenuates toxicity,[36–38] and kidneys from dietary-restricted live donors have improved function and decreased rejection in recipients.[39] Indeed (although likely for different reasons), DR shares with carbohydrate loading the important postoperative effect of increased insulin sensitivity,[40] one of the hallmarks of extended-longevity models.[32] DR is not, after all, entirely new to surgery: Over 10 years ago it was observed not only to facilitate bariatric operations, but also to be associated with fewer postoperative complications.[41]

Physical prehabilitation

Regarding the actual, physical exercise generally associated with the term "prehabilitation," several meta-analyses have shown improvements with formal prehabilitation protocols, including some showing improved exercise capacity (but not length of stay, morbidity, or readmission),[42,43] and others showing shorter length of stay (but not improved functional capacity or morbidity),[44] but the most recent systematic reviews and meta-analyses are largely negative.[45–48] Still as discussed above, as a part of the ERAS bundle, there is likely significant value in physical prehabilitation programs, and the ideal ones, given the underwhelming results in meta-analyses, would be low cost from a healthcare-resource perspective.

Multimodal anesthesia

The preoperative initiation of a multimodal, pain-medication bundle in the preop area typically includes a scopolamine patch, acetaminophen, magnesium, and celecoxib.[49] Caveats of scopolamine patches, which are used to prevent PONV, include a relative contraindication in patients with narrow-angle glaucoma or age >70, and the patch should be removed 24–72 h after surgery, if there is no nausea. Gabapentin had been included in many preoperative bundles, including in the authors', but now has been eliminated given recent data suggesting an unfavorable risk–benefit ratio, particularly regarding pulmonary complications.

Intraoperative ERAS elements

As shown in Table 8.1, the intraoperative ERAS elements typically include interventions both from the surgery and the anesthesiology teams. The primary goal of multimodal ERAS anesthesia, like all other ERAS elements, is to minimize surgical stress. Guidelines for ERAS anesthesia include avoiding long-acting anxiolytic and opioids; preventing and treating PONV; avoiding excessively deep anesthesia; maintaining normal glucose levels, normal arterial oxygen levels and saturations, and normothermia (e.g., forced-air heating blankets, warmed IVF, etc.); using balanced crystalloids (as opposed to 0.9% saline), and multimodal, opioid-sparing anesthesia, with generous use of regional techniques.[49–51]

Surgical elements include primarily the use of minimally invasive approaches, but also avoidance of oral bowel preparation and abdominal drains. Nasogastric and urinary tubes should be removed at the end of the operation when possible, or as soon as possible thereafter. Strict adherence to antimicrobial prophylaxis, including skin preparation, use of wound protectors, use of clean supplies for closing, and nasal decontamination, is essential. Irrigation with an antimicrobial agent such as Povidone-iodine has been shown to decrease rates of surgical-site infection.[52] All irrigation solution should be warmed, especially in open laparotomies.

Postoperative ERAS elements

Postoperatively, epidural anesthesia should be preferred over parenteral opioids, especially for open operations, given its association with faster recovery of gastrointestinal function, improved insulin sensitivity, and likely reduced cardiovascular and respiratory complications.[53] If hypotension occurs with the epidural, and the patient is normovolemic, then vasopressors may be considered as a first-line therapy.

Postoperative delirium should be avoided by avoiding offending medications (e.g., benzodiazepines, narcotics, anticholinergics) and disturbances in the sleep—wake cycle (and, as discussed above, excessively deep anesthesia and prolonged fasting).[53]

Early and aggressive ambulation, ideally in a structured, or "forced" way, reliably hastens return of gastrointestinal function and discharge from the hospital.[54,55]

Gum-chewing has been found in some[56–58] meta-analyses to decrease postoperative ileus, and, given its low risk and cost, should be used in addition to opioid avoidance, early ambulation, laxatives, and early feeding as tolerated (given the better toleration of liquid diets compared to solid diets, and the wide availability of nutrient-rich, liquid, dietary supplements, rushing to solid food may be counterproductive). When opioids are required, peripheral opioid-blocking agents may be useful to mitigate their adverse effects.

And, importantly, in addition to strict adherence to standard postoperative prophylaxes and continuation of the multimodal analgesia, the final and essential part of the postoperative ERAS protocol is an audit of the entire process. Audits should be at regular intervals, ongoing, and formally reviewed with the ERAS-implementing team, as evidence shows that even the best ERAS programs tend to lapse back into old patterns of behavior, with loss of the erstwhile, early benefits, which can be recouped as guided by audits.[18] There are several ways to audit an ERAS program, and excellent guidance is available through the ERAS Society[59] and through the ACS's Improving Surgical Care and Recovery (ISCR) Safety Program, which is funded and guided by the Agency for Healthcare Research and Quality (AHRQ) in collaboration with the Johns Hopkins Armstrong Institute for Patient Safety and Quality.[60]

Benefits of ERAS protocols
Clinical outcomes

The most obvious short-term benefits one would expect to see from minimizing surgical stress would be shorter lengths of stay and fewer complications, and indeed that is precisely what has been found, especially in studies of colorectal ERAS protocols, which are the most numerous studies. Several meta-analyses of randomized, controlled trials show that the short-term outcomes of length of stay and postoperative complications are significantly improved compared to traditional care.[61,62] There are fewer studies looking at long-term outcomes such as survival. Individual studies, in both malignant[63–65] and benign[66] diseases, suggest a long-term survival benefit associated with ERAS, but one of the most recent systematic reviews falls short of confirming this.[67] However, given that ERAS is associated with fewer complications, and therefore with on-time receipt of and completion of chemotherapy, confirmation of the finding of greater long-term survival would not be unexpected.

Economics

Given that long lengths of stay and postoperative complications are very expensive, it is unsurprising that the benefits of ERAS protocols are not limited to patients' clinical outcomes, but rather extend as well to the finances of the hospital. Many reports, from different countries, in different-sized hospitals, focusing different types of operations (predominantly colorectal, but also pancreatic and hepatobiliary, gynecologic, thoracic, bariatric, hernia, and vascular), have confirmed a favorable cost−benefit analysis associated with ERAS protocols.[68−75]

Implementation of an ERAS protocol

Getting started with an ERAS protocol de novo requires substantial preparation, and failing to prepare, as Ben Franklin (probably never) said, constitutes preparing to fail. As discussed above (*Why ERAS Works*), the key to success is the multimodality, which entails building a team and dismantling interdepartmental silos *prior to* implementation. Importantly, these two processes occur simultaneously during the preparation phase, and the key here, as in protean other situations in life, is communicating with people. The first and most important step is to assemble a team of supportive, enthusiastic, and available people. Ideally, an ERAS working group should include one or two surgeon-champions and representatives from disciplines and departments that interact with the surgical patient, including anesthesiology, nursing, physical therapy and rehabilitation, the operating and recovery rooms, pharmacy, nutrition, patient safety, information technology, and last but certainly not least, since their buy-in is essential, administration.

As a team is assembling, it is helpful to find an organization or institution to guide and support the process of implementing and running an ERAS program. We found it very helpful to enroll in the ACS's ISCR Safety Program (available in collaboration AHRQ and the Johns Hopkins Armstrong Institute for Patient Safety and Quality).[60] This program offers introductory recruitment webinars and regular, frequent, coaching calls. The ERAS Society also offers similarly useful support.[76] However, in addition to this formal support, identifying a friendly hospital in the same area, or in the same network, that has already successfully implemented an ERAS protocol will help avoid reinventing the wheel.

Conclusion

A multidisciplinary, multimodal bundle of care elements, ERAS is designed to minimize surgical stress and hasten postoperative recovery. The most important part is preparation—both of the ERAS protocol before implementation and of the patients for their perioperative journey once the ERAS program is implemented. Although each ERAS element is evidence based, it is really the combined effect of all the elements that provides the significant benefits of better outcomes for patients and therefore lower costs for hospitals. Furthermore, the team-building, silo-dismantling, culture-changing process that is required for a robust ERAS program produces a benefit to patients and to hospitals that is likely synergistic, not merely additive.

References

1. Engelman RM, Rousou JA, Flack 3rd JE, Deaton DW, Humphrey CB, Ellison LH, Allmendinger PD, Owen SG, Pekow PS. Fast-track recovery of the coronary bypass patient. *Ann Thorac Surg* 1994;**58**(6):1742−6.
2. Kehlet H, Mogensen T. Hospital stay of 2 days after open sigmoidectomy with a multimodal rehabilitation programme. *Br J Surg* 1999;**86**(2):227−30.
3. Bardram L, Funch-Jensen P, Jensen P, Crawford ME, Kehlet H. Recovery after laparoscopic colonic surgery with epidural analgesia, and early oral nutrition and mobilisation. *Lancet* 1995;**345**(8952):763−4.
4. Fearon KC, Ljungqvist O, Von Meyenfeldt M, Revhaug A, Dejong CH, Lassen K, Nygren J, Hausel J, Soop M, Andersen J, Kehlet H. Enhanced recovery after surgery: a consensus review of clinical care for patients undergoing colonic resection. *Clin Nutr* 2005;**24**(3):466−77.
5. ERAS Society Specialties. https://erassociety.org/specialties/ (accessed December 8, 2021).
6. ERAS Society ERAS Society History. https://erassociety.org/about/history/.
7. Watt DG, McSorley ST, Horgan PG, McMillan DC. Enhanced recovery after surgery: which components, if any, impact on the systemic inflammatory response following colorectal surgery? A systematic review. *Medicine (Baltim)* 2015;**94**(36):e1286.
8. Finlayson C, Arya J, Galandiuk S, Harken A. The meaning of surgery. *Surgery* 2000; **127**(4):361−2.
9. Petry JJ. Surgery and meaning. *Surgery* 2000;**127**(4):363−5.
10. Stewart MA. Effective physician-patient communication and health outcomes: a review. *CMAJ (Can Med Assoc J)* 1995;**152**(9):1423−33.
11. Teutsch C. Patient-doctor communication. *Med Clin* 2003;**87**(5):1115−45.
12. Balboni T, VanderWeele T, Doan-Soares S, Long K, Ferrell B, Fitchett G, et al. Spirituality in serious illness and health. *JAMA* 2022;**328**(2):184−97. https://doi.org/10.1001/jama.2022.11086. https://jamanetwork-com.proxy1.library.jhu.edu/journals/jama/fullarticle/2794049.35819420.
13. Vasconcelos A, Lucchetti A, Cavalcanti A, Conde S, Gonçalves L, Nascimento F, et al. Religiosity and spirituality of resident physicians and implications for clinical practice—the SBRAMER multicenter study. *J Gen Intern Med* 2020;**35**(12):3613−9. https://doi.org/10.1007/s11606-020-06145-x.32815055.
14. Cunningham SC. *It's Considerate to Be Literate about Religion*. Waukesha, WI: Orange Hat Publishing; 2022.
15. Thomsen T, Villebro N, Moller AM. Interventions for preoperative smoking cessation. *Cochrane Database Syst Rev* 2014;**3**:CD002294.

16. Egholm JW, Pedersen B, Moller AM, Adami J, Juhl CB, Tonnesen H. Perioperative alcohol cessation intervention for postoperative complications. *Cochrane Database Syst Rev* 2018;**11**:CD008343.
17. Kaye AD, Kucera I, Sabar R. Perioperative anesthesia clinical considerations of alternative medicines. *Anesthesiol Clin North Am* 2004;**22**(1):125—39.
18. Ljungqvist O, de Boer HD, Balfour A, Fawcett WJ, Lobo DN, Nelson G, Scott MJ, Wainwright TW, Demartines N. Opportunities and challenges for the next phase of enhanced recovery after surgery: a review. *JAMA Surg* 2021;**156**(8):775—84.
19. Chow WB, Ko CY, Rosenthal RA, Esnaola NF. ACS NSQIP/AGS best practice guidelines: optimal preoperative assessment of the geriatric surgical patient. In: *American College of Surgeons*. American College of Surgeons; 2012.
20. Fried LP, Tangen CM, Walston J, Newman AB, Hirsch C, Gottdiener J, Seeman T, Tracy R, Kop WJ, Burke G, McBurnie MA, Cardiovascular Health Study Collaborative Research G. Frailty in older adults: evidence for a phenotype. *J Gerontol A Biol Sci Med Sci* 2001;**56**(3):M146—56.
21. Bellera CA, Rainfray M, Mathoulin-Pelissier S, Mertens C, Delva F, Fonck M, Soubeyran PL. Screening older cancer patients: first evaluation of the G-8 geriatric screening tool. *Ann Oncol* 2012;**23**(8):2166—72.
22. Saliba D, Elliott M, Rubenstein LZ, Solomon DH, Young RT, Kamberg CJ, Roth C, MacLean CH, Shekelle PG, Sloss EM, Wenger NS. The vulnerable elders survey: a tool for identifying vulnerable older people in the community. *J Am Geriatr Soc* 2001; **49**(12):1691—9.
23. Thorell A, Nygren J, Ljungqvist O. Insulin resistance: a marker of surgical stress. *Curr Opin Clin Nutr Metab Care* 1999;**2**(1):69—78.
24. Hausel J, Nygren J, Thorell A, Lagerkranser M, Ljungqvist O. Randomized clinical trial of the effects of oral preoperative carbohydrates on postoperative nausea and vomiting after laparoscopic cholecystectomy. *Br J Surg* 2005;**92**(4):415—21.
25. Sato H, Carvalho G, Sato T, Lattermann R, Matsukawa T, Schricker T. The association of preoperative glycemic control, intraoperative insulin sensitivity, and outcomes after cardiac surgery. *J Clin Endocrinol Metab* 2010;**95**(9):4338—44.
26. Ljungqvist O, Jonathan E. Rhoads lecture 2011: insulin resistance and enhanced recovery after surgery. *JPEN - J Parenter Enter Nutr* 2012;**36**(4):389—98.
27. Gianotti L, Sandini M, Hackert T. Preoperative carbohydrates: what is new? *Curr Opin Clin Nutr Metab Care* 2020;**23**(4):262—70.
28. Wischmeyer PE, Carli F, Evans DC, Guilbert S, Kozar R, Pryor A, Thiele RH, Everett S, Grocott M, Gan TJ, Shaw AD, Thacker JKM, Miller TE, Hedrick TL, McEvoy MD, Mythen MG, Bergamaschi R, Gupta R, Holubar SD, Senagore AJ, Abola RE, Bennett-Guerrero E, Kent ML, Feldman LS, Fiore Jr JF. Perioperative quality initiative, W., American society for enhanced recovery and perioperative quality initiative joint consensus statement on nutrition screening and therapy within a surgical enhanced recovery pathway. *Anesth Analg* 2018;**126**(6):1883—95.
29. Weimann A, Braga M, Carli F, Higashiguchi T, Hubner M, Klek S, Laviano A, Ljungqvist O, Lobo DN, Martindale R, Waitzberg DL, Bischoff SC, Singer P. ESPEN guideline: clinical nutrition in surgery. *Clin Nutr* 2017;**36**(3):623—50.
30. Kaiser MJ, Bauer JM, Ramsch C, Uter W, Guigoz Y, Cederholm T, Thomas DR, Anthony PS, Charlton KE, Maggio M, Tsai AC, Vellas B, Sieber CC, Mini Nutritional Assessment International G. Frequency of malnutrition in older adults: a multinational perspective using the mini nutritional assessment. *J Am Geriatr Soc* 2010;**58**(9):1734—8.

31. Schiesser M, Kirchhoff P, Muller MK, Schafer M, Clavien PA. The correlation of nutrition risk index, nutrition risk score, and bioimpedance analysis with postoperative complications in patients undergoing gastrointestinal surgery. *Surgery* 2009;**145**(5):519−26.

32. Longchamp A, Harputlugil E, Corpataux JM, Ozaki CK, Mitchell JR. Is overnight fasting before surgery too much or not enough? How basic aging research can guide preoperative nutritional recommendations to improve surgical outcomes: a mini-review. *Gerontology* 2017;**63**(3):228−37.

33. Speakman JR, Mitchell SE. Caloric restriction. *Mol Aspect Med* 2011;**32**(3):159−221.

34. Roth GS, Ingram DK, Lane MA. Caloric restriction in primates and relevance to humans. *Ann N Y Acad Sci* 2001;**928**:305−15.

35. Mitchell JR, Beckman JA, Nguyen LL, Ozaki CK. Reducing elective vascular surgery perioperative risk with brief preoperative dietary restriction. *Surgery* 2013;**153**(4):594−8.

36. Zorn S, Ehret J, Schauble R, Rautenberg B, Ihorst G, Bertz H, Urbain P, Raynor A. Impact of modified short-term fasting and its combination with a fasting supportive diet during chemotherapy on the incidence and severity of chemotherapy-induced toxicities in cancer patients—a controlled cross-over pilot study. *BMC Cancer* 2020;**20**(1):578.

37. de Groot S, Vreeswijk MP, Welters MJ, Gravesteijn G, Boei JJ, Jochems A, Houtsma D, Putter H, van der Hoeven JJ, Nortier JW, Pijl H, Kroep JR. The effects of short-term fasting on tolerance to (neo) adjuvant chemotherapy in HER2-negative breast cancer patients: a randomized pilot study. *BMC Cancer* 2015;**15**:652.

38. Bauersfeld SP, Kessler CS, Wischnewsky M, Jaensch A, Steckhan N, Stange R, Kunz B, Bruckner B, Sehouli J, Michalsen A. The effects of short-term fasting on quality of life and tolerance to chemotherapy in patients with breast and ovarian cancer: a randomized cross-over pilot study. *BMC Cancer* 2018;**18**(1):476.

39. Jongbloed F, de Bruin RWF, Steeg HV, Beekhof P, Wackers P, Hesselink DA, Hoeijmakers JHJ, Dolle MET, JNM IJ. Protein and calorie restriction may improve outcomes in living kidney donors and kidney transplant recipients. *Aging (Albany NY)* 2020; **12**(13):12441−67.

40. Kip P, Sluiter TJ, Moore JK, Hart A, Ruske J, O'Leary J, Jung J, Tao M, MacArthur MR, Heindel P, de Jong A, de Vries MR, Burak MF, Mitchell SJ, Mitchell JR, Ozaki CK. Short-term pre-operative protein caloric restriction in elective vascular surgery patients: a randomized clinical trial. *Nutrients* 2021;**13**(11).

41. Van Nieuwenhove Y, Dambrauskas Z, Campillo-Soto A, van Dielen F, Wiezer R, Janssen I, Kramer M, Thorell A. Preoperative very low-calorie diet and operative outcome after laparoscopic gastric bypass: a randomized multicenter study. *Arch Surg* 2011;**146**(11):1300−5.

42. Michael CM, Lehrer EJ, Schmitz KH, Zaorsky NG. Prehabilitation exercise therapy for cancer: a systematic review and meta-analysis. *Cancer Med* 2021;**10**(13):4195−205.

43. Lau CSM, Chamberlain RS. Prehabilitation programs improve exercise capacity before and after surgery in gastrointestinal cancer surgery patients: a meta-analysis. *J Gastrointest Surg* 2020;**24**(12):2829−37.

44. Lambert JE, Hayes LD, Keegan TJ, Subar DA, Gaffney CJ. The impact of prehabilitation on patient outcomes in hepatobiliary, colorectal, and upper gastrointestinal cancer surgery: a PRISMA-accordant meta-analysis. *Ann Surg* 2021;**274**(1):70−7.

45. Smyth E, O'Connor L, Mockler D, Reynolds JV, Hussey J, Guinan E. Preoperative high intensity interval training for oncological resections: a systematic review and meta-analysis. *Surg Oncol* 2021;**38**:101620.

46. Liu C, Lu Z, Zhu M, Lu X. Trimodal prehabilitation for older surgical patients: a systematic review and meta-analysis. *Aging Clin Exp Res* 2021;**34**:485—94. https://doi.org/10.1007/s40520-021-01929-5.

47. Dewulf M, Verrips M, Coolsen MME, Olde Damink SWM, Den Dulk M, Bongers BC, Dejong K, Bouwense SAW. The effect of prehabilitation on postoperative complications and postoperative hospital stay in hepatopancreatobiliary surgery a systematic review. *HPB (Oxford)* 2021;**23**(9):1299—310.

48. Dagorno C, Sommacale D, Laurent A, Attias A, Mongardon N, Levesque E, et al. Prehabilitation in hepato-pancreato-biliary surgery: a systematic review and meta-analysis. A necessary step forward evidence-based sample size calculation for future trials. *J Vis Surg* 2021;**159**(5):362—72. https://doi.org/10.1016/j.jviscsurg.2021.07.003.

49. Grant MC, Pio Roda CM, Canner JK, Sommer P, Galante D, Hobson D, Gearhart S, Wu CL, Wick E. The impact of anesthesia-influenced process measure compliance on length of stay: results from an enhanced recovery after surgery for colorectal surgery cohort. *Anesth Analg* 2019;**128**(1):68—74.

50. Nygren J, Thacker J, Carli F, Fearon KC, Norderval S, Lobo DN, Ljungqvist O, Soop M, Ramirez J, Enhanced Recovery After Surgery S. Guidelines for perioperative care in elective rectal/pelvic surgery: enhanced recovery after surgery (ERAS(R)) society recommendations. *Clin Nutr* 2012;**31**(6):801—16.

51. Beverly A, Kaye AD, Ljungqvist O, Urman RD. Essential elements of multimodal analgesia in enhanced recovery after surgery (ERAS) guidelines. *Anesthesiol Clin* 2017;**35**(2):e115—43.

52. Buddensick TJ, Cunningham SC, Kamangar F. Updated literature on povidone-iodine for control of surgical site infections. *Ann Surg* 2012;**256**(1). e1—2; author reply e3.

53. Feldheiser A, Aziz O, Baldini G, Cox BP, Fearon KC, Feldman LS, Gan TJ, Kennedy RH, Ljungqvist O, Lobo DN, Miller T, Radtke FF, Ruiz Garces T, Schricker T, Scott MJ, Thacker JK, Ytrebo LM, Carli F. Enhanced recovery after surgery (ERAS) for gastrointestinal surgery, part 2: consensus statement for anaesthesia practice. *Acta Anaesthesiol Scand* 2016;**60**(3):289—334.

54. Ramos Dos Santos PM, Aquaroni Ricci N, Aparecida Bordignon Suster E, de Moraes Paisani D, Dias Chiavegato L. Effects of early mobilisation in patients after cardiac surgery: a systematic review. *Physiotherapy* 2017;**103**(1):1—12.

55. Ni CY, Wang ZH, Huang ZP, Zhou H, Fu LJ, Cai H, Huang XX, Yang Y, Li HF, Zhou WP. Early enforced mobilization after liver resection: a prospective randomized controlled trial. *Int J Surg* 2018;**54**(Pt A):254—8.

56. Roslan F, Kushairi A, Cappuyns L, Daliya P, Adiamah A. The impact of sham feeding with chewing gum on postoperative ileus following colorectal surgery: a meta-analysis of randomised controlled trials. *J Gastrointest Surg* 2020;**24**(11):2643—53.

57. Park SH, Choi MS. Meta-analysis of the effect of gum chewing after gynecologic surgery. *J Obstet Gynecol Neonatal Nurs* 2018;**47**(3):362—70.

58. Liu Q, Jiang H, Xu D, Jin J. Effect of gum chewing on ameliorating ileus following colorectal surgery: a meta-analysis of 18 randomized controlled trials. *Int J Surg* 2017;**47**:107—15.

59. ERAS Society Interactive Audit. https://erassociety.org/interactive-audit/.

60. American College of Surgeons AHRQ Safety Program for Improving Surgical Care and Recovery. https://www.facs.org/quality-programs/iscr (accessed December 13, 2021).

61. Varadhan KK, Neal KR, Dejong CH, Fearon KC, Ljungqvist O, Lobo DN. The enhanced recovery after surgery (ERAS) pathway for patients undergoing major elective open

colorectal surgery: a meta-analysis of randomized controlled trials. *Clin Nutr* 2010; **29**(4):434−40.

62. Ni X, Jia D, Chen Y, Wang L, Suo J. Is the enhanced recovery after surgery (ERAS) program effective and safe in laparoscopic colorectal cancer surgery? A meta-analysis of randomized controlled trials. *J Gastrointest Surg* 2019;**23**(7):1502−12.

63. Yang FZ, Wang H, Wang DS, Niu ZJ, Li SK, Zhang J, Lu L, Chen D, Li Y, Jiang HT, Han HD, Chu HC, Cao SG, Zhou YB. [The effect of perioperative ERAS pathway management on short-and long-term outcomes of gastric cancer patients]. *Zhonghua Yixue Zazhi* 2020;**100**(12):922−7.

64. Tian YL, Cao SG, Liu XD, Li ZQ, Liu G, Zhang XQ, Sun YQ, Zhou X, Wang DS, Zhou YB. Short- and long-term outcomes associated with enhanced recovery after surgery protocol vs conventional management in patients undergoing laparoscopic gastrectomy. *World J Gastroenterol* 2020;**26**(37):5646−60.

65. Pisarska M, Torbicz G, Gajewska N, Rubinkiewicz M, Wierdak M, Major P, Budzynski A, Ljungqvist O, Pedziwiatr M. Compliance with the ERAS protocol and 3-year survival after laparoscopic surgery for non-metastatic colorectal cancer. *World J Surg* 2019;**43**(10):2552−60.

66. Savaridas T, Serrano-Pedraza I, Khan SK, Martin K, Malviya A, Reed MR. Reduced medium-term mortality following primary total hip and knee arthroplasty with an enhanced recovery program. A study of 4,500 consecutive procedures. *Acta Orthop* 2013;**84**(1):40−3.

67. Pang Q, Duan L, Jiang Y, Liu H. Oncologic and long-term outcomes of enhanced recovery after surgery in cancer surgeries—a systematic review. *World J Surg Oncol* 2021; **19**(1):191.

68. Stowers MD, Lemanu DP, Hill AG. Health economics in enhanced recovery after surgery programs. *Can J Anaesth* 2015;**62**(2):219−30.

69. Paci P, Madani A, Lee L, Mata J, Mulder DS, Spicer J, Ferri LE, Feldman LS. Economic impact of an enhanced recovery pathway for lung resection. *Ann Thorac Surg* 2017; **104**(3):950−7.

70. Bogani G, Sarpietro G, Ferrandina G, Gallotta V, Ditto A, Pinelli C, Casarin J, Ghezzi F, Scambia G, Raspagliesi F. Enhanced recovery after surgery (ERAS) in gynecology oncology. *Eur J Surg Oncol* 2021;**47**(5):952−9.

71. Thiele RH, Rea KM, Turrentine FE, Friel CM, Hassinger TE, McMurry TL, Goudreau BJ, Umapathi BA, Kron IL, Sawyer RG, Hedrick TL. Standardization of care: impact of an enhanced recovery protocol on length of stay, complications, and direct costs after colorectal surgery. *J Am Coll Surg* 2015;**220**(4):430−43.

72. Stone AB, Grant MC, Pio Roda C, Hobson D, Pawlik T, Wu CL, Wick EC. Implementation costs of an enhanced recovery after surgery program in the United States: a financial model and sensitivity analysis based on experiences at a quaternary academic medical center. *J Am Coll Surg* 2016;**222**(3):219−25.

73. Roulin D, Donadini A, Gander S, Griesser AC, Blanc C, Hubner M, Schafer M, Demartines N. Cost-effectiveness of the implementation of an enhanced recovery protocol for colorectal surgery. *Br J Surg* 2013;**100**(8):1108−14.

74. Lee L, Mata J, Ghitulescu GA, Boutros M, Charlebois P, Stein B, Liberman AS, Fried GM, Morin N, Carli F, Latimer E, Feldman LS. Cost-effectiveness of enhanced recovery versus conventional perioperative management for colorectal surgery. *Ann Surg* 2015;**262**(6):1026−33.

75. Harryman C, Plymale MA, Stearns E, Davenport DL, Chang W, Roth JS. Enhanced value with implementation of an ERAS protocol for ventral hernia repair. *Surg Endosc* 2020; **34**(9):3949−55.

76. Ljungqvist O, Scott M, Fearon KC. Enhanced recovery after surgery: a review. *JAMA Surg* 2017;**152**(3):292−8.

Preoperative preparation of the surgical patient

Jerry Stonemetz, MD [1], John C. Evanko, MD MBA [2]

[1]*Medical Director, Perioperative Services, Anesthesia & Critical Care Medicine, Johns Hopkins University, Baltimore, MD, United States;* [2]*Executive Vice President & Chief Medical Officer, MCIC Vermont, LLC, New York, NY, United States*

Preparation of the surgical patient begins with a consideration of all phases of surgical care when preparing a patient for surgery. Classic preoperative, intraoperative, and postoperative phases should be on the mind of the surgeon when developing their recommended surgical therapy. Initial presentation of the patient often reveals considerable information about the physical and mental state of the patient and should help guide the surgeon in recommending the most appropriate therapy to achieve the desired therapeutic goal. Shared decision-making models should take into account concerns about the intraoperative and postoperative phases of care when a surgeon and patient decide upon the surgical options and desired treatment goals during the preoperative phase.

The preoperative phase should be considered as two distinct phases, each with a different goal and thought process. The surgical planning phase begins with the diagnostic workup, followed by the identification of pathology and the exploration of treatment options. During this phase, the surgeon and patient are engaged in continual dialogue about the patient's goals, the various treatment options, and their respective risks, benefits, and likelihood of successful treatment. Options of expectant management, medical, alternative, and surgical treatments, to name a few, should be explored with the patient. The patient's pathology, state of health, and comorbidities must be carefully considered and weighed against the considered treatments and resulting recovery period. If surgical intervention is necessary, open, minimally invasive, endoscopic, or endovascular surgical options should be weighed against overall procedure length, anesthesia considerations, and immediate postoperative care requirements. This entire process is considered shared decision-making and results in the informed consent of a patient when a treatment option is agreed upon.

The second phase of preoperative preparation begins once a recommended surgery is deemed necessary and agreed to by the patient. This phase includes the medical optimization and anesthesia evaluation of the patient undergoing the intended procedure and the subsequent interpretation and evaluation of appropriate preoperative testing deemed necessary. In a relatively healthy patient undergoing a minor low-risk procedure, the preparation or testing can be kept to a minimum and will be discussed later in this chapter. A patient with a more complex medical history undergoing a difficult and lengthy procedure with a significant anticipated recovery period may require medical optimization in order to stabilize their medical condition and enhance their physical condition prior to surgery. Complex medical conditions out of the scope of the surgeon's practice may necessitate consultations with various medical specialties to manage their conditions preoperatively and postoperatively. An evaluation of the patient's social habits may indicate a need for referral to appropriate counseling to enhance the recuperation period and overall compliance with medical recommendations. The patient's family and support resources should be evaluated to ensure adherence with postoperative restrictions and not place the patient in jeopardy during their anticipated recovery period. The results of these evaluations and considerations must be continually balanced against the original surgical recommendation, and when necessary, the surgeon should recommend altering the surgical plan to accommodate these realities in order to most safely achieve the goal of treatment. After all, the dictum, primum non nocere, compels us to do no harm and compels us to improve and not worsen the overall condition of the patient with our surgical therapy.

Preoperative preparation can be very complex and often the care coordination required to safely prepare a patient overwhelms the surgeon and their staff. The number of consultations and referrals can multiply very quickly and the resulting number of follow-up recommendations and options can confuse even the most experienced surgeon. Each of these interactions presents an opportunity for error, and lack of coordination and preparation which may contribute to potential patient harm and poor outcomes. Many healthcare systems and surgical programs are employing multidisciplinary surgical care conferences to discuss upcoming complex surgical cases in order to streamline the process and enhance teamwork among the various disciplines of medicine. Effective conferences will include surgeons, anesthesiologists, internists, hospitalists, physiatrists, consultants, nurses, social workers, care coordinators, patient navigators, and home care specialists in the discussion of complex cases to ensure a tailored, comprehensive, and coordinated care plan is developed addressing the needs of the patient. Risk calculators and other algorithms may be employed to risk stratify appropriate candidates to be reviewed at the conference if an institution decides not to review every case. Alternative treatment options and experienced opinions are often discussed culminating in the sharing of best practices to be followed and the potential surgical pitfalls to be avoided. Necessary hospital resources can be anticipated and properly resourced when discussed prior to the surgery. Anesthesia concerns could be discussed with the appropriate consultants to better understand the patient's physiology and medical condition to guide intraoperative monitoring and postoperative critical care needs. Medical comanagement can be arranged for immediate postoperative hospitalization to aid the surgeon and critical care teams in the medical management of the patient. Discharge planning and home care coordination can be arranged with a better understanding of the anticipated recovery status and limitations of the patient. The multidisciplinary conference enhances the preparation and coordination for all five phases of the surgical continuum: surgical planning, medical optimization, intraoperative, postoperative hospitalization, and posthospital recovery phase. Care pathways and standardized treatment protocols can easily be constructed and followed to improve care and decrease variability and overall cost when a mature multidisciplinary conference is established in the culture of an organization.

From the moment the patient and surgeon decide to proceed with surgery, the preoperative time frame represents a golden opportunity to proactively manage and optimize the patient for the upcoming surgery. These interventions include identification and prophylaxis of patients at risk for deep venous thrombosis and pulmonary embolism; preoperative administration of beta-blockers; appropriate selection of antibiotics; and better glycemic control of diabetic patients. We believe that the future of perioperative medicine will usher in advances in proactively reaching out to surgical patients during this preoperative time period and delivering disease-specific management. There exists today technology that utilizes patient health records and online questionnaires that are tied to decision support systems to guide preoperative testing. By correctly identifying and risk stratifying surgical patients, we can tailor clinical pathways that optimize their medical conditions as well as better prepare them for surgery.

These authors are proponents of the preoperative clinic based on our experience at our institutions as well as a plethora of published studies demonstrating enhanced patient safety, patient satisfaction, reduction of testing and expenses, as well as a significant reduction in cancellations and delays on the day of surgery.[1] We work together for our collective institutions in improving the Preoperative Processes, in an attempt to reduce malpractice claims and improve care. Our experience indicates that there are ample opportunities to reduce harm through better organization and preoperative preparation. Our patients who are "optimized" demonstrated fewer same-day cancellations, fewer day-of-surgery testing, and lower PSI-90 Complication rates. Time will indicate if this process also results in fewer malpractice claims.

However, not all patients should be required to make a separate trip to the hospital for an evaluation prior to surgery. At our institutions, we have created a Preoperative Roadmap that has been provided to our surgeons to give some guidance as to which patients should be selected to come to our clinic. Additionally, this roadmap provides some basic algorithms that indicate what testing should be done on patients deemed appropriate to bypass the clinic. This roadmap was developed based on principles defined by the American Society of Anesthesiologists (ASA) Task Force on Preoperative Testing convened in 2002 and updated based on new evidence regarding specific patient conditions.[1] Fig. 9.1 is a diagram of the algorithm we utilize in our Roadmap to illustrate how to triage the surgical patient. Essentially, we ask our surgeons to determine if their patients are medically "sick"or "healthy." Healthy patients only need to be seen in a preoperative clinic if they are having major surgery. We define major surgery as specified by the American Heart Association (AHA) as involving major blood vessels (vascular or cardiac) or extensive disruption of physiology such as an 8-hour Whipple procedure or major transplant procedure.

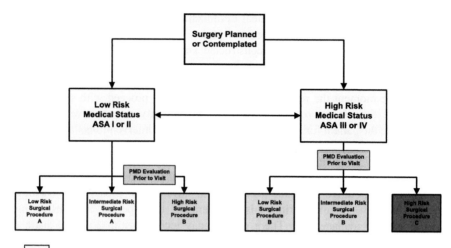

A – May have preanesthesia assessment done day of surgery

B – Recommend preanesthesia assessment with PEC visit at least 24 hours preoperatively. Should have an evaluation done prior to PEC visit by PMD.

C – Recommend Preanesthesia Consult scheduled in PEC at least 48 hours preoperatively. Should have an evaluation done prior to anesthesia consult by PMD.

FIGURE 9.1

Preoperative triage algorithm. Low-risk medical conditions: Healthy with no medical problems (ASA I) or well-controlled chronic conditions (ASA II). High-risk medical conditions: Multiple medical comorbidities not well controlled (ASA III) or extremely compromised function secondary to comorbidities (ASA IV). Low-risk surgical procedure: Poses minimal physiological stress (e.g., minor outpatient surgery). Intermediate-risk surgical procedure: Medium-risk procedure with moderate physiological stress and minimal blood loss, fluid shifts, or postoperative changes. High-risk surgical procedure: High-risk procedure with significant fluid shifts, possible blood loss, as well as perioperative stress anticipated.

PEC, preoperative evaluation clinic; *PMD,* primary medical doctor. **A**—May have preanesthesia assessment done day of surgery. **B**—Recommend preanesthesia assessment with PEC visit at least 24 h preoperatively. Should have an evaluation done prior to PEC visit by PMD. **C**—Recommend preanesthesia consult scheduled in PEC at least 48 h preoperatively. Should have an evaluation done prior to anesthesia consult by PMD.

From Johns Hopkins Preoperative Roadmap, available at http://www.hopkinsmedicine.org/anesthesiology/
Patient_Care/Preoperative_Roadmap.pdf.

For a healthy patient scheduled for minor surgery, there really are no indications for much preoperative testing. Routine CxR and ECG are not warranted for most patients. It is common to find a requirement for an ECG for all patients over the age of 50; however, that is based on local custom and there is no real good evidence that this should be required.[2] Additionally, laboratory testing should also be considered only for patient conditions or surgery that warrants the appropriate test. Minor outpatient surgery really only requires a hemoglobin level on menstruating females and possibly a urine pregnancy test, unless there is something in the history that stipulates further testing is indicated. A good example of a significantly oversubscribed preoperative test is coagulation studies.[3] At most institutions, a Prothrombin time (PT/INR) and Partial Thromboplastin tests (PTTs) are ordered on the vast majority of patients. There are several problems with ordering this test preoperatively. First, most labs have now split out the PT/INR from the PTT, and ordering a PTT adds an additional cost to the test. There are practically no preoperative patients that warrant a PTT. Exceptions are hemophilias, and these should be identified from a basic history and physical. The PTT test represents the intrinsic coagulation pathway and is routinely used to monitor heparin dosing. Obviously, preoperative patients are rarely on heparin, so this test is worthless to obtain. As for the PT/INR, there are patients where this test is indicated. They would be patients with a history of liver disease or bruising and prolonged bleeding. Ironically, we typically order a PT/INR on patients on anticoagulants such as Coumadin. Again, there is little rationale for ordering this test preoperatively. These patients will all have abnormal values for their INR. There is rationale for ordering the tests the morning of surgery, but not a few days prior to surgery. Both of these examples illustrate how we can reduce the significant expense of unnecessary preoperative testing without affecting outcomes.

Comorbidities

The roadmap also defines how to approach certain patient comorbidities as far as appropriate testing (Table 9.1). Of particular concern is the patient who is not able to achieve at least four metabolic equivalents (METs) of activity which is defined as being able to climb two flights of stairs without stopping or walking briskly for up to four city blocks. There are many reasons patients are not able to achieve this level of activity, such as arthritis or obesity, but without attaining this level of activity, we are not able to assess cardiac reserve. Consequently, we frequently will want a cardiac ECHO for these patients, in particular, if they are scheduled for intermediate or major surgery.[4]

The patient that represents one of our greatest challenges is the patient who is morbidly obese as defined by a body mass index (BMI) > 40. These patients are particularly prone to comorbidities that may seem unusual at an early age. The most concerning combination of comorbidities are the presence of morbid obesity and sleep apnea. This common combination may result in pulmonary hypertension

Table 9.1 Medical conditions that may warrant an ASA III or IV status and would benefit from a preoperative assessment at a PEC center.

General conditions:	• Medical condition inhibiting ability to engage in normal daily activity—unable to climb two flights of stairs without stopping. • Medical condition necessitating continual assistance or monitoring at home within the past 6 months. • Admission to a hospital within the past 2 months for acute or exacerbation of a chronic condition. • History of previous anesthesia complications or history of malignant hyperthermia.
Cardiocirculatory:	• History of angina, coronary artery disease, or myocardial infarction. • Symptomatic arrhythmias, particularly new onset A-fib. • Poorly controlled hypertension (systolic >160 and/or diastolic >110). • History of congestive heart failure. • History of significant valvular disease (aortic stenosis, mitral regurgitation, etc.).
Respiratory:	• Asthma/COPD requiring chronic medication or with acute exacerbation and progression within the past 6 months. • History of major airway surgery or unusual airway anatomy (history of difficult intubation in the previous anesthetic). • Upper or lower airway tumor or obstruction. • History of chronic respiratory distress requiring home ventilatory assistance or monitoring.
Endocrine:	• Insulin-dependent diabetes mellitus. • Adrenal disorders. • Active thyroid disease. • Morbid obesity.
Neuromuscular:	• History of seizure disorder or other significant CNS diseases (multiple sclerosis, muscular dystrophy, etc.). • History of myopathy or other muscular disorders.
Hepatic/renal/ heme:	• Any active hepatobiliary disease or compromise (hepatitis). • End-stage renal disease (dialysis). • Severe anemias (sickle cell, aplastic, etc.).

From Johns Hopkins Preoperative Roadmap, available at http://anesthesiology.hopkinsmedicine.org/ wp-content/uploads/2018/10/Preoperative-Roadmap_10.9.18.pdf.

that is undiagnosed but may result in perioperative death if not recognized and dealt with appropriately. These patients should have an ECHO to rule out pulmonary hypertension, but unfortunately, these patients also have a body habitus that precludes using the ECHO to assess right heart function. In this situation, the patient may need a right heart catheterization.

Medication management

Historically, implicit in our orders for nothing per os (NPO) after midnight, we are telling patients not to take their morning medications. Our thinking has changed dramatically based on recent evidence. Now, we realize that most patients who are on chronic medications really should continue those medications on the morning of surgery, and through the perioperative period. There are exceptions, and they are listed in Table 9.2. Specifically, we now realize that beta-blockers are important for

Table 9.2 Guidelines for preoperative medications.

As a general rule, for patients scheduled for surgery with anesthesia, we recommend all medications should be continued on the day of surgery.

In particular, it is very important for patients to take their morning dosage of the following medications:

- Beta-blockers and any antiarrhythmics such as Digoxin or Calcium Channel blockers.
- Asthmatic medications including inhalers, Theophylline, Singulair, and/or steroids.
- GERD medication.
- Statins such as Lipitor, Zocor, Crestor, etc.
- Aspirin — unless specifically told by their surgeon, patients should continue to take their ASA if they have cardiac stents.
- ACE/ARB—consider having patients take these if HTN is difficult to control without them.
- Consider starting patients on beta-blockers preoperatively who could be considered at risk for cardiac ischemia.

Exceptions to this recommendation are summarized below:

Class of medications	Medication	Recommendations
Oral hypoglycemic agents	Metformin/Glucophage Actos/ Glyburide/Tolinase/Avandia/ Amaryl/all others	Hold at least 8 h preop. Recommend holding morning dose, day of surgery.
Diuretics	Lasix/HCTZ	Hold morning day of surgery, *unless* prescribed for CHF—these patients should take their morning dose of diuretics.
ACE/ARB	Lisinopril/Lotrel/Captopril/ Lotensin/Monopril/Prinzide/ Atacand/Benicar/Diovan/Avalide	Hold morning day of surgery, *unless* prescribed for CHF—these patients should take their morning dose of meds.
Insulin	NPH, regular	Hold insulin morning day of surgery. Bring insulin with patient to hospital.
All herbal supplements		Stop all herbal supplements at least 24 h prior to surgery.
SGLT2 inhibitors	Canglifozin (Invokana)/ Dapagliflozin (Farxiga)/ Empaglifozin (Jardiance)/ Ertugliflozin (Steglatro)	For all surgeries, stop 3 days prior to surgery; for Ertuglifloxin, stop 4 days prior to surgery.

From Johns Hopkins Preoperative Roadmap, available at: https://anesthesiology.hopkinsmedicine.org/ wp-content/uploads/2022/08/FY23-Preoperative-Roadmap-7.22.pdf.

improved surgical outcomes and, in fact, have become one of the SCIP measures. This measure looks at whether a patient who is on a beta-blocker as a home medication has taken this medication within 24 h of surgery. Alternatively, a beta-blocker can be administered intraoperatively, but the preferred recommendation is to have the patient take their medicine orally preoperatively. This brings into question the NPO status. We now feel that sips of water immediately prior to surgery are not a problem, and there is some evidence to suggest that clear liquids taken within 2 h of surgery may actually reduce postoperative nausea and vomiting. This recommendation has taken on new light as it pertains to ERAS (Enhanced Recovery After Surgery), which typically recommends up to 20 ounces of a carbohydrate drink, such as Gatorade. It is the clear fluids and the carbohydrate loading that promotes a more rapid return of bowel function.

Conversely, medications that are recommended to be held are listed below:

- **Oral hypoglycemic agents:** These should be held for at least 8 h preoperatively, which means that patients who take them in the evening should be allowed to continue these medications the night before surgery. One exception may be Metformin for patients who are concomitantly going to receive contrast dye as part of their procedure. These patients should have this medication stopped at least 24 h prior to the procedure in an attempt to reduce the risk of renal failure. The rationale for holding oral hypoglycemic comes from reports of profound lactic acidosis in patients who received the medication preoperatively and were undergoing major surgery. There have been no studies to date that look at the consequences of taking these medications preoperatively in minor surgery; however, we continue to recommend holding in light of a lack of evidence of their safety.
- **Insulin:** Currently we recommend that all patients hold their morning dose of short-acting insulin since they are not taking any oral glucose preoperatively. Typically, we recommend they bring their morning insulin with them to the hospital and once a blood sugar level is assessed, we can determine the appropriate dosing of this medication. We also recommend that long-acting agents such as Lantus be reduced by half the evening before surgery, although we are not aware of any studies that demonstrate a problem with standard dosing. We are seeing more patients taking long-acting insulin in the morning, and we are recommending these patients take half of that dose prior to surgery. Finally, we also try to counsel insulin diabetic patients that if they begin to feel hypoglycemic preoperatively that they can take 8–10 ounces of clear apple juice. Not orange juice or anything with pulp—just clear apple juice. This should not affect their ability to proceed with surgery.
- **ACE Inhibitors/ARB:** Today many patients are started on ACE inhibitors or ARBs as the preferred therapy for hypertension. There are adequate studies to illustrate that these patients have a high propensity to develop hypotension that is unresponsive to normal pressors with the induction of general anesthesia. It has been demonstrated that this hypotension is more responsive to vasopressin

presumably because this drug activates the rennin—angiotensin pathway that is suppressed by these inhibitors. Exceptions to this recommendation are those patients who are prescribed these medications as therapy for congestive heart failure. These patients should take their medications in the morning of the day of surgery. Of note, there are some studies that have indicated that continuation of these medications may have benefit as renal protection in patients undergoing major vascular or cardiac surgery; however, the current recommendations are to hold these medicines the morning of surgery.[5]

- **Anticoagulants:** Depending upon the specific anticoagulant prescribed and the indications, stopping these drugs preoperatively will have variable time frames.[6] Typically, we recommend stopping Warfarin for 5 days and Clopidogrel for 7 days preoperatively. Some patients will require anticoagulant bridging with Lovenox which can be stopped 12—24 h preoperatively. One aspect to consider is whether the patient is a reasonable candidate for regional anesthesia rather than general anesthesia. For these patients, Warfarin must be stopped for at least 5 days, Clopidogrel must be stopped for 7 days, and Lovenox must be stopped for at least 24 h. Aspirin is not a contraindication to regional anesthesia. Many surgeons want ASA stopped 7—10 days preop; however, there is mounting evidence that we should reconsider this approach except in a very few select types of surgery. The rationale for this recommendation will be discussed below.

- **Herbal medications:** In general, since there is so little control over what constitutes herbal medications, we generally recommend that these medicines be stopped at least 24 h preoperatively.[7] There are some specific supplements that should be considered to be held even longer. Examples are fish oil and vitamin E because of reported problems with bleeding, and most importantly any supplements that contain ephedra—a major ingredient in dietary supplements such as Metabolife and Ma-Huang. This drug has been shown to cause cardiomyopathy similar to Fen-Phen which was taken off the market years ago.

Aspirin

Aspirin affects platelet function secondary to changes to platelets that occur during their synthesis. Consequently, while on aspirin, a patient's platelet function is affected for the life of the platelets. Studies have demonstrated that for the vast majority of patients, essentially all antiplatelet activity will cease if aspirin is stopped for 7 days. This also means that the platelets are primarily replaced within this time frame as well. This explains the rationale for discontinuing aspirin 7 days prior to surgery, despite the obvious benefits to patients who need this antiplatelet therapy. Unfortunately, this current practice has now been shown to have absolute detrimental effects on a specific subset of patients, and that represents patients who have cardiac stents in place.

The most recent recommendations from the AHA discuss patients who have had stents placed recently, as well as patients who are past this initial critical window.[8]

To summarize these recommendations, it is important to understand that patients who have just had cardiac stents placed are at high risk of thrombosis of these stents, and consequently that is why they are maintained on antiplatelet therapy. That therapy is currently clopidogrel and aspirin. Essentially, patients who receive bare metal stents should not have surgery unless life or limb-threatening for 6 months after placement, and that is primarily because this dual antiplatelet therapy should not be discontinued. For patients who receive drug-eluting stents, this dual therapy should continue for at least 1 year. Obviously, any emergency surgery requires a thorough discussion of benefits and risks between the patient, the surgeon, and typically their cardiologist.

Our major concern now, however, is the patient who is past this window of dual antiplatelet therapy. The AHA does recommend life-long aspirin therapy in all of these patients. Additionally, their recommendations are that aspirin is continued up to the day of surgery except for neurosurgery and retinal surgery where the risk of bleeding is so significant. Possibly even more important is the resumption of antiplatelet therapy. Ideally, these patients should resume their medications the day after surgery. For patients who are dual therapy, we do recommend stopping clopidogrel 7 days prior to surgery but maintaining the 81 mg dosage of aspirin.

It is essential to understand some of the differences between clopidogrel and aspirin in order to understand our recommendations. Clopidogrel affects platelet function in a different manner than aspirin and is based on the circulating platelet versus the synthesis of the platelet. As long as clopidogrel is in circulation, it will negatively affect platelet function. Consequently, we cannot reverse this antiplatelet activity by administering new platelets as we can with aspirin. That is why we recommend stopping clopidogrel 7 days prior to surgery but continuing the low-dose aspirin which seems to be an effective dosage to prevent thrombosis of these stents. What we frequently see are cardiologists recommending stopping both 5 days prior to surgery in order to preserve some antiplatelet therapy. Our problem with this approach is that it provides a scenario where we are unable to reverse the antiplatelet activity by administering new platelets, whereas we can if they are simply on aspirin. It is also important to realize that in order to prevent stent thrombosis, we need antiplatelet therapy, not anticoagulation. Hence, warfarin or heparin is not an appropriate substitution.

Pacemakers

We are seeing an ever-increasing volume of patients with pacemakers inserted who are now coming to surgery after the pacemaker has been implanted. One of the primary reasons for this increase is the rationale that patients with extremely low cardiac function (ejection fractions of less than 30%) benefit substantially from pacemaker insertions, and in general, these will be implantable cardioversion devices (ICDs). It is important to understand how to manage these pacemakers preoperatively. The anesthesiologist will want documentation as to the type and function of these pacemakers as well as a recent interrogation of this device.

Our recommendations based on recent studies are that routine pacemakers need interrogations within 6 months of surgery. Exceptions to this are pacer-dependent patients and ICDs wherein both of these situations the pacemaker should have been interrogated within 3 months of surgery.[9]

Additionally, it will be important to have a discussion with the anesthesiologist as to the recommendation on how to handle the pacemaker during surgery. Their concern will be the effect of electrocautery (Bovie) interference on the normal pacemaker function. Essentially, a pacemaker will frequently sense such interference as cardiac function, and the results will depend upon what type of pacemaker is implanted. Routine pacemakers will likely sense Bovie interference as heartbeats and suppress any discharges. This will be particularly problematic in the pacer-dependent patient since this Bovie interference may result in no pacemaker discharge causing asystole. An alternative method of dealing with pacer-dependent patients will likely be to have the pacemaker reprogrammed into an asynchronous mode which means there will be no sensing of the pacemaker. This results in the constant firing of the pacemaker at the predetermined rate. Once the surgery is completed, the pacemaker can be reprogrammed back to a sensing mode.

An ICD views Bovie interference differently. This device is looking for signs of cardiac dysrhythmias such as ventricular fibrillation (VFib) or ventricular tachycardia (VTach). After sensing one of these tachyarrhythmias, the ICD will attempt cardioversion internally by emitting a shock. If it senses the Bovie instead and emits this shock, the pacemaker may in fact generate VFib or VTach. Consequently, we generally require the ICD function to be turned off prior to surgery and turned back on once the case is completed.

There may be opportunities to place a magnet over the pacemaker or ICD to accomplish these goals; however, without proper documentation of what will happen with a magnet, it is not prudent to use the magnet since not all pacemakers function the same with a magnet. This functionality should be defined in the interrogation report. Additionally, the type of surgery may also preclude the use of a magnet and consequently require reprogramming. We advise a discussion between the anesthesiologist and surgeon prior to surgery in order to avoid last-minute cancellations or delays.

Conclusion

As the severity and acuity of medical problems increase in our surgical patients, it will become ever more important to assess these patients prior to the day of surgery. For hospitals that cannot afford a preoperative clinic, they must begin to explore methods of proactively getting patient information so that rules-based logic can be applied to their preoperative management. We feel online preoperative questionnaires represent great opportunities to better capture significant patient information that is relevant to the appropriate triage for evaluations. For patients who are not able to use the computer, the surgeon's office staff can guide them through the questionnaire. This technology can significantly reduce cancellations and delays at any institution.

Finally, we strongly recommend that the anesthesia department be engaged in assisting to define these preoperative protocols and management since this information is changing rapidly. We do not believe the typical surgeon should attempt to remain current on the nuances of preoperative management and should come to rely on their colleagues in anesthesia and other clinical specialties in a multidisciplinary manner to establish effective clinical guidance.

References

1. Pasternak LR, Arens JF, Caplan RA, et al. Practice advisory for preoperative evaluation: report by task force on preoperative evaluation. *Anesthesiology* 2002;**96**(2):485−96.
2. Fleisher L. The preoperative electrocardiogram: what is the role in 2007? *Ann Surg* 2007; **246**(2):171−2.
3. Chee YL, Crawford JC, Watson HG, et al. Guidelines on the assessment of bleeding risk prior to surgery or invasive procedures. British Committee for Standards in Haematology. *Br J Haematol* 2008;**140**(5):496−504.
4. Fleisher L, Beckman J, Brown K, et al. ACA/AHA 2007 guidelines on perioperative cardiovascular evaluation and care for noncardiac surgery. *Circulation* 2007;**116**(17).
5. Comfere T, Sprung J, Kumar MM, et al. Angiotensin inhibitors in the general surgical population. *Anesth Analg* 2005;**100**(3):636−44.
6. Di Minno MN, Prisco D, Ruocco A, et al. Perioperative handling of patients on antiplatelet therapy with need for surgery. *Intern Emerg Med* 2009;**4**(4):279−88.
7. Adusumilli PS, Ben-Porat L, Pereira M, et al. The prevalence and predictors of herbal medicine use in surgical patients. *J Am Coll Surg* 2004;**198**(4):583−90.
8. Brilakis E, Banerjee S, Berger P. Perioperative management of patients with coronary stents. *J Am Coll Cardiol* 2007;**49**(22):2145−50.
9. Zaidan JR, Atlee JL, Belott P, Briesacher KJ, et al. Practice advisory for perioperative management of patients with cardiac rhythm management devices: pacemakers and implantable cardioverter−defibrillators. *Anesthesiology* 2005;**103**:186−98.

Designing safe procedural sedation: adopting a resilient culture

10

Vera Meeusen, PhD, CHM, MA, RN, FACPAN, AFACHSM [1,2],
Paul Barach, B.Med.Sci, MD, MPH, Maj (ret.), AUA [3,4,7],
André van Zundert, MD, PhD, FRCA, EDRA, FANZCA [5,6]

[1]*CNC Endoscopy Unit, Princess Alexandra Hospital, Woolloongabba, QLD, Australia;* [2]*Associate Professor, Faculty of Medicine, The University of Queensland, Brisbane, QLD, Australia;* [3]*Honorary Professor, Faculty of Medicine, The University of Queensland, Brisbane, QLD, Australia;* [4]*Faculty, Thomas Jefferson University, Philadelphia, PA, United States;* [5]*Professor & Chair Anesthesiology, Faculty of Medicine, The University of Queensland, Brisbane, QLD, Australia;* [6]*Department of Anaesthesia and Perioperative Medicine, Royal Brisbane and Women's Hospital, Herston, QLD, Australia;* [7]*Honorary Professor, University of Birmingham, Birmingham, United Kingdom*

GLOSSARY OF TERMS

AGA	American Gastroenterological Association
ANZCA	Australian and New Zealand College of Anaesthetists
ASA	American Society of Anesthesiologists
ASGE	American Society for Gastrointestinal Endoscopy
BIS	Bispectral Index
BMI	Body mass index
BPS	Balanced propofol sedation
CAD	Coronary artery disease
CO	Carbon monoxide
CO_2	Carbon dioxide
COPD	Chronic obstructive pulmonary disease
DM	Diabetes mellitus
ECG	Electrocardiogram
ED	Emergency department
EDNAPS	Endoscopist-directed, nurses-administered propofol sedation
EDP	Endoscopist-directed propofol
ERCP	Endoscopic retrograde cholangiopancreatography
ESA	European Society of Anaesthesiologists
ESRD	End-stage renal disease
$EtCO_2$	End-tidal carbon dioxide
EUS	Endoscopic ultrasound
GABA	γ-Aminobutyric acid
GERD	Gastroesophageal reflux disease

HR	Heart rate
HTN	Hypertension
ICU	Intensive care unit
ISAS	Iowa Satisfaction with Anesthesia Scale
IV	Intravenous
MAC	Monitored anesthesia care
MET	Metabolic equivalent for task
MI	Myocardial infarction
NAAP	Nonanesthetist-administered propofol
NAPS	Nurse-administered propofol sedation
PROSAS	Procedural sedation assessment survey
QoR	Quality of Recovery
RCRI	Revised Cardiac Risk Index
RHSMD	Ratio of height to sternomental distance
RHTMD	Ratio of height to thyromental distance
RR	Respiratory rate
SCOPE	Stratifying Clinical Outcomes Prior to Endoscopy
SMD	Sternomental distance
TIA	Transient ischemic attack
TMD	Thyromental distance
ULBT	Upper lip bite test

Introduction

While millions of patients receive sedation every day, high-profile cases have brought medical errors in sedation to the public's attention. Alleviating pain and anxiety is a key component of the care provided to hospitalized and ambulatory patients. While reassurance, distraction, and behavioral strategies may offer relief, pharmacologic interventions are often required, especially in acute care settings. Sedation in the operating room and increasingly outside the operating rooms has been a growing industry due to the increase in the volume and types of procedures outside the operating room, an increase in the demand for special conditions to produce better image and results (i.e., MRI and dentistry), and an increase in the complexity of cases due to an increase in survival rates with complex pathology.

Sedation for gastrointestinal endoscopy has revolutionized the diagnosis, treatment, and prognosis of gastrointestinal tract diseases. Worldwide, a growing number of endoscopies (of increasing complexity and duration) for gastroenterology are performed each year, of which a large part requires sedation or anesthesia. The goal of sedation is to guard the patient's safety, provide comfort, control behavior, and minimize its impact on normal physiology. The practice of (endoscopic) sedation requires a thorough understanding of preprocedural assessment and preparation, sedation pharmacology, practical airway training, monitoring, adverse event management, and postprocedural care. The purpose of sedation is to relieve the patient's discomfort and anxiety while simultaneously reducing disruptive movements so that an adequate examination may be performed. Patient safety needs to be ensured while procedural efficacy is maintained.

A clinical microsystem is a group of clinicians and staff working together with a shared clinical purpose to provide care for a population of patients.[1] The clinical purpose and setting define the microsystem's essential components, which include the clinicians and support staff, information and technology, the specific care processes, and the behaviors required to provide care to its patients. Examples of clinical microsystems include a cardiovascular surgical care team, a community-based outpatient care center, neonatal intensive care, and a pediatric sedation service. The clinical microsystem provides a conceptual and practical framework for approaching organizational learning and delivery of safe sedation care. To understand the functioning of these healthcare microsystems, and to improve their perioperative patient safety, it is necessary to study the components that make up the system—humans, technologies, and their complex interactions. In healthcare, the premium placed on practitioner autonomy, the drive for productivity, and the economics of the system may lead to severe safety constraints and adverse medical events.[2]

The focus on the actions of individuals, without addressing the underlying microsystem, as the sole cause of adverse events, inevitably results in continued system failures and the resultant injuries and deaths of patients. Strategies to make sedation care more resilient and even safer might include the adoption of reliability engineering principles; setting up robust near-miss reporting systems [3]; applying critical event analysis tools such as trigger tools and failure mode and effects analysis (FMEA) when adverse incidents occur[147]; wide adoption of simulation and sedation team training; adopting checklists[151]; deploying standardized medication—doses, concentration, sets, implementing robust handoff protocols, and patient identification checklists [4]; and adherence to safe sedation practice standards.

Adequate pain control and sedation ensures the patient's comfort and cooperation, can influence the procedure's success, and can affect future attitudes toward healthcare providers and medical care. This chapter will describe key developments in sedation safety, safety research, risk and reliability management approaches, the role of human factors, and organizational practice models.

Preprocedural assessment

Sedation preparation involves performing an adequate risk assessment and determining when to enlist the assistance of anesthesia professionals. This should be done congruently with other pre-endoscopic evaluations, such as the need for antibiotic prophylaxis and bleeding tendency. The person administering sedation needs to assess for a previous adverse reaction to sedatives, symptoms of obstructive sleep apnea, and a history of alcohol overuse or drug abuse. These risk factors are associated with sedation complications. The physical examination should focus on vital signs, mental status, and the presence of pathologic anatomic features associated with a greater risk of airway obstruction and sedation difficulties.

Several distinct examinations must be performed based on an initial medical and surgical history review: firstly, a general exam to identify any underlying undiagnosed pathology present, looking closely for any obvious cardiovascular, respiratory, or abdominal signs; secondly, a thorough airway examination to predict the difficulty of airway management; and thirdly, detailed investigations may be required depending on comorbidities, age, and the nature of the procedure. Finally, there are standardized and validated score cards or tools available that can be used to document the assessment findings effectively, which not only facilitates day-of procedural review but also allows for benchmarking and quality improvements.

There is a well documented large variability[5] in the: (1) level of experience and the scope of practice of clinical providers administering sedation and/or general anesthesia, i.e., gastrointestinal specialists, endoscopy-trained nurses, nurse anesthetists, physician assistants, and anesthesiologists and each has to know their limitations; (2) drugs administered during the procedure (sedatives, pain killers, anesthetic drugs); (3) airway techniques used (there is an extensive range of devices available for airway management requiring different levels of skills); (4) level of monitoring (including cardiovascular and respiratory monitoring); (5) duration and difficulty level of the procedure; (6) depth of sedation/anesthesia; (7) hospital (major teaching hospital vs. rural hospital) and the number of procedures performed, and (8) patients, each with their risk factors (e.g., obesity, hypoventilation, obstructive sleep apnea).

Medical history

A full past medical history review is important to obtain good insights into the patient's risk factors for procedural sedation. Previous surgical operations, medical procedures or diagnosis and anesthesia experiences, and allergies should be reviewed. Screening questions may also elucidate undiagnosed disease and prompt further investigation.

Respiratory diseases can limit the patient from lying flat for an extended period, or the patient can suffer from a chronic cough or snoring. An assessment of the cardiovascular status is necessary to establish the overall exercise tolerance (cardiovascular fitness), hypertension, exertional chest pain, syncopal episodes, or orthopnea. For patients with renal, liver, endocrine, and gastrointestinal diseases, baseline functions and management need to be assessed, especially as they can interfere with sedation medication usage and airway management, e.g., active gastroesophageal reflux disease (GERD) has a high aspiration risk.

While most hereditary conditions relating to anesthesia are extremely rare, such as malignant hyperthermia, it is vital to ask about any known family history of problems with anesthesia. Also, issues like postoperative nausea and vomiting, delirium, and awareness must be addressed.

Medication usage

The use of medications prescribed and nonprescribed, herbal medicine,[148] and vitamin and mineral supplements need to be reviewed in detail, including what, indication, when, dosage, and effect (including side effects). Asking the patient about social factors like smoking history, alcohol intake, and any recreational drug use can have their influence on the sedative medication choice and dosaging. Other critical social factors to take note of include language spoken and the need for an interpreter. This is especially important if the patient will undergo a procedure under conscious sedation as they must be able to communicate clearly with the healthcare team. The personal living situation of patients can impact the hospitalization process as the patient may require additional support before or after the sedation.

Deconditioning

The level of deconditioning of a patient before undergoing a procedure refers to the changes in the body that occur during a period of inactivity. The changes happen in the heart, lungs, and muscles and cause tiredness and fatigue. The three stages of deconditioning include mild deconditioning with changes in the ability to do the usual exercise activities, moderate deconditioning with changes in the ability to do everyday activities, and severe deconditioning when the patient is no longer able to do a minimal activity or usual self-care. Deconditioning symptoms include weakness and tiredness, shortness of breath with minor physical effort (exertion), a faster heart rate than normal, pain or discomfort with activity, decreased strength, endurance, and balance. People at high risk for deconditioning are older adults; hospitalized or bedridden patients; patients who have cancer, obesity, or poor nutrition; and those patients with an illness or injury that affects movement and activity.

Frailty

Frailty is another indication of high risk for postprocedural sedation complications. It is not an inevitable part of aging. Frailty is associated with poor mobility, increased falls, hospitalizations, admission to residential care and mortality, poor quality of life, depression, cognitive decline, and reported loneliness. Different validated frailty score cards are available, and they all help document a person's physical performance, nutritional status, cognition, mental health, and health supports.

Assessing the metabolic equivalent for task level (Table 10.1)

One way of determining patients' activity levels is using the metabolic equivalent for task (MET) level score. The MET is a unit that estimates the amount of energy used by the body during physical activity as compared to resting metabolism. The MET is the oxygen used by a person in milliliters per minute per kilogram body mass divided by 3.5. One metabolic equivalent (MET) is the amount of oxygen consumed while sitting at rest, equal to 3.5 mL O_2 per kg body weight $\times$ min. The MET level is an easy way to describe the physical activity tolerance of a patient. Wahid et al.[6] performed a systematic review of physical activity and major chronic diseases. They

Table 10.1 Metabolic equivalents for tasks (METs).

MET	Activity	Perioperative cardiac risk
1–3 MET	Taking care of yourself, eating, drinking, desk work, walking one or two blocks	High
4–9 MET	Climb stairs, walk briskly, running short distances, moderate sports	Intermediate to low
10 ≤ MET	Vigorous active sports	Low

found that 150 minutes of moderate-intensity aerobic activity per week compared to inactivity resulted in a 23% lower risk of mortality (related to cardiovascular disease), 17% lower incidence of cardiovascular diseases, and 26% lower incidence of type 2 diabetes mellitus.

Revised cardiac risk index

Lee Goldman published the Goldman Risk Index (GRI) in 1977, which was updated in 1999 and published as the Revised Cardiac Risk Index (RCRI) to estimate a patient's risk of perioperative cardiac complications in noncardiac surgery.[7] If a patient scores positive for two or more out of the six factors, a patient is defined as "high-risk." The first factor "high-risk surgery (intraperitoneal, intrathoracic, or suprainguinal vascular procedures)" is irrelevant for our patient undergoing sedation. The other five factors are: history of ischemic disease, congestive heart failure or cerebrovascular disease, perioperative treatment with insulin or preoperative serum creatinine levels >2.0 mg/dL.

ASA classification (Table 10.2)

The American Society of Anesthesiologists (ASA) physical status classification system is a widely accepted and validated risk stratification system for assessing the fitness of patients before surgery. It was developed in the 1940s and is used to assess and communicate a patient's pre-surgical medical comorbidities.

Smoking

Smoking habits can have an important impact on risks of sedation care. Patients should be instructed to stop smoking at least 3–4 weeks before the procedure. Smoking increases airway reactiveness, inhibits ciliary motility to remove secretions, causes poor wound healing, and increases the rate of complications after surgery. The maximal beneficial effects occur if smoking is stopped for at least 8 weeks prior to surgery. However, carboxyhemoglobin (carbon monoxide—CO) levels decrease in

Table 10.2 ASA classification levels.[8]

	Definition	Adult examples, including, but not limited to:
ASA I	A normal healthy patient	Healthy, non-smoking, no or minimal alcohol use
ASA II	A patient with mild (systemic) disease, without substantive functional limitations	Current smoker, social alcohol drinker, pregnancy, obesity (30 < BMI < 40), well-controlled DM or HTN, mild lung disease
ASA III	A patient with severe systemic disease, substantive functional limitations, or one or more moderate to severe diseases	Poorly controlled DM or HTN, COPD, morbid obesity (BMI ≥ 40), active hepatitis, alcohol dependence or abuse, implanted pacemaker, moderate reduction of ejection fraction, ESRD undergoing regularly scheduled dialysis, history (>3 months) of MI, CVA, TIA, or CAD/ stents
ASA IV	A patient with severe systemic disease that is a constant threat to life	Recent (<3 months) MI, CVA, TIA, or CAD/stents, ongoing cardiac ischemia or severe valve dysfunction, severe reduction of ejection fraction, shock, sepsis, disseminated intravascular coagulation, ascites reinfusion dialysis, or ESRD not undergoing regularly scheduled dialysis
ASA V	A moribund patient who is not expected to survive without the operation	Ruptured abdominal/thoracic aneurysm, massive trauma, intracranial bleed with mass effect, ischemic bowel in the face of significant cardiac pathology, or multiple organ/system dysfunction
ASA VI	A declared brain-dead patient whose organs are being removed for donor purposes	

the first 12−24 hours after quitting smoking (improves oxygenation). Both nicotine and CO have negative effects on the heart (increased oxygen demand, decreased contractility). It should be noted that in some patients, airway reactiveness and secretions might increase paradoxically for about a week after smoking cessation.

Fasting guidelines

Fasting guidelines for sedation are similar to general anesthesia. Although each country has its own fasting guidelines for elective interventions, there is consensus about fasting for adults: 2 hours is enough for clear fluids, but 6 hours is required for solid food or cow's milk.[11–15] The Canadian and American anesthesiologist's societies[16–18] differentiate between 6 hours for a light meal and 8 hours for heavy meal with meat, fried, or fatty foods. Chewing gum is often considered similar to the risk of having clear fluids.

In conclusion, nowadays most reviews take place via video, phone call, or online self-assessment tools. After a complete review of all data, the person performing the sedation must develop and communicate a plan with the patient and obtain their consent for the sedation. This plan should entail management of medications, smoking or drug use, fasting guidelines, potential complications, and the admission process. Also, a preliminary airway management plan can be included but a complete airway assessment is only possible during a direct face-to-face contact. On the day of the sedation, a quick review of the assessment is advisable as conditions may have changed and a final ASA classification is made after evaluating the patient. Increased ASA scores and especially class III or higher positively correlate with a higher rate of sedation complications and a requirement for high recovery e strategies.

Preprocedural airway assessment

This section will concentrate on how best to predict difficulties in maintaining adequate oxygenation either with face-mask ventilation or with advanced airway management during (gastrointestinal) endoscopic procedures under sedation, whereby the patient's ventilation should be continuously observed by clinical assessment and monitoring of oxygen saturation (measured by pulse oximetry), and ventilation (with end-tidal carbon dioxide through noninvasive waveform capnography).

Airway management remains one of the most important responsibilities of the clinician administering sedation. Complications can occur even during conscious sedation procedures. Prediction of a difficult airway allows a management plan to be developed, time for proper patient selection, and proper selection of equipment, devices and techniques and support from others.

Difficult airway management remains a significant cause of morbidity and mortality and is generally encountered during unexpected clinical conditions. It is usually defined as difficulties with either performing adequate bag-mask ventilation, problems with visualizing the glottis with a direct laryngoscope (failed laryngoscopy), or difficulties with the insertion of a supraglottic airway device or the endotracheal tube leading to challenges or even failed endotracheal intubation. Furthermore, even a good view of the glottis does not necessarily translate into easy control of the airway.

Correctly predicting difficulties during airway management (i.e., difficulties with a facemask, OPAs, NPAs, SADs, ETTs) contributes to safer airway management. Therefore, a preoperative assessment of every patient's airway is recommended. Many countries have produced their own guidelines for preoperative airway assessment, although there does not exist a specific overall recommendation about what exactly needs to be evaluated, nor what is the most optimal selection of metrics that provide an accurate identification for predictors of difficult airways. No single test has shown to be an accurate predictor of difficult airway management, and none of the current tests are both highly sensitive and highly specific. Yet there is a clear need for a more accurate, simple, and clinically applicable airway assessment tools for predicting difficulties. Several predictive scores for difficult airway use different anthropometric features as simple preprocedural bedside tests19−31; Honarmand 2014,[32,33] (Table 10.3).

Other criteria that may cause a difficult airway are buck teeth, snoring/CPAP, oral infections, abscesses or tumors, posterior neck fat pad, cervical spine mobility, and loose or missing teeth. Patients with bushy beards can be difficult to manually ventilate via bag mask ventilation.

Combinations of these tests result in better prediction scores of anatomically difficult airways as reported by Wilson and El Ganzouri. Other factors can contribute to difficulties in airway management, i.e., obesity, protruding incisors, single canines. However, numerous studies have demonstrated the limited ability to reliably and accurately predict a difficult airway. Alessandri et al.[34] showed the relationship between ultrasound assessment of the anterior soft tissues of the neck, difficult laryngoscopy, and difficult mask ventilation. Ultrasound neck screening provides quick, relatively easy, and accurate information, with diagnostic and therapeutic relevance. Longer skin-to-larynx distances appears predictive for both difficult mask ventilation and difficult laryngoscopy.[35]

The prediction of airway difficulties remains a challenging task, and the results of all studies underline the importance of being constantly prepared for unexpected challenges. None of the airway screening tests seems to perform well alone, and different combinations are suggested to improve accuracy and higher predictability. The STOP-BANG acronym (for Snoring, Tiredness, Observed aPnea, hypertension, high Body mass index, Age, Neck circumference, and Gender) questionnaire is an instrumental screening tool and a good predictor for airway complications in patients with undiagnosed obstructive sleep apnea. The choice of assessment is ultimately at the discretion of the individual sedation provider. Even large cohort studies,[36−39] including hundreds of thousands of patients in Denmark, showed that the accuracy of clinical prediction of a difficult airway is poor. However, the recommended preoperative airway assessment is the way forward using a combination of presurgery metrics. These researchers demonstrate an overall prevalence of difficult/impossible facemask ventilation of 1.1%,[36] which may be particularly important in conscious sedation.

Routine physical evaluation of the airway is generally done by the healthcare professional responsible for the sedation. However, during the COVID-19 pandemic, to reduce unnecessary exposure of healthcare professionals, virtual airway assessment was done via remote telemedicine, as part of the preprocedural evaluation of the patient, providing a valid alternative to direct physical consultation.[25] Simple tests are: Can you fit three fingers in your mouth when fully opened? Can you place

Table 10.3 Predictors of Airway difficulties.

Management predictor	High-risk score	Definition and measurement
Mallampati classification	Grades 3 and 4	Identifies potential obstructive sleep apnea and predicts difficulty with any endotracheal intubation. This classification is based on the structures visualized with maximal mouth opening and tongue protrusion in the sitting position. Class 1: Soft palate, fauces, uvula, anterior and posterior pillars visible Class 2: Soft palate, fauces, uvula visible Class 3: Soft palate, base of uvula visible Class 4: Soft palate not visible at all
Interincisor gap	<3 cm	Rigid ruler, measuring in the midline
Upper lip bite test (ULBT)	Classes 2 and 3	Place bottom teeth in front of upper teeth. Move mandibular – incisors—as high on the upper lip as possible. Class 1: Lower incisor can bite upper lip above vermilion line Class 2: Incisor can bite upper lip below vermilion line Class 3: Cannot bite upper lip
Thyromental distance (TMD)	<6 cm	Rigid ruler from lower border of thyroid notch to bony point of mentum with patient's head extended and mouth closed.
Ratio of height to thyromental distance (RHTMD)	>23.5	Predictor for difficult laryngoscopy. RHTMD = height in cm/TMD in cm
Sternomental distance (SMD)	<13.5 cm	Indicator of head and neck mobility. The straight distance between the upper border of the manubrium sterni and the bony point of the mentum with the head in full extension and the mouth closed.
Ratio of height to sternomental distance (RHSMD)	>12.5	Predictor for difficult laryngoscopy. RHSMD = height in cm/SMD in cm
Neck mobility	<90°	Normal >90°
Neck circumference	>43 cm	
BMI	>30 kg/m^2	

your lower teeth in front of your upper teeth? Can you fit three fingers between your chin and your Adam's apple? Do you have any problems with neck movements? What is your neck circumference? These are some of the questions that can easily provide valuable information even from a remote distance.

It's key is to focus on unanticipated airway compromise and obstruction by pre-procedural airway assessment and preparation. The inability to maintain an open airway and adequate oxygenation is one of the most feared complications during deep sedation, such as gastrointestinal endoscopic procedures, which can result in catastrophic outcomes, such as anoxic brain injury and death.

Levels of sedation

Procedural sedation is a drug-induced depression of consciousness. Depending on the level of sedation, patients will be able to respond purposefully to verbal or tactile stimuli and may lack memory. Although we may aim for a certain level of sedation, sedation is a continuum of consciousness states, ranging from near awake to deep sedation, and can be obtained by using a variety of drugs and administration routes.

The level of sedation required to perform the procedure successfully and with high patient satisfaction depends on several factors. The healthcare professionals consenting and providing sedation need to consider the level of the patient's anxiety, gender, age, pain tolerance, existing pain, bowel sensitivity, and the use of medication and illicit drugs. Procedural considerations may be the complexity of the procedure and the therapeutic maneuvers necessary to reach the optimal therapeutic result and also strongly depends on the endoscopist's technical expertise, patience, and speed. After considering all factors, it is essential to discuss the most suitable level of sedation and to bring these in line with the patient's expectations. The clinician providing sedation should not be distracted by other responsibilities and is responsible for safe sedation and monitoring.

Different definitions were used to describe varying sedation levels, and they may differ for patients in the ICU, ED, and general anesthesia. In anesthesia, the most commonly used definitions for sedation were originally developed by the ASA in 1999 and was last updated in 2019 (Table 10.4).

Minimal and moderate sedation can still leave the patient with the ability to respond purposefully to actions and commands while cardiovascular and ventilation functions are still preserved. Deep and general sedation represents a continuum in which patients may require assistance with maintaining the airway or cardiovascular function or full ventilation support.

The Ramsay sedation scale was developed to promote adequate sedation in the intensive care unit (ICU), and it was slightly modified for anesthesia 40 (Table 10.5).

The Modified Observer's Assessment of Alertness/Sedation (MOAA/S) scale is directed at determining the degree of suppression of consciousness and is widely used in the anesthesia research literature for quantifying the hypnotic effects of drugs (Table 10.6).

Healthcare professionals providing sedation need to recognize the different sedation levels and be alert to changes with deepening sedation levels and be able to rescue a patient in respiratory failure from a deep level of sedation or even unconsciousness. Deep sedation and general anesthesia should strictly be overseen by anesthesia specialists who can maintain adequate respiration and cardiovascular function.

Table 10.4 ASA sedation levels.

	Minimal sedation anxiolysis	Moderate sedation (conscious sedation)	Deep sedation	General anesthesia
Responsiveness	Normal response to verbal stimulation	Purposeful response to verbal or tactile stimulation	Purposeful response following repeated or painful stimulation	Unrousable even with painful stimulus
Airway	Unaffected	No intervention required	Intervention may be required	Intervention often required
Spontaneous ventilation	Unaffected	Adequate	May be inadequate	Frequently inadequate
Cardiovascular function	Unaffected	Adequate	May be inadequate	May be impaired

Table 10.5 Ramsay sedation scale.

Response	Level
Fully awake	1
Drowsy	2
Apparently asleep but rousable by normal speech	3
Apparently asleep but responding to standardized physical stimuli (e.g., glabellar tap)	4
Asleep, but not responding to strong physical stimuli (comatose)	5

Table 10.6 MOAA/S scale.

Response	Score
Agitated	6
Responds readily to name spoken in normal tone (alert)	5
Lethargic response to name spoken in normal tone	4
Responds only after name is called loudly and/or repeatedly	3
Responds only after mild prodding or shaking	2
Does not respond to mild prodding or shaking	1
Does not respond to a deep stimulus	0

Quality measurements

Clinicians are mainly concerned about the safety of the sedation and levels of comfort. Leffler et al.[41] developed a procedural sedation assessment survey (PROSAS) measuring the quality of moderate sedation. Procedural sedation quality was defined as the absence of any sedation-related adverse event, and patient satisfaction was within the predetermined threshold. Patient satisfaction is directly influenced by the side effects of the sedation, control over the sedation level, level of comfort, and adverse events of the sedation.

The Iowa Satisfaction with Anesthesia Scale (ISAS) is a similar tool as the PROSAS, but the ISAS measures patient satisfaction after deep sedation 42 (Table 10.7). The items in the survey tool are very similar but do not include the experience of adverse events during the procedure, as patients will not be aware of them during deep sedation. The PROSAS can often be completed during the first phase of recovery whereas the ISAS tool needs to be completed during the second stage recovery—such as the day after the procedure (via phone call). The items are rated on a positive to negative scale: agree very much — disagree very much[42] (Table 10.8). Post anesthesia satisfaction studies done days after the procedure reveal as much as 6% of patients report minor events such as postoperative nausea and vomiting, significant sore throat, and hoarseness, and are significantly associated with patient dissatisfaction.[149]

Patient selection and screening

The selection of appropriate patients for minimal and moderate sedation is crucial to the safety and success of sedation. Minimal and moderate sedation can be provided by nonanesthetists depending on the healthcare professional training and competency levels and on local legal requirements.

Table 10.7 Iowa satisfaction with anesthesia survey (ISAS).

I threw up or felt like throwing up
I would want to have the same anesthetic again
I itched
I felt relaxed
I felt pain
I felt safe
I was too cold or too hot
I was satisfied with my anesthetic care
I felt pain during the procedure
I felt good
I hurt

Table 10.8 Procedural Sedation Assessment survey (PROSAS)[a].

Patient	
How much discomfort did you experience during the procedure?	Scale 0–10: None – slight discomfort – moderate discomfort – significant discomfort – sever pain
If having this procedure again in the future, how much sedation would you prefer to have?	Scale –5–0 +5: Markedly less sedation – somewhat less sedation – same amount of sedation – somewhat more sedation – markedly more sedation
On a scale of 0–10, how much pain were you feeling before the procedure?	Scale 0–10: None – slightly pain – moderate pain – significant pain – severe pain
On a scale of 0–10, how much pain are you feeling now?	Scale 0-10: None – slightly pain – moderate pain – significant pain – severe pain
Do you have any nausea now?	Yes - No
Do you have any dizziness now?	Yes - No
Do you have any fatigue/tiredness now?	Yes - No
Clinician administering sedation	
Any episodes of O_2 desaturation <90% or leading to intervention?	Yes - No
Any problematic changes in heart rate or blood pressure during intervention? (Systolic blood pressure <90 mm hg, >160 mm hg; heart rate <50 bpm, >120 bpm)	Yes - No
Any hemodynamic or respiratory conditions that interrupted the procedure?	Yes - No
What level of sedation best describes the case overall?	Scale -5 – 0 + 5: Markedly undersedated – somewhat undersedated – appropriate sedation – somewhat oversedated – markedly oversedated
How much discomfort did the patient experience during the procedure?	Scale 0–10: None – slight discomfort – moderate discomfort – significant discomfort – sever pain
Please rate the patient's cooperation during the procedure:	• procedure aborted due to lack of cooperation • procedure delayed/interrupted due to lack of cooperation • adequately cooperative
Endoscopist	
Was the exam interrupted in any way due to patient discomfort?	Yes – No
Recovery nurse	
How did procedural sedation impact patient recovery?	Scale -5–0 + 5: Persistent pain due to undersedation – minor discomfort due to undersedation – optimal recovery - slightly sedated: Slow and minor difficulty in attaining awareness and consciousness - sedated: Difficulty in attaining awareness and consciousness
Did the patient report any pain during recovery?	Yes - No
Did the patient complain of any nausea during recovery?	Yes - No

[a] 41,43.

Important criteria to consider in patients that will likely require anesthesia support include:

- Younger than 18 years old
- Gravidity
- ASA class III of cardiac cause or higher
- Advanced therapeutic endoscopy (e.g., ERCP, balloon dilatation)
- Morbid obesity (BMI >35 kg/m^2)
- Severe sleep apnea (based on clinical diagnosis)
- Difficult airway
- Previously experienced anesthesia issues
- Allergy to propofol or soy oil
- Interventions requiring (intermittent) deep sedation
- Anticipated intolerance to standard sedatives and opioids
- Chronic use of significant amounts of pain medication
- Patients with previous high sedation needs

In 2014, Braunstein et al. developed a scoring system to risk-stratify patients for high sedation needs during gastroscopy and colonoscopy who could benefit from anesthesia support. Based on the patient's characteristics, a SCOPE score was established, which correlates well with the patient's estimated risk for high sedation needs (Tables 10.9 and 10.10).[146]

Table 10.9 Stratifying Clinical Outcomes Prior to Endoscopy (SCOPE) scoring system.

Gastroduodenoscopy		Colonoscopy	
Characteristics	**Points**	**Characteristics**	**Points**
Ages 18–29	10	Ages 18–29	10
Ages 30–39	9	Ages 30–39	10
Ages 40–49	7	Ages 40–49	6
Ages 50–59	3	Ages 50–59	2
Ages 60–69	0	Ages 60–69	0
Indication for reflux[a]	2	Diagnostic indication	3
Indication not for reflux[a] or abdominal pain	1	Female gender	3
Male gender	1	BMI <25	2
Psychiatric history	1	Tobacco use	1
Benzodiazepine use	2	Benzodiazepine use	6
Opioid use	2	Opioid use	4
Fellow present	1	Other psychoactive medication use	1

[a] Includes GERD, esophagitis, and Barrett's esophagus.

Table 10.10 Estimate a patient's risk of high sedation needs based on their SCOPE score.

Gastroscopy		Colonoscopy	
SCOPE score	Risk %	SCOPE score	Risk %
I	10	I	10
II	20	II	15
III	25	III	20
IV	30	IV	30
V	50	V	75

Medications used for sedation (Table 10.11)

The factors to be considered when choosing effective sedation medications include the type and expected duration of the procedure, but also patient-specific considerations, drug interactions, side effects, and intolerance. The induction and maintenance of sedation is a dynamic process that requires the clinician providing sedation to continuously evaluate the depth of sedation and assess how the patient is tolerating the procedure. Before starting the procedure, reliable venous access should be obtained and intravenous fluids (crystalloids) can be administered.

Table 10.11 Sedation drug recommended doses.

Drug	Initial dosage (IV bolus)	Repeat dosage	Maximum dose
Midazolam	1–2.5 mg (0.05–0.1 mg/kg)	Repeated every 3–5 min	None
Diazepam	5–10 mg	None	30 mg/8 h
Remimazolam	2.5–5 mg	1.25–2.5 mg	None
Propofol	20–40 mg	10–20 mg every 60 s	None
Alfentanil	3–8 mcg/kg	3–5 mcg/kg	3 - 40 mcg/kg
Fentanyl	50–100 mcg	25–50 mcg	None
Epinephrine (1:1000)	1 mg (arrest) 100–500 mcg (anaphylaxis)	See ALS and anaphylaxis guideline	None
Atropine	0.5–0.6 mg	Every 3–5 min	3 mg
Flumazenil	200 mcg	100 mcg	3 mg/hour
Naloxone	0.4–2 mg	Every 2–3 min	10 mg

Propofol

Propofol **increases GABA-mediated inhibatory tone in the CNS**, and has hypnotic, amnesic, and antiemetic effects but does not provide analgesia. Propofol's favorable pharmacodynamic and pharmacokinetic profile has led to its widespread use in procedural sedation. Propofol as monotherapy in basic, and advanced sedation has been shown to induce moderate sedation more rapidly than the midazolam and fentanyl or alfentanil combinations improving recovery time and patient satisfaction. The depth of sedation increases in a predictable, dose-dependent manner. Propofol has a narrow therapeutic window between moderate sedation and general anesthesia. There is no reversal agent if oversedation or loss of protective airway reflexes occurs. The pharmacokinetics are affected by weight, sex, age, and concomitant disease. Respiratory depression is aggravated by coadministration with benzodiazepines and opioids. Myoclonic movements or abnormal posturing may also be seen during recovery but are short-lived and resolve spontaneously.

Benzodiazepines

Benzodiazepines, particularly midazolam, are widely used for procedural sedation, often in combination with opioids. Benzodiazepines are sedatives that decrease anxiety and can cause antegrade amnesia, muscle relaxation, and anticonvulsant but do not cause analgesia.

Midazolam is a short-acting benzodiazepine with an onset of 2−5 min with a maximum effect after about 5−10 min, a duration of 30−60 min, and an elimination half-time of 1.5−2.5 h. Usual sedation dosage is 0.02−0.03 mg/kg with repeated doses accumulating in adipose tissues, which can prolong sedation. The most important side effects of midazolam are dose-dependent respiratory depression, which is potentiated by opioids and propofol use.

Sometimes *midazolam* can cause a paradoxical reaction, and a patient may experience agitation, confusion, inconsolable hysteria, and aggression. This is more common in young and advanced ages, alcoholics, and patients with psychiatric or personality disorders. In these situations, *midazolam* can be reversed with *flumazenil*.

Diazepam is comparable to midazolam but has a slower onset of 1−3 min, a much longer elimination half-time (20−40 h), and active metabolites. Enterohepatic recirculation may cause peak plasma concentrations and feelings of sedation 6−8 h and 12 h after injection. The anterograde amnesia effect is less compared to midazolam.

Remimazolam is a new ultra-short-acting benzodiazepine with recovery times comparable to propofol due to its rapid conversion into inactive metabolites.[44] Its onset time is similar to *midazolam* (1−3 min) but reaches peak sedation within 3−5 min. *Remimazolam* has an elimination half-time of 7−8 min without prolonged or residual effects due to its organ-independent elimination, allowing similar dosage in liver or renal disease patients.[45] *Remimazolam* has less cardiovascular or respiratory depression than propofol.[44,46] Due to its onset time of 1–3 min, propofol may still be the preferred sedation agent for short diagnostic gastroscopic procedures. *Remimazolam* is not approved in all countries, yet more studies are necessary to obtain insights into full potential and behavior compared to other medications.

Opioids

Opioids like *fentanyl* and *alfentanil* are synthetic derivatives of morphine. They rarely cause cardiovascular depression (e.g., hypotension) and respiratory depression in typical sedation doses but are potentiated by sedatives. In the elderly and patients with liver and renal diseases, its effect can be more prolonged and profound, including leading to respiratory depression.

Fentanyl is highly lipophilic, allowing rapid penetration of the blood–brain barrier, causing a rapid onset (2–3 min), and has a short duration action of 30–60 min. It is 75–100 times more potent than morphine and has no amnestic properties. Fentanyl may cause a brief, self-limiting cough after bolus intravenous administration.

Alfentanil has a quicker onset of action (within 1 min) than fentanyl and a shorter duration of action than fentanyl. In addition, alfentanil has a shorter half-life and may produce less respiratory depression than fentanyl, but its metabolism is less predictable than fentanyl.

Because of their potentiated effect on sedatives, it is recommended to dose the sedative first, wait 1–2 min, observe the response, and then administer the opioid. Elderly patients with reduced liver and renal function require smaller doses and longer dosing intervals.

Reversal agents

Flumazenil is a selective GABA$_A$ receptor antagonist and can reverse benzodiazepines. It has a rapid onset within 1–2 min with a peak effect after 6–10 min. Because of the longer half-life of most benzodiazepines, including midazolam, the patient should be carefully monitored for recurrent sedation when the initial dose of flumazenil wears off.

Naloxone is a nonselective and competitive opioid receptor antagonist and can rapidly reverse opioids. It has a high affinity for μ-opioid receptors (fentanyl and alfentanil).

Sedation therapy

The use of *propofol* for gastrointestinal endoscopy is preferable because of its fast onset and rapid patient recovery.[47,48] Complications are almost 40% less likely than sedation with traditional sedative agents [41,49] in sedation with fentanyl and midazolam. The addition of an opioid is preferable during more painful, often interventional, endoscopic procedures and should lead to the need for decreased sedation dosages.[50]

Studies have shown varied approaches to dosing *propofol* as a monosedation therapy:

—Intermittent intravenous bolus titration to the necessary level of moderate-to-deep sedation as clinically judged.

—30—50 mg of propofol at the beginning of the endoscopic procedure, followed by single boluses of 20—30 mg based on sedation depth.[51]

—An initial IV bolus of propofol (0.5—1 mg/kg) is administered intravenously, followed by a repeated bolus (10—20 mg) according to the patient's condition, or a continuous propofol infusion (2—6 mg/kg/h, with an additional bolus administered as needed).[52]

—Propofol initial bolus injection of 40 mg for patients <70 years old, 30 mg for patients aged 70—89, and 20 mg for those aged 90 years or older. When the target sedation level was not obtained, additional injections of 20 mg propofol were given.[53]

—Propofol bolus of 50 mg for patients younger than 70 years of age, or 30 mg for older patients, in combination with a strong short-acting opioid analgesic, alfentanil, 1 mg or 0.5 mg. Supplement bolus 20 mg per bolus for patients younger than 70 years of age, 10 mg for older patients for a refractory period of 1 min.[54]

—Initial doses of propofol are 50 mg or less. In small, elderly, or frail patients and those with multiple comorbidities, initial boluses were commonly 20—30 mg. After the initial bolus, no more than 20 mg of propofol is administered at an interval no shorter than every 20 s.[55]

Intermittent deep sedation with propofol monotherapy can provide sufficient sedation for the gag-free introduction of the endoscope with a dose of 100 mg minus the patient's age in years, but no more than 60 mg (hence, an 80-year-old would receive 20 mg). Additional doses of half the initial dose every 45—60 s can be required until the patient is unresponsive to verbal and light tactile stimulation. Deep sedation can be maintained with intermittent doses of 10—20 mg if the patient shows signs of discomfort, sound, or movement, or every 1—2 min if the patient is asleep with stable cardiopulmonary status. Unfortunately, studies with intermittent deep sedation demonstrated high rates of hypoxia and hypotension.[56]

Other studies used a combination of *propofol* and *midazolam and recommend*:

- 2—3 mg of midazolam together with 10—20 mg propofol followed by single propofol boluses of 20—30 mg based on sedation depth[51]
- 1—2 mg of midazolam, followed by a slow induction bolus of 0.3—0 mg/kg to 75 mg/kg of propofol. Top-up doses of 10—20 mg of propofol (Sathananthan)
- During balanced propofol sedation (BPS), doses of fentanyl are 50—75 mg, and midazolam doses are 1—2 mg. Following the initial dose of opioid and/or benzodiazepine, all further doses are with propofol [57]

Alternative approaches

Other drugs like ketamine, dexmedetomidine, and opioids such as remifentanil and sufentanil may be used in combination with propofol with varied outcomes. Most randomized controlled trials studies have had a limited number of participants (around 25–35 per group) and were conducted in a specific patient group.

Dexmedetomidine is an alpha-2 adrenoreceptor agonist with sedative, anxiolytic, and analgesic properties and is mainly used in intensive care units. Patients can experience hypotension and bradycardia, which can be treated with atropine or ephedrine.[51] The patient satisfaction levels scores are significantly lower as compared with propofol[52] and midazolam[58] but show a faster recovery time.[58]

Etomidate is a hypnotic commonly used for patients with a high risk of hemodynamic instability. Its main side effect is myoclonus which can be prevented by an initial dose of midazolam.[59]

Ketamine has analgesic and hypnotic properties with high safety profile and is sometimes used with propofol to increase hemodynamic stability and lower respiratory depression.[9,50,60] Ketamine, however, increases saliva secretion, which can cause laryngospasm and airway obstruction.

Some clinicians offer self-inhaled nitrous oxide/oxygen mixture (Entonox) as an adjunct to intravenous medication when necessary for short procedures, including colonoscopy. Although Entonox is also used recreationally, there are some safety concerns as it can cause paresthesia in the extremities (80%), unsteady gait or walking difficulties (58%), weakness (43%), fallings or equilibrium disorders (24%), Lhermitte's sign (15%), and ataxia (12%).[61]

Methoxyflurane has been extensively used during general anesthesia since the mid-last century. Nowadays, methoxyflurane portable inhalers (also called "green whistle") are available and widely used by paramedics in the community, wound dressing in burn patients, and bone marrow biopsies. It has a strong analgesic effect without significant sedative effects, no respiratory depression but slightly impaired psychomotor skills (10% reduction), and cognitive performance up to 30 min after the dosage.[62] Nguyen et al. demonstrated that it is also safe and effective to use during colonoscopy even in morbidly obese patients with obstructive sleep apnea.[63] Methoxyflurane has a rapid recovery profile,[64] resulting in an early return of psychomotor skills, and ability to drive home and resume (work) activities safely within a few hours after the procedure.[65]

When using Entonox or methoxyflurane, extra safety measures, e.g., nonreturn valves in the supply system and an antihypoxic alarm, should be used. Exposure of healthcare professionals to these gases could be a concern, and scavenger systems should be used to decrease occupational exposure.

Oxygen administration can be considered during mild to moderate sedation[66] and is recommended for most patients unless contraindicated for the patient.[10,67–69]

Monitoring

Patients undergoing sedation should constantly be monitored for changes in vital parameters. The clinician must be able to interpret and respond to changes in pulse oximetry, heart rate (HR), electrocardiogram (ECG), end-tidal CO2, respiratory rate (RR), and noninvasive blood pressure values and must understand the importance of continuous low- and high-flow supplemental oxygen via nasal, facemask, or oral routes.

According to ANZCA, monitoring is "Observing and checking progress and quality over a period of time." 70 Monitoring is used to measure parameters, observations, plan and avoid trouble, understanding diagnosis, and treatment of complications. Clinical patient observations can inform clinicians about the quality and frequency of patient breathing by observing airflow at nostrils and chest movements. Visual cardiovascular observations include skin and mucosal color, capillary refill, distension of jugular or central veins, clammy, red, or pale skin, and rate, volume, and rhythm of the pulse. Sweaty skin and pupil size may indicate the depth of sedation, but this can be misleading when using opioids. A stethoscope should always be available for chest auscultations.

Anesthesia and gastroenterological societies have their standards and guidelines for monitoring patients during sedation. In the United Kingdom, the monitoring guideline for sedation is the same as for general anesthesia (Klein 2021). The European Society of Anaesthesiologists[71] and the Australian and New Zealand College of Anaesthetists[69] have specific guidelines for sedation, including monitoring requirements. The ASA has particular guidelines for moderate sedation[67,68] and a separate one for deep sedation.[10]

Vital signs should be recorded before administration of the sedation, at regular intervals during the procedural sedation, during the recovery phase, and before discharge home (Table 10.12).

Other monitoring and equipment that need to be available in case of adverse events or emergencies are neuromuscular function monitoring (e.g., Train of Four) in case muscular blocking agents are to be used. Extensive cardiovascular monitoring in the very sick or ASA >3 patients or emergencies may include central venous pressure, invasive arterial blood pressure, transesophageal echocardiogram, and cardiac output monitors. In closed breathing circuits, e.g., endotracheal tube or supraglottic airway devices, ventilation alarms for disconnection, and inspiratory low O_2 levels need to be available with potential spirometry.

Human error, performance limitations, and complications

Human errors form a significant portion of preventable mishaps in healthcare. Even the most competent clinicians are not immune to this. Although there was little research in the field of healthcare safety until the mid-1980s, in other fields (e.g.,

Table 10.12 Vital signs monitoring during sedation.

Consciousness	Levels should be monitored continuously. This can be done by asking the patient to respond to verbal commands or a tactile stimulus.[67–69,71]
Discomfort	This is also recommended by ASGE, but it is not clear how this needs to be measured or whether this is the same measurement as the level of consciousness.[66]
Electrocardiogram (ECG)	The american guideline recommends ECG monitoring only in patients with clinically significant cardiovascular diseases during moderate sedation[66–68] and continuously during deep sedation.[10] Other societies recommend continuous ECG monitoring.[71]
Noninvasive blood pressure	Almost all societies recommend at least every 5-minute interval for noninvasive blood pressure and heart rate[10,67–69,71] except for ASGE which recommends noninvasive blood pressure measurements at least once during the procedure.[66]
Waveform capnography	Most societies recommend continuous monitoring for moderate and deep sedation[10,11,67,68,71] but not ASGE[66]. Although capnography monitoring of respiratory activity reduces episodes of hypoxemia, the clinical impact is controversial. Some recommend only using capnography in patients who are at high risk for hypoxemia,[72] but others see a benefit of measuring $EtCO_2$ as it is an early warning signal.[56,73]
Pulse oximetry and heart rate	Continuous monitoring is recommended by all societies.[10,66–69,71]
Temperature	Measurements are recommended by the american Societies only during deep sedation[67,68] and in the United Kingdom during all procedures (Klein 2021). Other societies recommend this as a baseline measurement and monitoring during the procedure when active patient warming devices are used.
Electroencephalogram	Monitoring (bispectral index or cerebral oximetry) is controversial. Some studies have demonstrated higher satisfaction among patients and endoscopists. None of the societies have included BIS as a requirement or recommendation during sedation in any patient group. BIS monitoring does not reduce the dose of propofol required but does result in higher satisfaction scores among patients and endoscopists and better titration possibilities. BIS should be considered in high-risk patients or those undergoing planned deep sedation.[72]

aviation, road and rail travel, nuclear power, chemical processing), the field of safety science, human error, and intensive accident investigations have been well developed for several decades.[74,75] The rapidly rising rate of litigation in the 1980s, and increasing interest from the media, brought medical accidents to the attention of doctors and the general public. In parallel with these changes, researchers from several disciplines have developed methods for analyzing accidents of all kinds.[76] Although theories of error and accident causation have evolved and are applicable across many human activities, they have not yet been widely used in medicine.[77] These developments have led to a much broader understanding of accident causation, with less focus on the individual who makes an error and more on preexisting organizational and system underlying factors that provide the context in which errors occur. An essential consequence of this has been the realization that the accident analysis may reveal deep-rooted, unsafe system's features of organizations. Reason's "Swiss cheese" model captures these relationships very well.[78] Understanding and predicting safe sedation performance in ambulatory, emergency department or perioperative room settings requires a detailed knowledge of both the setting and the human factors that influence the performance of the sedation team.

Three universal ingredients of accidents

All human endeavors involve some measures of risk. In many cases, the local hazards are well understood and can be guarded against by various technical or procedural countermeasures. There are three reasons for adverse events during sedation.[79] Regardless of their skills, abilities, and specialist training, all human beings make fallible decisions and commit unsafe acts. This human propensity for committing errors and violating safety procedures during sedation can be moderated by selection, training, well-designed equipment, and good management and oversight. Still, it can never be eliminated.[80] No matter how well designed, constructed, operated, and maintained they might be, all man-made systems possess latent failures to some degree. These unseen failures are analogous to resident pathogens in the human body that combine with local triggering factors (i.e., life stress, toxic chemicals, etc.) to overcome the immune system and produce disease.[81] These three ubiquitous accident ingredients reveal something important about the nature of making care safer. We can mitigate the risk of adverse events during sedation by process improvement, standardization, and an in-depth understanding of the constant safety degrades in systems. Still, we cannot prevent all risks.[82,83]

Each procedure will have unique moments that may require extra attention as they are prone to trigger physiological perturbation, adverse events, or need an abrupt increase in the level of sedation. The gastroscope insertion is very stimulating and may require higher doses of propofol or lidocaine spray, although lidocaine spray itself causes a higher risk of regurgitation. Progression of the endoscope through the esophagus may trigger cardiac arrhythmias like tachycardia and premature ventricular or atrial contractions. Endoscope looping or bowel distension during colonoscopy can be very painful, but pushing the colonoscope with too much force or into the sigmoid and transverse colon is a potent stimulus. Vasovagal episodes are both possible during upper gastrointestinal endoscopy and colonoscopy.

Clinicians administering sedation should be aware of the rescue techniques for each commonly encountered adverse effect like hypoxemia, hypotension, cardiac arrhythmias, and apnea. Transient hypoxemia and hypotension represent the most common problems that occur in 5-10% of patients during endoscopic sedation, [49,51,54,56,84,85] but also bradycardia, tachycardia, arrhythmia, and other cardiopulmonary complications have been reported.[51,54,84,86,87]; The most frequent significant events included laryngospasm[51] and aspiration.[84] Serious cardiovascular complications such as myocardial infarction are rare and occur in less than 0.5% of patients.[86] Respiratory depression and arrest are often related to overmedication, especially in frail, low body weight, and elderly patients.

Patients with a BMI >30 have a higher incidence of hypoxia and upper airway obstruction and require more often airway rescue maneuvers like chin lift and bag mask ventilation.[88,89]

Bellolio et al.[90] performed a systematic review and meta-analysis exploring the incidence of adverse events during procedural sedation in adults. They found an overall incidence per 1000 patients with 95% CI for agitation of 9.8, apnea 12.4, aspiration 1.2, bradycardia 6.5, hypotension 15.2, hypoxia 40.2, intubation 1.6, laryngospasm 4.2, and nausea/vomiting 16.4. Cardiovascular events were the most likely to occur due to propofol or midazolam/opioid sedation, apnea with midazolam or midazolam/opioid sedation, while vomiting mainly occurred when using sedations with ketamine.

Depending on the severity of the adverse event or complication, a patient who experienced minor transient complications such as nausea, faint, and transient oxygen desaturations can be managed in the clinic and discharged home safely on the same day. More moderate complications such as oversedation, allergic reactions, and pronounced changes in vital signs may require a longer recovery period with additional medical oversight but can still be discharged home. Severe complications often require abortion of the procedure, medical intervention, and admission to hospital. Examples of severe complications are aspiration, laryngo- or broncho-spasm, anaphylaxis, etc.

Inadequate sedation level

Despite good preparations and intentions, sedation may become insufficient or too risky. Based on the content of the consent provided, there are few options. Depending on the healthcare professional's scope of practice, the sedation level can be increased to deep sedation or even to general anesthesia, or the level can be decreased to minimal or even without sedation. The use of local anesthetic spray is another option during gastroscopies. If the consent does not mention these options, it is important to cease the procedure, discuss alternative options, obtain consent, and rebook the procedure.

Constant monitoring of the level of consciousness is crucial and may fluctuate during the procedure. Adequate sedation is provided when there is a good tolerance of the procedure, the patient is calm and cooperative, meaningful communication between patient and healthcare professional is possible, and the pain level is acceptable and manageable. If a patient is anxious, agitated, experiences pain, and/or has any signs of hypertension, hypoxia, hypercapnia, and tachycardia, sedation levels may be inadequate. Retroflexion at the rectum during colonoscopy may arouse the patient but a reactionary bolus of a sedative is unnecessary as the remaining part of the procedure should be almost pain free.

Oversedation can be dangerous, and the healthcare professional needs to be able to manage the side effects effectively and bring the patient back to an appropriate level of sedation. Oversedation can be recognized by poor cough, respiratory depression, hypotension and/or bradycardia, gastrointestinal tract paralysis, and immobility.

Cardiovascular complications

Hypotension

Hypotension is often caused by propofol or midazolam/opioid blunting sympathetic response, vasovagal response, or dehydration, especially after prolonged fasting and bowel preparation. Although the hypotension is rarely significant, it can be managed by ceasing or delaying the next propofol bolus, placing the patient in Trendelenburg, or administration of intravenous fluid boluses (crystalloids). If this is insufficient, an alpha-1 receptor agonist vasoconstrictor like metaraminol (0.5−1.0 mg) or ephedrine (3−9 mg) can be administered (every 2−5 min).[73] Ephedrine may be preferred as metaraminol can cause reflex bradycardia. Hypotension can also be the first sign of the more severe complication of anaphylaxis.

Bradycardia

Bradycardia is often a symptom of vasovagal stimulation and can be managed by removing the vasovagal trigger, e.g., stop progressing the colonoscope, and control loops. Administration of atropine 0.4−0.6 mg is advisable if the heat rate gets below 40 bpm or correlates with hypotension. If untreated, it can result in asystole.

Tachycardia

Sinus tachycardia is often a sign of discomfort but can also be a sign of dehydration. The patient's comfort level should be checked, and the level of sedation or analgesia may need to be increased. In case of dehydration, an intravenous bolus of crystalloids may be beneficial. If this is not feasible, consider aborting the procedure.

Pulmonary complications

A major responsibility for clinicians using sedation is quick realization of adequate ventilation and oxygenation by securing the patient's airway. It is paramount that the provider is vigilant and skilled in managing the oversedated patient and avoiding or rectifying airway complications. The deeper the sedation, the more comfortable it will be for the patient. However, that comes at a price as it increases the risk of respiratory complications proportionately.

The upper airway is an extraordinarily complex anatomical region. Both endoscopists and anesthesiologists sometimes must compete for oral access. Anticipating and preparing for difficulty in airway management is crucial to avoiding airway catastrophes and can enhance patient safety by detecting the patient with an increased likelihood of difficult intubation.

Tremendous efforts have been made to reduce adverse events resulting from difficult airway management during gastrointestinal procedures, producing systematic evaluations of the airway in the preprocedural period, the use of airway assessment scores, evidence-based guidelines produced by scientific societies, skill and team training, and the development of technically advanced airway equipment.[91]

Hypoventilation

Hypoventilation often occurs at the beginning of the procedure after induction or after bolus injection of a sedative or opioid and will often resolve when the patient receives a pain stimulus like scope looping or insertion of the colonoscope into the sigmoid and transverse colon. Hypoventilation and hypoxia can be managed by ceasing the administration of the sedative drugs, increasing the oxygen therapy, and maintaining a patent airway. If the patient does not respond adequately to these measures, the endoscopy should be stopped and advanced airway techniques may be necessary or even a medical emergency call may be required.

Apnea can be caused by the sedation drugs that were administered, and one or more airway rescue interventions such as vigorous tactile stimulation and application of positive pressure or ventilation with bag mask may be needed. Other options are the administration of reversal agents such as naloxone in case of an expected opioid overdose and flumazenil in case of an overdose of benzodiazepines. Tracheal intubation should be a last resort option.

Hypoventilation can also be caused by a partial or complete airway obstruction. Partial or incomplete obstruction to air can be recognized by stridor, snoring, chest wall, and suprasternal retraction and can be managed by visual inspection of the patient's airway, repositioning of the airway, manual airway maneuvers, suctioning, and placement of an oro- or nasopharyngeal airway. Other actions may involve manual ventilation of the patient and reversal of the sedative drugs. During a complete upper airway obstruction there is ventilatory effort but with no air exchange. This requires immediate action by repositioning of the airway, suctioning, insertion of oro- or nasopharyngeal airway, positive pressure manual bag mask ventilation, and potentially tracheal intubation with administration of neuromuscular blocking agents.

Laryngospasm

Laryngeal spasm is a prolonged form of vocal cord adduction causing a partial or complete inspiratory airway obstruction. It can be a closure of the true vocal cords alone or the true and false vocal cords. This prolonged intense glottic closure is a response to direct glottic or supraglottic stimulation airway irritation caused by inhaled agents (cold oxygen!), secretions, or the presence of a foreign body. Laryngospasm most often occurs during induction or emergence of anesthesia or moderate-to-deep sedation. Patients classified as ASA III or higher and chronic smokers and patients with upper airway tract infections or with GERD are at higher risk of developing laryngospasm.

Signs of an inspiratory obstruction can range from high-pitched squeaky sounds to total absence of sounds and cannot be relieved by applying routine airway rescue maneuvers. Symptoms of a partial obstruction are suprasternal retraction, use of accessory muscles, intercostal retraction, body movements, engorged neck veins, tracheal tug, paradoxical movement of chest and abdomen, and potential desaturation. The absence of breathing sounds is a sign of a complete airway obstruction causing bradycardia and cyanosis and requires immediate action.

Laryngospasm is an airway crisis, and the initiation of a medical emergency call and preparation for a rescue airway are necessary. The initial stimulus causing the spasms needs to be removed, and 100% oxygen needs to be administered via a non-rebreathing mask or positive pressure ventilation. Airway maneuvers such as jaw trust and the insertion of an oro- or nasopharyngeal airway may be required. Application of Larson's maneuver, applying firm digital pressure between the posterior ramus of the mandible and anterior to the mastoid process, can be helpful as well.[92]

Further steps may involve the administration of anxiolysis or hypnotic, nebulizing lidocaine 2% with 100% oxygen, injection of propofol 0.25−1 mg/kg, lidocaine 2%, and steroids. If the spasm is not resolved, propofol and a neuromuscular blocking agent like succinylcholine or rocuronium with potentially tracheal intubation may be necessary. Be mindful that the laryngospasm can reoccur when the neuromuscular blocking agents wear off.

Bronchospasm

Bronchospasm is a spasm of the bronchial smooth muscles causing a narrowing of the bronchi. It is often caused by mechanical or chemical irritants combined with underlying hyperactivity of the airway, such as upper airway tract infection and smoking. Triggers that may induce bronchospasm are airway irritation, anaphylaxis, aspiration, pulmonary edema, allergies, acute exacerbation of asthma, a misplaced endotracheal tube, or extubation spasm. Signs and symptoms of bronchospasm are expiratory wheezes, rash, increased peak airway pressure, desaturation, increased EtCO$_2$, and 'shark-fin' curve appearance on the capnogram. When suspecting bronchospasm, abort the procedural intervention, apply 100% oxygen, ventilate manually, exclude laryngospasm and aspiration, stop the administration of potential allergy or anaphylaxis triggering suspected drugs, potentially deepen sedation, and perform endotracheal intubation.

Pulmonary aspiration

Pulmonary aspiration is the passive process of oropharyngeal or gastric contents entering the trachea. During sedation, the pharyngeal function is impaired, and the peak pressure in the upper esophageal sphincter is decreased. This will cause a force reduction to propel content during swallowing and may lead to content penetrating the trachea.[93] The aspiration risk is increased in older or obese patients,

patients experiencing impaired swallowing, esophageal strictures or impaired motility, COPD, seizures, immunosuppression, and neurologic diseases (e.g., multiple sclerosis), and patients who receive enteral feeding.[94,95] Park et al.[96] found eight predictors for the occurrence of pulmonary aspiration after gastric endoscopic submucosal resection and developed a risk scoring system (Table 10.13).

Gastric emptying times and residual gastric volume may vary in any patient and can depend on previously mentioned factors. Performing a gastric ultrasound pre-procedure can give a good prediction of the aspiration risks.[97,98] If there is any suspicion of aspiration, the procedure should be stopped, and visual inspection and airway access assessment is required. The appearance of any respiratory signs and symptoms that were not present before sedation may indicate aspiration. Other physical signs may include cough, crackles/rales, wheezing or rhonchi, decreased breath sounds, tachypnea, and/or respiratory distress with a decrease in the patient's oxygen saturation and requirement of supplemental oxygen. Treatment may include endotracheal intubation and bronchoscopy with lavage. Pulmonary aspiration needs to be confirmed with a chest X-ray which will typically show focal infiltrate, consolidation, or atelectasis.

Anaphylaxis

Anaphylaxis is the most severe form of an allergic reaction, is life-threatening, and needs immediate treatment. Anaphylaxis is a serious allergic response that often involves swelling, skin rash, hives, nausea, vomiting, difficulty breathing, unresponsive hypotension or bronchospasm, cardiac arrest (PEA), and shock. If anaphylactic shock is not treated immediately, it can be fatal, e.g., massive swelling of the tongue makes breathing impossible. A major difference between anaphylaxis and other allergic reactions is that anaphylaxis typically involves more than one system of the body. The reaction can occur within seconds or minutes of exposure to an allergen. Symptoms usually start within 5–30 min of encountering an allergen to which an individual is allergic. In some cases, however, it may take more than an hour to notice anaphylactic symptoms. If not treated right away, usually with epinephrine, it can result in unconsciousness or death.

Table 10.13 Aspiration probability and risk prediction.

Variable	Score	Probability	
Age ≥70	4	0–5 points	0.17%
Male	8	6–10 points	0.38%
BMI ≥27 kg/m²	4	11–15 points	0.85%
Procedure time ≥80 min	5	16–20 points	1.86%
Lower third of esophagus	5	21–25 points	4.06%
Tumor size ≥10 mm	3	26–30 points	8.62%
Desaturation during procedure	9	≥31 points	≥17.4%
Recovery time ≥35 min	4		

Rapid diagnosis and response are essential, and many departments have an anaphylaxis emergency box with cognitive aids available for these situations. The treatment of anaphylaxis consists of removal of the trigger, securing the airway and breathing, and applying 100% oxygen. As airway edema may develop quickly, intubate early and resuscitate by using epinephrine, fluids, and elevation of the legs. Once the patient is stabilized, consider the use of steroids and antihistamines, determine tryptase levels at 1, 4, and 24 hours, screen coagulation screen, monitor the patient closely for an extended period, and consider ICU admission. Performing a differential diagnosis may involve the exclusion of e.g., vasovagal responses, flush syndromes, excess histamine production, shock, and acute respiratory syndrome.

Neuromuscular complications

Seizures

Generalized motor seizures can cause sustained (tonic) or repeated (clonic) muscle contractions. The most common triggers are fatigue, stress, stroboscopic lights or chronic use of sedatives, mood-stabilizing or antiepileptic drugs, or excessive amounts of alcohol. Seizures can also be an adverse effect of flumazenil and rapid induction of propofol or benzodiazepines. Seizures most commonly occur during induction or emergence from sedation/anesthesia when the drug concentration of the hypnotic or sedative is relatively low. To confirm an actual seizure, an electroencephalogram may be required. Myoclonic epilepsy is a type of seizure described as shocklike jerks and involuntary, brief contractions of some muscle fibers or muscle or different muscle groups. Hiccups are a form of myoclonus seizures.

Muscle rigidity

Muscle rigidity is an involuntary muscle stiffening in extension and can be associated with shaking. Its most common cause is pain with the muscles unable to relax normally. A more serious but rare cause is the use of ketamine. Muscle rigidity can be treated with the administration of benzodiazepines. When seizures or muscle rigidity occurs, it can interfere with the procedure and cause serious damage to tissues and organs, and the administration of drugs (sedatives) may be required.

Delayed return of consciousness

A delayed return to consciousness is defined as a slower return of consciousness than what normally would be expected considering the amount and time of the last and total dose of sedative and analgesia drugs given during the procedure. This can be caused by metabolic issues such as hypo- or hyperglycemia or hypo- or hypernatremia, serotonin, or anticholinergic syndrome but also by more severe issues like myxedema or functional coma and brainstem stroke.

Risk factors for a delayed return of consciousness are a reduced respiratory central drive (COPD, obstructive sleep apnea, obesity hypoventilation syndrome), neuromuscular disorders (myasthenia gravis, motor neuron disease, muscular dystrophy), mismatch in pulmonary ventilation—perfusion ratios, hepatic and renal failure, or hypothyroidism.

Postprocedural care

Applying standardized criteria to assess recovery status after sedation is needed to facilitate a safe and efficient discharge. Monitoring used during the intervention can be continued during the initial recovery phase. Depth of sedation scales can continue to be applied during this period as well. Serious adverse effects of sedation may occur up to 30 min after administration of certain medications (Table 10.14). Bloating and abdominal pain are common unpleasant side effects after endoscopy and may be relieved by passing wind and early mobilization. Most procedural complications will be visible and managed during the procedure, but sometimes an adverse event may be present within minutes, hours, or even days after the procedure. Although the complication rates after gastrointestinal endoscopic procedures are very low, most frequently observed complications involve bleeding, especially after sphincterotomy, perforation (polypectomy), and pancreatitis after endoscopic retrograde cholangiopancreatography (ERCP) of endoscopic ultrasound (EUS) with fine needle aspiration.[99–101] All adverse events need to be fully disclosed to the patients.[102]

Besides the procedural complications, the recovery after sedation has many similar complications to those in patients recovering from general anesthesia. Shirota[103] found that 1.1% of the patients experience hypoxia ($SpO_2 < 90\%$) during the recovery period after esophagogastroduodenoscopy even among patients without risk factors for hypoxia. Other adverse events may be pain, nausea, vomiting, and dizziness. Clark et al.[104] demonstrated that positioning patients in a sitting position

Table 10.14 Post-sedation complications.

Complication	Symptoms
Esophageal perforation	Retrosternal chest pain, dyspnea, sepsis
Colonic perforation	Persistent and increased abdominal pain, absence of flatus, abdominal distension, and tenderness
Bleeding	Melena, symptomatic anemia, hematemesis, hematochezia, hypovolemic shock
Pancreatitis	Nausea, abdominal pain, increased level of amylase and lipase values

Based on Adler DG. Consent, common adverse events, and post—adverse event actions in endoscopy. Gastrointest Endosc Clin N Am. 2015;25(1):1—8; Parker BK, Manning S. Postprocedural gastrointestinal emergencies. Emerg Med Clin. 2021;39(4):781—794; Yoshida N, Mano Y, Matsuda T, Sano Y, Inoue K, Hirose R, Dohi O, Itoh Y, Goto Y, Sobue T, Y Takeuchi, Nakayama T, Muto M. Complications of colonoscopy in Japan: an analysis using large-scale health insurance claims data. J Gastroenterol Hepatol. 2021;36(10):2745—2753.

facilitated a speedy recovery and discharge compared to patients left in a supine or semisupine position.

Miles et al. [105] introduced the Quality of Recovery score (QoR-40) in 2000 to evaluate the recovery after surgery up to 24 h after the procedure (Table 10.15). In 2013, they published a shorter form, the QoR-15, which can be completed within 2.5 min. The QoR-15 was evaluated among mainly surgical inpatients, but also demonstrated good validity and reliability for ambulant patients.[106] Barber et al. demonstrated the suitability of the QoR-15 among patients recovering from sedation with propofol (21%) or propofol in combination with opioids and/or midazolam (79%). They found a clear improvement over the first 24 hours after the sedation. Unfortunately, they did not differentiate the recovery improvements between patients with monosedation with propofol and propofol in combination with other drugs.[107]

Standardized discharge criteria from the initial recovery phase like the Modified Aldrete score will reduce discharge delays, provide consistency in care, and improve safety.[108–111] The anesthesia department should develop a local discharge policy with measurable criteria suitable for the patient population and interventions performed at that location. Several discharge tools are available to meet the requirements set by the American Joint Commission and meet the Standards set by the American Society of PeriAnesthesia Nurses (ASPAN) Standards (Table 10.16).

It is still common practice that patients are advised not to drive heavy machinery or sign legal documents in the first 24 hours after sedation. Horiuchi, however, demonstrated that 1 hour after propofol sedation, psychomotor skills, including driving skills, has returned to normal.[112,113] Psychomotor skills can adequately be

Table 10.15 Post Sedation Quality of Recovery score (QoR-15).

1. Able to breath easily
2. Been able to enjoy food
3. Feeling rested
4. Have had a good sleep
5. Able to look after personal toilet and hygiene unaided
6. Able to communicate with family or friends
7. Getting support from hospital: doctors and nurses
8. Able to return to work or usual home activities
9. Feeling comfortable and in control
10. Having a feeling of general well-being
11. Moderate pain
12. Severe pain
13. Nausea or vomiting
14. Feeling worried or anxious
15. Feeling sad or depressed

All items are scored on a VAS: None of the time (0) — All the time (10).

Table 10.16 Hospital and Recovery Room Post Sedation Discharge criteria.[108]

	Aldrete	PARSAP	Steward	White	Chung
Oxygenation	X	X		X	
Respiration	X	X	X	X	X
Circulation	X	X			X
Consciousness	X	X	X	X	
Activity	X	X	X	X	X
Pain		X		X	
Nausea/vomiting				X	X
Intake/output		X			X
Feeding		X			
Ambulation		X			
Hemodynamic stability				X	

tested by asking the patient to walk in a straight line, turn, and walk back to the starting position.[104] Whereas Willey[114] demonstrated that patients with a maximum Aldrete score still can have significant psychomotor impairment, they advised incorporating a psychomotor test, e.g., Letter Cancellation test into the discharge criteria. These results demonstrate that to increase patient satisfaction, safety, and comfort; there is a need to review postprocedural instructions and customize them based on the sedation medications used and the outcomes of a psychomotor test.

Applying human factors in the clinical environment

The study of human factors is an integral part of current safety research.[115] Human factors (also called ergonomics) is the study of human interactions with tools, devices, and systems with the goal of enhancing safety, efficiency, and user satisfaction.[116] Human error in medicine can range from medication errors while selecting and loading a medication syringe, programming an infusion pump, or recovering the patient after sedation. Knowledge about how people interact with each other and with technology has been productively applied to enhance human performance in a wide range of domains, from fighter planes to kitchens, to operating rooms to emergency departments. One must carefully consider the impact of the many "performance shaping factors" that are known to play a role in optimizing sedation.[117,118] However, even though most errors can be traced to the action (or inaction) of an individual, the root causes of error always go beyond a single action by one individual.[119]

Factors that influence the sedation microsystem's effectiveness include the performance of individual team members, the equipment they use, the care environment (e.g., established care process and procedures), and the underlying organizational and cultural factors. For example, distracters such as information overload, noise, and key team member absence can be a danger to both patients and healthcare professionals. Patient safety human factors research has expanded to study team interaction and collaborative decision-making,[120] the interaction of humans and technology,[121] the importance of technology,[122] and organizational issues,[123] institutional functions, role of accreditors,[150] and national regulations.

Environment and equipment

Safety procedures, optimal equipment, and safe nondistracting environments are key to high-quality and safe patient care. Emergency equipment to provide advanced life support and rescue patients from obstructed or difficult airway problems should always be readily available and be managed by healthcare professionals properly trained to apply them.

Emergency equipment may include but is not limited to:

—sedation reversal and neuromuscular drugs
—emergency airway equipment, including positive airway bag mask, advanced airway equipment, and "can't intubate can't oxygenate" equipment and devices
—intravenous access and fluids
—suction
—defibrillator

Before the start of each procedural sedation session, a thorough standardized check of the environment needs to take place, and the completion of the check should be documented on a checklist. This should entail checking the availability and adequate functioning of monitoring and emergency equipment, cognitive aids, emergency call alarms, rescue medication, stethoscope, suction, oxygen, and oxygen supply devices.

Oxygen supply devices

Hypoxemia or hypoxic periods with desaturation of the patient is one of the most common and fortunately transient complications during endoscopy. Traditionally, nasal prongs are the oxygen supply device that is used both during gastroscopy and colonoscopy. The aim of any oxygen supply device is to maintain oxygen flow into the airway and decrease the dead space.

High-flow nasal cannulas can provide continuous oxygen flows up to 70 L/min. These devices offer actively heated and humidified oxygen via a nasal cannula and can be used during gastroscopy and colonoscopy. They reduce dead space and can provide a positive end-expiratory pressure effect.[124] This positive pressure creates a flow in the lungs, causing a passive removal of CO_2. Monitoring of SpO_2 and capnography are crucial as patients may stop breathing and accumulate high levels of CO_2 before desaturation appears. Although the device may be more expensive than other oxygen devices, they are very effective in patients with obstructive sleep apnea, morbid obesity, chronic obstructive pulmonary diseases, or prolonged procedures. Some high-flow nasal cannulas sample CO_2 as well. Nay et al. compared high-flow nasal oxygen with conventional nasal oxygen therapy and found that high-flow nasal oxygen showed 20% less incidence of hypoxemia compared to a conventional nasal cannula or when using a nasopharyngeal tube.[125]

Some bite blocks offer the possibility of connecting an oxygen tube with an oxygen outlet on the inside of the bite block. Some of the models even have the possibility to sample CO_2. The maximal flow of these devices is often 10 L/min, and they provide dry cold oxygen directly from the wall or bottle.

For upper endoscopies, procedural facemasks offer the convenience of a simple facemask or non-rebreathing mask with a separate opening for the endoscopy to pass through and a connection for a CO_2 sample line. The masks offer the possibility for intermittent positive pressure ventilation.

Gastro supraglottic airway devices are second-generation supraglottic airway devices where the second channel is extra-large so you can pass an endoscope through. The administration of oxygen is similar to other second-generation cuffed supraglottic airway devices. The insertion of these devices requires deep sedation.

Specially designed nasopharyngeal airway devices can be used to provide jet ventilation (Wei nasal jet tube)[126] or connect to a Mapleson breathing system to decrease the desaturation incidence. Their disadvantage is the high risk of nasal bleedings, and enough lubrication needs to be used to avoid this.[124]

Healthcare team members

Legislation, licensure, the scope of practice, credentialing, etc., must be considered when establishing a procedural sedation team. Training and credentialing requirements for nonanesthetists providing sedation are available in America,[127] Europe (ESGE, ESGENA), and Australia[69] (GESA). Using propofol for sedation by nurses requires extra intense training.[128–130] Healthcare professionals who are competent in rescuing a patient from deep sedation and potential cardiovascular instability and can establish a patent airway and adequate ventilation are essential.

In most countries, minimal and moderate sedation with, for instance, benzodiazepines and opioids can be provided by any medical officer who is trained and deemed competent in providing this level of sedation. In some countries, this is also the case for specifically trained nurses or nurse practitioners.

The administration of propofol by nurses is allowed in Europe and Asia, but in other countries, this is restricted to anesthesiologists and specifically trained nonanesthesiologists. However, there is an overwhelming amount of evidence that specifically trained nurses can safely administer propofol used for sedation with direct or indirect supervision of a medical officer.[55,86,87,131]

The nonanesthetist-administered propofol (NAAP) model describes the administration of propofol by a nurse under the direction of a nonanesthesiologist physician.[132] Monitored anesthesia care (MAC) involves moderate-to-deep sedation without airway reflexes or even general anesthesia and is provided by an anesthesia-trained professional. A level of moderate-to-deep sedation is targeted, and propofol can be administered as a single agent (nurse-administered propofol sedation, NAPS) or in combination with other agents as BPS.[66,145] NAPS and BPS are also referred to as endoscopist-directed propofol (EDP) or endoscopist-directed, nurses-administered propofol sedation (EDNAPS).[131]

Several large studies have demonstrated similar complication rates between non-anesthesia propofol sedation providers and anesthesia providers for ASA I–II adult patients with a BMI lower than 35 undergoing diagnostic or low-complex interventional, nonemergency gastrointestinal interventions that take less than 1 hour.[9,51,85–87,131,133,134] Both 30-day mortality rate and mortality rate after complications (failure-to-rescue) were lower when anesthesiologists directed anesthesia care as opposed to nurse providers in patients with ASA III levels and higher[144].

Teamwork, culture, and communication

Engineering a culture of safety

National cultures arise largely from shared norms and values; an organizational culture is shaped mainly by shared practices. How do we create an optimal organizational climate that fosters safe sedation outcomes? Culture can be defined as the collection of individual and group values, attitudes, and practices that guide the behavior of group members.[135] Acquiring a safety and resilience culture is a process of collective learning that recognizes the inevitability of error and proactively seeks to identify latent threats. Characteristics of a strong safety and resilient culture includes a commitment of the leadership to discuss and learn from errors, communications founded on mutual trust and respect, shared perceptions of the importance of safety, encouraging and practicing teamwork, and incorporating nonpunitive systems for reporting and analyzing near-miss and adverse events.[136]

Acquiring a safety culture is a process of collective learning and trust building. When the usual reaction to an adverse incident is "Write another procedure" and "more training," this does not make the system more resistant to future organizational accidents. Still, it may deflect the blame from the organization as a whole. There is a long tradition in medicine of examining past practices to understand how things might have been done differently. However, morbidity and mortality conferences, grand rounds, and peer reviews often share many of the same shortcomings[137]:

- lack of human factors and systems thinking;
- a narrow focus on individual performance, excluding analysis of contributory team factors and larger social issues;
- retrospective bias;
- a tendency to search for errors as opposed to the myriad causes of error induction; and
- lack of multidisciplinary integration into organization-wide safety culture, thus perpetuating a "code of silence."

Safe sedation requires coordinated and introspective teamwork. If clinicians deliver sedation are not empowered by managerial leadership to be honest and reflective on their practice, rules and regulations will have a limited impact on enabling safer outcomes. Healthcare administrators need to understand the fundamental dynamics that lead to adverse events. Event Analyses tools such as root cause analysis (RCA) and FMEA can help clinicians and others better understand how adverse events occur and design resilience into the system.[138]

The role of effective teamwork in repeatedly accomplishing complex tasks safely is well accepted in many domains.[139] Teamwork during sedation care can be characterized in several different ways, and multiple deficiencies may interact to impair team success and patient outcomes.[140] The team evaluation must include the review of the secondary management, including careful delineation of team structure, ongoing team training, effective support structures, and continuous quality improvement based on practice and immersive learning opportunities. Valuable tools for training the sedation team include using simulation, standardized patients, and videotape-based analysis and debrief.

Sedation teams seem to make fewer mistakes than individuals, especially when each team member knows his or her responsibilities, as well as that of the other team members. However, simply bringing individuals together to perform sedation on a child task does not automatically ensure that they will function as a team. A safe sedation team depends on the willingness of clinicians from diverse backgrounds to cooperate toward a shared goal, communicate, work together effectively, and improve.[141] Each team member must be able to: (1) anticipate the needs of the others; (2) adjust to each other's actions and to the changing environment; (3) monitor each other's activities and distribute workload dynamically; and (4) have a shared understanding of accepted processes, and how events and actions should proceed.

Turning physician and nurse experts into an expert sedation team requires substantial planning and practice around explicit teamness competencies.[142] For example, conducting a "time-out" immediately before starting the procedure as described in the Universal Protocol with fail-safe preoperative verification of the correct patient, procedure, site, and implant.[143] This requires active discussion among all members of the sedation/procedure team, consistently initiated by a designated member of the team; that is, the procedure is not started until all questions or concerns are resolved.

During sedation, patient complications are possible. Effective communication within the team is paramount to managing the patient in a timely and efficient manner. It is always a two-way process, and team members should feel empowered to question, assert, and speak up when concerns are identified. The environment can also play a role in communication failures, e.g., noise. Different strategies can be used to increase effective communication. Closed-loop communication will limit misinterpretations as the receiver of the message interprets the message, then acknowledges its receipt, and communicates it back to the sender. The sender then confirms that the intended message is received, and the receiver reports back when the message has been actioned.

Example of closed-loop communication:

- *Sender: "Leanne, give 1 mg adrenaline IV followed by a 20 mL normal saline push bolus."*
- *Receiver: "OK, Gerald, I am going to give 1 mg adrenaline IV followed by a 20 mL normal saline push bolus."*
- *Sender: "That's correct, Leanne."*
- *Receiver: "Gerald, 1 mg adrenaline IV with a 20 mL normal saline flush has been given."*

Team crisis communication

Team crisis communication requires a good understanding of situational awareness and is a key nontechnical skill for effective crisis management. The message must be sent to somebody specific by using their name and must be explicit (what, when, who, how) and needs to clearly state the required actions. Before you send a message, think about whether this is the right time to communicate this now, and do not interrupt other key activities unnecessarily unless it is important to the situation and truly urgent.

One can facilitate the "teamwork" process by:

- fostering a shared awareness of each member's tasks and role on the team through cross-training and other team training modalities;
- Training members in specific teamwork skills such as communication, situation awareness, leadership, followership, resource allocation, and adaptability;
- Conducting team training in simulated scenarios with a focus on both team behaviors and technical skills;
- Training anesthesia team leaders in the necessary leadership competencies to build and maintain effective teams; and
- Establishing and consistently utilizing reliable methods of team performance evaluation and rapid feedback.

Graded assertiveness allows team members to avoid conflict or triggering defensiveness and allows escalation if required. It also gives the other team members a chance to correct any mistakes or misunderstandings and to save face. Different methods can be used for graded assertiveness, e.g., CUSS approach (concern − unsure - safety − stop), PACE approach (probe - alert - challenge − emergency), or the 5-step advocacy (getting attention - state concern - state the problem as you see it - state a solution - obtain an agreement).

Example using the PACE approach:

- *Situation: airway event during endoscopy. The endoscopist administered the initial sedation dose, and the sedation nurse noticed an airway apnea.*
- *Sedation nurse **probes**: 'Is the chest rising?'*
- *The sedation nurse **alerts**, speaking louder and using the endoscopist's name: 'Andrew, I cannot see the chest rising.'*

- *Sedation nurse **challenges**: Andrew, the chest is not rising, and the saturations are not improving. I am concerned and do not think this is working. Can you remove the scope so I can take over and access the airway?'*
- *Sedation nurse calls the **emergency**: Andrew, the chest is not rising, the saturations are not growing. I will put out an emergency 666 call for the MET team.'*

Example of 5-step advocacy:

- *Getting attention: "Excuse me, Doctor."*
- *State your concern: "The patient is hypotensive."*
- *State the problem as you see it: "I think we need to get help now."*
- *State a solution: "I'll phone ICU to arrange the transfer."*
- *Obtain an agreement: "Does that sound good to you?"*

Documentation

Complete documentation is vital for several reasons. Firstly, it is an essential communication tool for healthcare providers involved in the patient's care to share their planning, monitoring, and management of the patient's progress. Secondly, documentation decreases potential misdiagnosis or harm to the patient. Complete, clear, and concise documentation is also beneficial for reviews required for improvement and quality management, education, revenue processes, or liability issues.

Documentation should include but is not limited to:

- Preprocedural assessment including ASA score, BMI, medical history, allergies, medication
- Telehealth and phone call notes
- Multidisciplinary team meetings, time-out procedures
- Vital signs assessed during all periprocedural phases
- Drugs (name, dosage), IV fluids (type, quantity), cannulation side
- Oxygen therapy (type and flow) administered
- Sedation-associated complications and their management
- Completed checklists
- Fulfillment of discharge criteria
- Discharge instructions for the patient
- Names and roles of staff members attending the procedure

References

1. Barach P, Johnson J. Safety by Design: understanding the dynamic complexity of redesigning care around the clinical microsystem. *Qual Saf Health Care* 2006;**15**(Suppl. 1): i10−6.
2. Mohr J, Batalden P, Barach P. Integrating patient safety into the clinical microsystem. *Qual Saf Health Care* 2004;**13**:34−8.

3. Barach P, Small DS. Reporting and preventing medical mishaps: lessons from non-medical near miss reporting systems. *Br Med J* 2000;**320**:753–63.

4. Bagian JP, Paull DE. Handovers during anesthesia care: patient safety risk or opportunity for improvement? *JAMA* 2018;**319**(2):125–7. https://doi.org/10.1001/jama.2017.20602.

5. Vaessen HH, Knape JT. Considerable variability of procedural sedation and analgesia practices for gastrointestinal endoscopic procedures in Europe. *Clin Endosc* 2016;**49**(1):47–55. https://doi.org/10.5946/ce.2016.49.1.47.

6. Wahid A, Manek N, Nichols M, Kelly P, Foster C, Webster P, Kaur A, Friedemann-Smith C, Wilkins E, Rayner M, Roberts N, Scarborough P. Quantifying the association between physical activity and cardiovascular disease and diabetes: a systematic review and meta-analysis. *J Am Heart Assoc* 2016;**5**(9):e0024959. https://doi.org/10.1161/JAHA.115.002495. PMC 5079002. PMID 27628572.

7. Lee TH, Marcantonio ER, Mangione CM, Thomas EJ, Polanczyk CA, Cook EF, Sugarbaker DJ, Donaldson MC, Poss R, Ho KKL, Ludwig LE, Pedan A, Goldman L. Derivation and prospective validation of a simple index for prediction of cardiac risk of major noncardiac surgery. *Circulation* 1999;**100**(10):1043–9.

8. Doyle DJ, Goyal A, Garmon EH. American society of anesthesiologists classification. October 9, 2021. In: StatPearls [internet]. Treasure Island (FL): StatPearls Publishing; PMID: 28722969. Available from: https://www.ncbi.nlm.nih.gov/books/NBK441940/.

9. Akbulut UE, Saylan S, Sengu B, Akcali GE, Erturk E, Cakir M. A comparison of sedation with midazolam–ketamine versus propofol–fentanyl during endoscopy in children: a randomized trial. *Eur J Gastroenterol Hepatol* 2017;**29**:112.

10. American Society of Anesthesiologists (ASA). Standards for basic anesthetic monitoring. December 13, 2020. https://www.asahq.org/standards-and-guidelines/standards-for-basic-anesthetic-monitoring.

11. Australian and New Zealand College of Anaesthetists (ANZCA). *Guideline on pre-anaesthesia consultation and patient preparation, PG07.* 2021. Available at: https://www.anzca.edu.au/getattachment/d2c8053c-7e76-410e-93ce-3f9a56ffd881/PS07-Guideline-on-pre-anaesthesia-consultation-and-patient-preparation. [Accessed 8 September 2021].

12. Association of Anaesthetists of Great Britain and Ireland. Pre-operative assessment and patient preparation - the role of the anaesthetist. Available at: https://anaesthetists.org/Home/Resources-publications/Guidelines/Pre-operative-assessment-and-patient-preparation-the-role-of-the-anaesthetist-2 (Accessed on October 8, 2021).

13. Smith I, Kranke P, Murat I, Smith A, O'Sullivan G, Søreide E, Spies C, In't Veld B, European Society of Anaesthesiology. Perioperative fasting in adults and children: guidelines from the European Society of Anaesthesiology. *Eur J Anaesthesiol* 2011;**28**:556.

14. Søreide E, Eriksson LI, Hirlekar G, Eriksson H, Henneberg SW, Sandin R, Raeder J. (Task force on Scandinavian Pre-operative Fasting Guidelines, Clinical Practice Committee Scandinavian Society of Anaesthesiology and Intensive Care Medicine). Pre-operative fasting guidelines: an update. *Acta Anaesthesiol Scand* 2005;**49**:1041.

15. Verbandsmitteilung DGAI. Praeoperatives Nuechternheitsgebot bei elektiven Eingriffen. *Anaesthesiol Intensivmed* 2004;**12**:722.

16. American Society of Anesthesiologists (ASA). Practice guidelines for preoperative fasting and the use of pharmacologic agents to reduce the risk of pulmonary aspiration: application to healthy patients undergoing elective procedures: an updated report by the American Society of Anesthesiologists task force on preoperative fasting and the

use of pharmacologic agents to reduce the risk of pulmonary aspiration. *Anesthesiology* 2017;**126**:376.

17. Dobson G, Chow L, Filteau L, et al. Guidelines to the practice of anesthesia - revised edition 2020. *Can J Anaesth* 2020;**67**:64.

18. Rosen D, Gamble J, Matava C, Canadian Pediatric Anesthesia Society Fasting Guidelines Working Group. Canadian Pediatric Anesthesia Society statement on clear fluid fasting for elective pediatric anesthesia. *Can J Anaesth* 2019;**66**:991.

19. Amornyotin S, Kongphlay S. Complication rate of propofol-based deep sedation for colonoscopy in marked obesity patients. *J Gastroenterol Hepatol Res* 2015;**4**(8). Available from: http://www.ghrnet.org/index.php/joghr/article/view/1285/1474.

20. Bray R, Knapp H. Identifying predictors of airway complications during conscious sedation procedures. *Gastroenterol Nurs* 2021;**44**(5):310−9. https://doi.org/10.1097/SGA.0000000000000574. PMID: 34319934.

21. Faramarzi E, Soleimanpour H, Khan ZH, Mahmoodpoor A, Sanaie S. Upper lip bite test for prediction of difficult airway: a systematic review. *Pakistan J Med Sci* 2018;**34**(4):1019−23. https://doi.org/10.12669/pjms.344.15364.

22. Flores KS, Choi JA, Johnson KN, Vaneenenaam Jr DP, Harris HM, Forest DJ, Bryan YF. Airway complications during gastrointestinal endoscopies using propofol in a rural hospital. *Anaesth Pain Intensive Care* 2020;**24**:40−425.

23. Harjai M, Alam S, Bhaskar P. Clinical relevance of mallampati grading in predicting difficult intubation in the era of various new clinical predictors. *Cureus* July 14, 2021;**13**(7):e16396. https://doi.org/10.7759/cureus.16396.

24. Honarmand A, Safavi M, Yaraghi A, Attari M, Khazaei M, Zamani M. Comparison of five methods in predicting difficult laryngoscopy: neck circumference, neck circumference to thyromental distance ratio, the ratio of height to thyromental distance, upper lip bite test and Mallampati test. *Adv Biomed Res* June 4, 2015;**4**:122. https://doi.org/10.4103/2277-9175.158033. PMID: 26261824; PMCID: PMC4513312.

25. Hrishi AP, Prathapadas U, Praveen R, Vimala S, Sethuraman M. A comparative study to evaluate the efficacy of virtual versus direct airway assessment in the preoperative period in patients presenting for neurosurgery: a quest for safer preoperative practice in neuroanesthesia in the backdrop of the COVID-19 pandemic. *J Neurosci Rural Pract* September 28, 2021;**12**(4):718−25. https://doi.org/10.1055/s-0041-1735824. PMID: 34737506; PMCID: PMC8558970.

26. Kang SH, Hyun JJ. Preparation and patient evaluation for safe gastrointestinal endoscopy. *Clin Endosc* May 2013;**46**(3):212−8. https://doi.org/10.5946/ce.2013.46.3.212. Epub 2013 May 31. PMID: 23767028; PMCID: PMC3678055.

27. Kopanaki E, Piagkou M, Demesticha T, Anastassiou E, Skandalakis P. Sternomental distance ratio as a predictor of difficult laryngoscopy: a prospective, double-blind pilot study. *Anesth Essays Res* 2020;**14**:49−55. https://www.aeronline.org/text.asp?2020/14/1/49/280461.

28. Payne E, Ragheb J, Jewell ES, Huang BP, Bailey AM, Fritsch LM, Engoren M. Are physician assistant and patient airway assessments reliable compared to anesthesiologist assessments in detecting difficult airways in general surgical patients? *Perioperat Med* November 22, 2017;**6**:20. https://doi.org/10.1186/s13741-017-0077-0. PMID: 29201360; PMCID: PMC5700753.

29. Shobha D, Adiga M, Rani DD, Kannan S, Nethra SS. Comparison of upper lip bite test and ratio of height to thyromental distance with other airway assessment tests for predicting difficult endotracheal intubation. *Anesth Essays Res* January−March 2018;

12(1):124−9. https://doi.org/10.4103/aer.AER_195_17. PMID: 29628567; PMCID: PMC5872848.

30. Torino A, Martino DD, Fusco P, Collina U, Marullo L, Ferraro F. Hot topics in airway management during gastrointestinal endoscopy. *J Gastrointest Dig Syst* 2016;**6**:377. https://doi.org/10.4172/2161-069X.1000377.

31. Workeneh SA, Gebregzi AH, Denu ZA. Magnitude and predisposing factors of difficult airway during induction of general anaesthesia. *Anesthesiol Res Pract* 2017;**2017**: 5836397. https://doi.org/10.1155/2017/5836397. Epub 2017 Jul 11. PMID: 28781593; PMCID: PMC5525083.

32. Hirmanpour A, Safavi M, Honarmand A, Jabalameli M, Banisadr G. The predictive value of the ratio of neck circumference to thyromental distance in comparison with four predictive tests for difficult laryngoscopy in obstetric patients scheduled for caesarean delivery. *Adv Biomed Res* September 30, 2014;**3**:200. https://doi.org/ 10.4103/2277-9175.142045. PMID: 25337530; PMCID: PMC4202503.

33. Vidhya S, Sharma B, Swain BP, Singh UK. Comparison of sensitivity, specificity, and accuracy of Wilson's score and intubation prediction score for prediction of difficult airway in an eastern Indian population-A prospective single-blind study. *J Fam Med Prim Care* March 26, 2020;**9**(3):1436−41. https://doi.org/10.4103/ jfmpc.jfmpc_1068_19. PMID: 32509629; PMCID: PMC7266177.

34. Alessandri F, Antenucci G, Piervincenzi E, Buonopane C, Bellucci R, Andreoli C, Alunni FD, Ranieri MV, Bilotta F. Ultrasound as a new tool in the assessment of airway difficulties. *Eur J Anaesthesiol* 2019;**36**(7):509−15. https://doi.org/10.1097/ EJA.0000000000000989.

35. Abraham S, Himarani J, Mary Nancy S, Shanmugasundaram S, Krishnakumar Raja VB. Ultrasound as an assessment method in predicting difficult intubation: a prospective clinical study. *J Maxillofac Oral Surg* 2018;**17**(4):563−9. https://doi.org/10.1007/ s12663-018-1088-1.

36. Lundstrøm LH, Rosenstock CV, Wetterslev J, Nørskov AK. The DIFFMASK score for predicting difficult facemask ventilation: a cohort study of 46,804 patients. *Anaesthesia* October 2019;**74**(10):1267−76. https://doi.org/10.1111/anae.14701. Epub 2019 May 20. PMID: 31106851.

37. Nørskov AK, Rosenstock CV, Wetterslev J, Astrup G, Afshari A, Lundstrøm LH. Diagnostic accuracy of anaesthesiologists' prediction of difficult airway management in daily clinical practice: a cohort study of 188 064 patients registered in the Danish Anaesthesia Database. *Anaesthesia* March 2015;**70**(3):272−81. https://doi.org/ 10.1111/anae.12955. Epub 2014 Dec 16. PMID: 25511370.

38. Nørskov AK, Wetterslev J, Rosenstock CV, Afshari A, Astrup G, Jakobsen JC, Thomsen JL, Lundstrøm LH, Collaborators. Prediction of difficult mask ventilation using a systematic assessment of risk factors vs. existing practice - a cluster randomised clinical trial in 94,006 patients. *Anaesthesia* March 2017;**72**(3):296−308. https:// doi.org/10.1111/anae.13701. Epub 2016 Nov 24. PMID: 27882541.

39. Danish Anaesthesia Database Rosenstock CV, Nørskov AK, Wetterslev J, Lundstrøm LH. Emergency surgical airway management in Denmark: a cohort study of 452 461 patients registered in the Danish Anaesthesia Database. *Br J Anaesth* September 2016;**117**(Suppl. 1):i75−82. https://doi.org/10.1093/bja/aew190. Epub 2016 Jul 28. PMID: 27468737.

40. Hinkelbein J, Lamperti M, Akeson J, Santos J, Costa J, De Robertis E, Longrois D, Novak-Jankovic V, Petrini F, Struys MMRF, Veyckemans F, Fuchs-Buder T,

Fitzgerald R. European Society of Anaesthesiology and European Board of Anaesthesiology guidelines for procedural sedation and analgesia in adults. *Eur J Anaesthesiol* January 2018;**35**(1):6–24. https://doi.org/10.1097/EJA.0000000000000683. PMID: 28877145.

41. Leffler DA, Bukoye B, Sawhney M, Berzin T, Sands K, Chowdary S, Shah A, Barnett S. Development and validation of the PROcedural Sedation Assessment Survey (PRO-SAS) for assessment of procedural sedation quality. *Gastrointest Endosc* January 2015;**81**(1):194–203.e1. https://doi.org/10.1016/j.gie.2014.07.062. Epub 2014 Oct 5. PMID: 25293829; PMCID: PMC4272880.

42. Dexter F, Aker J, Wright WA. Development of a measure of patient satisfaction with monitored anesthesia care: the Iowa Satisfaction with Anesthesia Scale. *Anesthesiology* 1997;**87**(4):865–73.

43. Simopoulos T, Leffler D, Barnett S, Campbell D, Lian SJ, Gill JS. Prospective assessment of pain and comfort in chronic pain patients undergoing interventional pain management procedures. *Pain Med* 2018;**19**(2):336–47. https://doi.org/10.1093/pm/pnx064.

44. Kilpatrick GJ. Remimazolam: non-clinical and clinical profile of a new sedative/anesthetic agent. *Front Pharmacol* July 20, 2021. https://doi.org/10.3389/fphar.2021.690875.

45. Goudra BG, Singh PM. Remimazolam: the future of its sedative potential. *Saudi J Anaesth* July 2014;**8**(3):388–91. https://doi.org/10.4103/1658-354X.136627. PMID: 25191193; PMCID: PMC4141391.

46. Zhang X, Li S, Liu J. Efficacy and safety of remimazolam besylate versus propofol during hysteroscopy: single-centre randomized controlled trial. *BMC Anesthesiol* 2021;**21**: 156. https://doi.org/10.1186/s12871-021-01373-y.

47. Riphaus A, Gstettenbauer T, Frenz MB, et al. Quality of psychomotor recovery after propofol sedation for routine endoscopy: a randomized and controlled study. *Endoscopy* 2006;**38**:677–83.

48. Vargo JJ, Bramley T, Meyer K, Nightengale B. Practice efficiency and economics. *J Clin Gastroenterol* 2007;**41**(6):591–8. https://doi.org/10.1097/01.mcg.0000225634.52780.0e.

49. Wadhwa V, Issa D, Garg S, Lopez R, Sanaka MR, Vargo JJ. Similar risk of cardiopulmonary adverse events between propofol and traditional anesthesia for gastrointestinal endoscopy: a systematic review and meta-analysis. *Clin Gastroenterol Hepatol* 2017; **15**:194–206.

50. Fabbri LP, Nucera M, Marsili M, Al Malyan M, Becchi C. Ketamine, propofol and low dose remifentanil versus propofol and remifentanil for ERCP outside the operating room: is ketamine not only a "rescue drug"? *Med Sci Mon Int Med J Exp Clin Res* September 2012;**18**(9):CR575–C580. https://doi.org/10.12659/msm.883354. PMID: 22936194; PMCID: PMC3560648.

51. Sieg A, Beck S, Scholl SG, Heil FJ, Gotthardt DN, Stremmel W, Rex DK, Friedrich K. Safety analysis of endoscopist-directed propofol sedation: a prospective, national multicenter study of 24 441 patients in German outpatient practices. *J Gastroenterol Hepatol* 2014;**29**:517–23. https://doi.org/10.1111/jgh.12458.

52. Nishizawa T, Suzuki H, Hosoe N, Ogata H, Kanai T, Yahagi N. Dexmedetomidine vs propofol for gastrointestinal endoscopy: a meta-analysis. *United Eur Gastroenterol J* 2017;**5**(7):1037–45. https://doi.org/10.1177/2050640616688140.

53. Horiuchi A, Nakayama Y, Hidaka N, et al. Low-dose propofol sedation for diagnostic esophagogastroduodenoscopy: results in 10,662 adults. *Am J Gastroenterol* 2009;**104**: 1650−5.

54. Poinclouxa L, Laquièrea A, Bazina J, Monzya F, Artiguesa F, Bonnya C, Abergela A, Dapoignya M, Bommelaer G. A randomized controlled trial of endoscopist vs. anaesthetist-administered sedation for colonoscopy. *Dig Liver Dis* 2011;**43**:553−8.

55. Rex DK. Endoscopist-directed propofol. *Gastrointest Endoscopy Clin N Am* 2016;**26**: 485−92. https://doi.org/10.1016/j.giec.2016.02.010.

56. Jensen JT, Hornslet P, Konge L, Møller AM, Vilmann P. High efficacy with deep nurse-administered propofol sedation for advanced gastroenterologic endoscopic procedures. *Endosc Int Open* 2016;**04**:E107−11. https://doi.org/10.1055/s-0041-107899.

57. Amornyotin S. Sedation and monitoring for gastrointestinal endoscopy. *World J Gastrointest Endosc* February 16, 2013;**5**(2):47−55. https://doi.org/10.4253/wjge.v5.i2.47.

58. Samson S, George SK, Vinoth B, Khan MS, Akila B. Comparison of dexmedetomidine, midazolam, and propofol as an optimal sedative for upper gastrointestinal endoscopy: a randomized controlled trial. *J Dig Endosc* 2014;**05**(02):051−7.

59. Kim JH, Byun S, Choi YJ, Kwon HJ, Jung K, Kim SE, Park MI, Moon W, Park SJ. Efficacy and safety of etomidate in comparison with propofol or midazolam as sedative for upper gastrointestinal endoscopy. *Clin Endosc* September 2020;**53**(5):555−61. https://doi.org/10.5946/ce.2019.210. Epub 2020 Mar 31. PMID: 32229801; PMCID: PMC7548146.

60. Yin S, Hong J, Sha T, Chen Z, Guo Y, Li C, Liu Y. Efficacy and tolerability of sufentanil, dexmedetomidine, or ketamine added to propofol-based sedation for gastrointestinal endoscopy in elderly patients: a prospective, randomized, controlled trial. *Clin Therapeut* 2019;**41**(9):1864−77.

61. Oussalah A, Julien M, Levy J, Hajjar FC, Stephan C, Laugel E, Wandzel M, Filhine-Tresarrieu P, Green R, Guéant JL. Global burden related to nitrous oxide exposure in medical and recreational settings: a systematic review and individual patient data meta-analysis. *J Clin Med* April 23, 2019;**8**(4):551. https://doi.org/10.3390/jcm8040551.

62. Nguyen NQ, Toscano L, Lawrence M, Moore J, Holloway RH, Bartholomeusz D, Lidums I, Tam W, Roberts, Thomson IC, Mahesh VN, Debreceni TL, Schoeman MN. Patient-controlled analgesia with inhaled methoxyflurane versus conventional endoscopist-provided sedation for colonoscopy: a randomized multicenter trial. *Gastrointest Endosc* 2013;**78**(6):892−901.

63. Nguyen NQ, Toscano L, Lawrence M, Phan VA, Singh R, Bampton P, Fraser RJ, Holloway RH, Schoeman MN. Portable inhaled methoxyflurane is feasible and safe for colonoscopy in subjects with morbid obesity and/or obstructive sleep apnea. *Endosc Int Open* 2015;**3**:E487−93.

64. Jephcott XC, Grummet J, Nguyen N, Spruyt O. A review of the safety and efficacy of inhaled methoxyflurane as an analgesic for outpatient procedures. *Br J Anaesth* 2018; **120**(5):1040−8.

65. Nguyen NQ, Burgess J, Debreceni TL, Toscano L. Psychomotor and cognitive effects of 15-minute inhalation of methoxyflurane in healthy volunteers: implication for post-colonoscopy care. *Endosc Int Open* 2016;**4**:E1171−7.

66. American Society of Gastrointestinal Endoscopy (ASGE). Guidelines for sedation and anesthesia in GI endoscopy. *Gastrointest Endosc* 2018;**87**(2):327−37.

67. American Society of Anesthesiologists (ASA). Committee on economics. Position on monitored anesthesia care. October 17, 2018. https://www.asahq.org/standards-and-guidelines/position-on-monitored-anesthesia-care.

68. American Society of Anesthesiologists (ASA). Practice guidelines for moderate procedural sedation and analgesia 2018: a report by the American society of anesthesiologists task force on moderate procedural sedation and analgesia, the American Association of Oral and Maxillofacial Surgeons, American College of Radiology, American Dental Association, American Society of Dentist Anesthesiologists, and Society of Interventional Radiology. *Anesthesiology* 2018;**128**:437−79. https://doi.org/10.1097/ALN.0000000000002043.

69. Australian and New Zealand College of Anaesthetists (ANZCA). Guidelines on sedation and/or analgesia for diagnostic and interventional medical, dental or surgical procedures. July 2014. Available from: https://www.anzca.edu.au/getattachment/c64aef58-e188-494a-b471-3c07b7149f0c/PS09-Guideline-on-sedation-and-or-analgesia-for-diagnostic-and-interventional-medical,-dental-or-surgical-procedures#page=.

70. Australian and New Zealand College of Anaesthetists (ANZCA). *Guideline on monitoring during anaesthesia, PG18*. 2017. Available at: https://www.anzca.edu.au/getattachment/0c2d9717-fa82-4507-a3d6-3533d8fa844d/PG18(A)-Guideline-on-monitoring-during-anaesthesia.pdf.

71. European Society of Gastroenterology and Endoscopy Nurses and Associates (ESGENA). Core curriculum for endoscopy nursing. ESGENA education working group (EEWG) planning group. September 2008. https://esgena.org/sitedata/wp-content/uploads/2018/09/esgena_st_core_curriculum_2008.pdf.

72. Lee TH, Lee CK. Endoscopic sedation: from training to performance. *Clin Endosc* 2014;**47**:141−50. https://doi.org/10.5946/ce.2014.47.2.141.

73. Sathananthan D, Young E, Nind G, George B, Ashby A, Drummond A, Redel K, Green N, Singh R. Assessing the safety of physician-directed nurse-administered propofol sedation in low-risk patients undergoing endoscopy and colonoscopy. *Endosc Int Open* 2017;**05**:EE110−5. https://doi.org/10.1055/s-0042-121667.

74. Rasmussen J. The role of error in organizing behavior. *Ergonomics* 1990;**33**:1185−99.

75. Sagan SD. *The limits of safety: organizations, accidents, and nuclear weapons*. Princeton, NJ: Princeton University Press; 1994.

76. Turner BA, Pidgeon NF. *Man-made disasters*. London: Butterworth and Heinemann; 1997.

77. Reason J. *Managing the risks of organizational accidents*. Aldershot, UK: Ashgate; 1997.

78. Reason J. *Human errors*. New York: Cambridge University Press; 1990.

79. Leape LL, Brennan TA, Laird N, et al. Incidence of adverse events and negligence in hospitalized patients: results of the Harvard Medical Practice Study. *N Engl J Med* 1991;**324**:370−6.

80. Committee on Quality of Health Care in America, Institute of Medicine. *To err is human: building a safer health system*. Washington, DC: National Academy Press; 1999.

81. Baker SP, O'Neill B, Ginsburg M, Guohua L. *The injury fact book*. 2nd ed. New York: Oxford University Press; 1992.

82. Bernstein P. *Against the gods; the remarkable story of risk*. John & Wiley Sons; 1996.

83. Perrow C. *Normal accidents: living with high-risk technologies*. NY: Basic Books; 1984.

84. Kozarek R. Are gastrointestinal endoscopic procedures performed by anesthesiologists safer than when sedation is given by the endoscopist? *Clin Gastroenterol Hepatol* 2020; **18**:1935−8.

85. Nishizawa T, Suzuki H. Propofol for gastrointestinal endoscopy. *United European Gastroenterology Journal* 2018;**6**(6):801−5. https://doi.org/10.1177/2050640618767 594.

86. Behrens A, Kreuzmayr A, Manner H, et al. Acute sedation-associated complications in GI endoscopy (ProSed 2 Study): results from the prospective multicentre electronic registry of sedation-associated complications. *Gut* 2019;**68**(3):445−52.

87. Leslie K, Allen ML, Hessian EC, Peyton PJ, Kasza J, Courtney A, Dhar PA, Briedis J, Lee S, Beeton AR, Sayakkarage D, Palanivel S, Taylor JK, Haughton AJ, O'Kane CX. Safety of sedation for gastrointestinal endoscopy in a group of university-affiliated hospitals: a prospective cohort study. *Br J Anaesth* January 2017;**118**(1):90−9. https://doi.org/10.1093/bja/aew393. PMID: 28039246.

88. Amornyotin S. Registered nurse-administered sedation for gastrointestinal endoscopic procedure. *World J Gastrointest Endosc* July 10, 2015;**7**(8):769−76. https://doi.org/10.4253/wjge.v7.i8.769. PMID: 26191341; PMCID: PMC4501967.

89. Flores A, Achécar-Justo LM, Del Río-Izquierdo M, Blázquez-Gómez I, Perez J, González-Pino A, Pichiule M, Van Domselaar M. Tu1082 Impact of obesity on the frequency of sedation-related complications endoscopist-directed. *Gastrointestinal* 2018; **87**(6). https://doi.org/10.1016/j.gie.2018.04.2142. SUPPLEMENT:AB525.

90. Bellolio MF, Gilani WI, Barrionuevo P, Murad MH, Erwin PJ, Anderson JR, Miner JR, Hess EP. Incidence of adverse events in adults undergoing procedural sedation in the emergency department: a systematic review and meta-analysis. *Acad Emerg Med* February 2016;**23**(2):119−34. https://doi.org/10.1111/acem.12875. Epub 2016 Jan 22. PMID: 26801209; PMCID: PMC4755157.

91. Terblanche NCS, Middleton C, Choi-Lundberg DL, Skinner M. Efficacy of a new dual channel laryngeal mask airway, the LMA®gastro™ airway, for upper gastrointestinal endoscopy: a prospective observational study. *Br J Anaesth* 2018;**120**:353−60.

92. Larson PC. Laryngospasm-the best treatment. *Anesthesiology* 1998;**89**:1293−4. https://doi.org/10.1097/00000542-199811000-00056.

93. Sundman E, Witt H, Sandin R, Kuylenstierna R, Bodén K, Ekberg O, Eriksson L. Pharyngeal function and airway protection during subhypnotic concentrations of propofol, isoflurane, and sevoflurane. *Anesthesiology* 2001;**95**(5):1125−32.

94. Mandell LA, Niederman MS. Aspiration pneumonia. *N Engl J Med* 2019;**380**:651−63. https://doi.org/10.1056/NEJMra1714562.

95. Schlam I, Dixon S, South C, Brook B. Endoscopy related pulmonary aspiration: 2623. *Am J Gastroenterol* 2016;**111**:S1322−3. https://doi.org/10.1038/ajg.2016.394.

96. Park K, Kim N, Kim K, Oh C, Chae D, Kim S. A simple risk scoring system for predicting the occurrence of aspiration pneumonia after gastric endoscopic submucosal dissection. *Anesth Analg* 2022;**134**(1):114−22. https://doi.org/10.1213/ANE.0000000000005779.

97. Sabaa MAA, Amer GF, Saleh AEAA, Elrahman MA, Elbakery AE. Comparative study between El-Ganzouri airway risk index alone and in combination with upper airway ultrasound in preoperative airway assessment. *Egypt J Hosp Med* 2019;**77**:5621−32.

98. Venkata K, Kalagara H, Ahmed A, Pierce A, Kaehler R, Mitchell R, Harrison D, Baig K, Peter S. S980 Point of care gastric ultrasound for predicting residual gastric content and risk of aspiration in ambulatory patients for advanced endoscopy

procedures. *Am J Gastroenterol* 2021;**116**:S468−9. https://doi.org/10.14309/01.ajg.0000777452.65402.c0.

99. Adler DG. Consent, common adverse events, and post−adverse event actions in endoscopy. *Gastrointest Endosc Clin N Am* 2015;**25**(1):1−8.

100. Parker BK, Manning S. Postprocedural gastrointestinal emergencies. *Emerg Med Clin* 2021;**39**(4):781−94.

101. Yoshida N, Mano Y, Matsuda T, Sano Y, Inoue K, Hirose R, Dohi O, Itoh Y, Goto Y, Sobue T, Takeuchi Y, Nakayama T, Muto M. Complications of colonoscopy in Japan: an analysis using large-scale health insurance claims data. *J Gastroenterol Hepatol* 2021;**36**(10):2745−53.

102. Cantor M, Barach P, Derse A, Maklan C, Woody G, Fox E. Disclosing adverse events to patients. *Joint Comm J Qual Saf* 2005;**31**:5−12.

103. Shirota Y, Hirase Y, Suda T, Miyazawa M, Hodo Y, Wakabayashi T. More than half of hypoxemia cases occurred during the recovery period after completion of esophagogastroduodenoscopy with planned moderate sedation. *Sci Rep* 2020;**10**:4312. https://doi.org/10.1038/s41598-020-61120-0.

104. Clark M, Wilson KE, Girdler NM, Stassen LFA. Effect of dexter patient positioning and verbal interaction or recovery following intravenous sedation. *Oral surgery* 2013;**6**(4):193−9. https://doi.org/10.1111/ors.12045.

105. Myles PS, Weitkamp B, Jones K, Melick J, Hensen S. Validation and reliability of a postoperative quality of recovery score: the QoR-40. *Br J Anaesth* 2000;**84**(1):11−5.

106. Stark PA, Myles PS, Burke JA. Development and psychometric evaluation of a postoperative quality of recovery score. *Anesthesiology* 2013;**118**(6):1332−40. https://doi.org/10.1097/ALN.0b013e318289b84b.

107. Barber R, Allen M, Leslie K. Quality of recovery from sedation for endoscopy. *Anaesth Intensive Care* 2016;**44**:4.

108. Dowling LP. Aldrete discharge scoring: appropriate for post anesthesia phase I discharge?. Master's Theses and Capstones. 14. 2015. https://scholars.unh.edu/thesis/14; https://www.apicareonline.com/index.php/APIC/article/view/1314/2160.

109. Jain A, Muralidhar V, Aneja S, Sharma AK. A prospective observational study comparing criteria-based discharge method with traditional time-based discharge method for discharging patients from post-anaesthesia care unit undergoing ambulatory or outpatient minor surgeries under general anaesthesia. *Indian J Anaesth* January 2018; **62**(1):61−5. https://doi.org/10.4103/ija.IJA_549_17. PMID: 29416152; PMCID: PMC5787893.

110. Phillips NM, Kent B, Haesler E, Cadeddu M. Post-anaesthetic discharge scoring criteria: key findings from a systematic review. *Int J Evid Base Healthc* 2013;**11**(4):275−84.

111. Robert C, Soulier A, Sciard D, Dufour G, Alberti C, Boizeau P, Beaussier M. Cognitive status of patients judged fit for discharge from the post-anaesthesia care unit after general anaesthesia: a randomized comparison between desflurane and propofol. *BMC Anesthesiol* 2021;**21**:76. https://doi.org/10.1186/s12871-021-01287-9.

112. Horiuchi A, Nakayama Y, Fujii H, Katsuyama Y, Ohmori S, Tanaka N. Psychomotor recovery and blood propofol level in colonoscopy when using propofol sedation. *Gastrointest Endosc* 2012;**75**(3):506−12.

113. Horiuchi A, Nakayama Y, Katsuyama Y, Ohmori S, Ichise Y, Tanaka N. Safety and driving ability following low-dose propofol sedation. *Digestion* 2008;**78**:190−4.

114. Willey J, Vargo JJ, ConnorJT, Dumot JA, Conwell DL, Zuccaro G. Quantitative assessment of psychomotor recovery after sedation and analgesia for outpatient EGD. *Gastrointest Endosc* 2002;**56**(6):810−6.

115. Weinger M, Englund C. Ergonomic and human factors affecting anesthetic vigilance and monitoring performance in the operating room environment. *Anesthesiology* 1990;**73**:995−1021.

116. Woods D, Johannesen L, Cook RI, et al. *Behind human error: cognitive systems, computers and hindsight*. Dayton, OH: WPAPB; 1994.

117. Lundstrom T, Pugliese G, Bartley J, et al. Organizational and environmental factors that affect worker health and safety and patient outcomes. *Am J Infect Control* 2002;**30**: 93−106.

118. Wears RL, Perry SJ. Human factors and ergonomics in the emergency department. *Ann Emerg Med* 2002;**40**:206−12.

119. Barach P, Weinger M. Trauma team performance. In: Wilson WC, Grande CM, Hoyt DB, editors. *Trauma: emergency resuscitation and perioperative anesthesia management*, Vol 1. NY: Marcel Dekker, Inc.; 2007. p. 101−13.

120. Patel VL, Cytrn KN, Shortliffe EH, et al. The collaborative Health Care team: the role of individual and group expertise. *Teach Learn Med* 2000;**12**:117−32.

121. Laxmisan A, et al. The multitasking clinician: decision-making and cognitive demand during and after team handoffs in emergency care. *Int J Med Inform* 2006:2336−45.

122. Bates D, Cohen M, Leape L, et al. Reducing the frequency of errors in medicine using information technology. *J Am Med Inform* 2005;**38**:200−12.

123. Mohr J, Abelson H, Barach P. Leadership strategies in patient safety. *Journal of Quality Management in Health Care* 2003;**11**(1):69−78.

124. Goudra B, Gouda G, Singh PM. Recent developments in devices used for gastrointestinal endoscopy sedation. *Clin Endosc* March 2021;**54**(2):182−92. https://doi.org/10.5946/ce.2020.057. Epub 2021 Mar 18. PMID: 33730777; PMCID: PMC8039741.

125. Nay MA, Fromont L, Eugene A, Marcueyz JL, Mfam WS, Baert O, Remerand F, Ravry C, Auvet A, Boulain T. High-flow nasal oxygenation or standard oxygenation for gastrointestinal endoscopy with sedation in patients at risk of hypoxaemia: a multicentre randomised controlled trial (ODEPHI trial). *Br J Anaesth* 2021;**127**(1):133−42.

126. Shao LJZ, Liu SH, Liu FK, et al. Comparison of two supplement oxygen methods during gastroscopy with intravenous propofol anesthesia in obese patients: study protocol for a randomized controlled trial. *Trials* 2018;**19**:602. https://doi.org/10.1186/s13063-018-2994-8.

127. Society of Gastroenterology Nurses of America (SGNA). Sedation administration. https://www.sgna.org/Practice-Resources/GI-Nurse-Sedation, accessed 16 February 2021.

128. Da B, Buxbaum J. Training and competency in sedation practice in gastrointestinal endoscopy. *Gastrointest Endosc Clin N Am* 2016;**26**(3):443−62.

129. Dumonceau JM, Riphaus A, Aparicio JR, Beilenhoff U, Knape JTA, Ortmann M, Paspatis G, Ponsioen CY, Racz I, Schreiber F, Vilmann P, Wehrmann T, Wientjes C, Walder B. European curriculum for sedation training in gastrointestinal endoscopy: position statement of the European Society of Gastrointestinal Endoscopy (ESGE) and European Society of Gastroenterology and Endoscopy Nurses and Associates (ESGENA). *Endoscopy* 2013;**45**:496−504. https://doi.org/10.1055/s-0033-1344142.

130. Vargo JJ, DeLegge MH, Feld AD, Gerstenberger PD, Kwo PY, Lightdale JR, Nuccio S, Rex DK, Schiller LR, The American Association for Study of Liver Diseases;

American College of Gastroenterology; American Gastroenterological Association Institute; American Society for Gastrointestinal Endoscopy; Society for Gastroenterology Nurses and Associates. Multisociety sedation curriculum for gastrointestinal endoscopy. *Gastrointest Endosc* July 2012;**76**(1):e1−25. https://doi.org/10.1016/j.gie.2012.03.001. Epub 2012 May 22. PMID: 22624793.

131. Gururatsakul M, Lee R, Ponnuswamy SK, Gilhotra R, McGowan C, Whittaker D, Ombiga J, Boyd P. Prospective audit of the safety of endoscopist-directed nurse administered propofol sedation in an Australian referral hospital. *J Gastroenterol Hepatol* 2020. https://doi.org/10.1111/jgh.15204.

132. Dumonceau J, Riphaus A, Schreiber F, Vilmann P, Beilenhoff U, Aparicio JR, Vargo JJ, Manolaraki M, Wientjes C, Rácz I, Hassan C, Paspatis G. Non-anesthesiologist administration of propofol for gastrointestinal endoscopy: European Society of Gastrointestinal Endoscopy, European Society of Gastroenterology and Endoscopy Nurses and Associates Guideline − updated June 2015. *Endoscopy* 2015;**47**(12):1175−89. https://doi.org/10.1055/s-0034-1393414. Available from: https://www.thieme-connect.de/products/ejournals/html/10.1055/s-0034-1393414.

133. Rex DK, Deenadayalu VP, Eid E, Imperiale TF, Walker JA, Sandhu K, Clarke AC, Hillman LC, Horiuchi A, Cohen LB, Heuss LT, Peter S, Beglinger C, Sinnott JA, Welton T, Rofail M, Subei I, Sleven R, Jordan P, Goff J, Gerstenberger PD, Munnings H, Tagle M, Sipe BW, Wehrmann T, Di Palma JA, Occhipinti KE, Barbi E, Riphaus A, Amann ST, Tohda G, McClellan T, Thueson C, Morse J, Meah N. Endoscopist-directed administration of propofol: a worldwide safety experience. *Gastroenterology* October 2009;**137**(4):1229−37. https://doi.org/10.1053/j.gastro.2009.06.042. quiz 1518-9. Epub 2009 Jun 21. PMID: 19549528.

134. Stevens T, Zuccaro G. Quality control strategies for sedation in gastrointestinal endoscopy. *Tech Gastrointest Endosc* 2004;**6**:78−82.

135. Helmreich RL, Merritt AC. *Culture at work in aviation and medicine.* Burlington: England: Ashgate; 2001.

136. Pronovost PJ, Weast B, Holzmueller CG, et al. Evaluation of the culture of safety: survey of clinicians and managers in an academic medical center. *Qual Saf Health Care* 2003;**12**:405−10.

137. Small DS, Barach P. Patient safety and health policy: a history and review. *Hematol Oncol Clin N Am* 2002;**16**(6):1463−82.

138. Dekker S. *Ten questions about human error: a new view of human factors and system safety.* Lawrence Erlbaum Associates; 2004.

139. Salas E, Dickenson TL, Converse SA, Tannenbaum SI. Toward an understanding of team performance and training. In: Swezey RW, Salas E, editors. *Teams: their training and performance. Norwood.* New Jersey: Ablex Publishing; 1992.

140. Schull MJ, Ferris LE, Tu JV, et al. Problems for clinical judgement: thinking clearly in an emergency. *Can Med Assoc J* 2001;**164**:1170−5.

141. Entin E, Lei F, Barach P. Teamwork skills training for patient safety in the perioperative environment: a research agenda. *Surg Innovat* 2006;**3**:3−13.

142. Baker D, Salas E, Barach P, et al. The role of teamwork in the professional education of physicians: current status and assessment recommendations. *Joint Comm J Qual Saf* 2005;**31**(4):185−202.

143. Seiden S, Barach P. Wrong-side, wrong procedure, and wrong patient adverse events: are they preventable? *Arch Surg* 2006;**141**:1−9.

144. Silber JH, Kennedy SK, Even-Shoshan O, Chen W, Koziol LF, Showan AM, et al. Anesthesiologist direction and patient outcomes. *Anesthesiology* 2000;**93**:152−63. https://doi.org/10.1097/00000542-200007000-00026.

145. Vargo JJ, Cohen LB, Rex DK, Kwo PY. Position statement: Nonanesthesiologist administration of propofol for GI endoscopy. *Am J Gastroenterol* 2009 Dec;**104**(12):2886-92. doi: 10.1038/ajg.2009.607. PMID: 19956113.

146. Braunstein ED., Rosenberg R, Gress F, Green PHR, Lebwohl B. Development and validation of a clinical prediction score (the SCOPE score) to predict sedation outcomes in patients undergoing endoscopic procedures. *Aliment Pharmacol Ther* 2014;**40**: 72−82. doi:10.1111/apt.12786.

147. Parretti C, Tartaglia R, Regina M, Venneri F, Sbrana G, Mandò M, Barach P. Improved FMEA methods for proactive healthcare risk assessment of the effectiveness and efficiency of COVID-19 remote patient telemonitoring. *Am J Med Qual* 2022 Oct 18. doi: 10.1097/JMQ.0000000000000089. Epub ahead of print. PMID: 36250651.

148. Ang-Lee MK, Moss J, Yuan C. Herbal medicines and perioperative care. *JAMA* 2001; **286**(2):208−16. https://doi.org/10.1001/jama.286.2.208.

149. Lehmann M, Monte K, Barach P, Kindler CH. Postoperative patient complaints: a prospective interview study of 12,276 patients. *J Clin Anesth* 2010 Feb;22(1):13-21. doi: 10.1016/j.jclinane.2009.02.015. PMID: 20206846.

150. Leyshon S, Listyowarodojo Bach T, Turk E, Orr A, Ray-Sannerud BN, Barach P. How regulators assess and accredit safety and quality in surgical services. In Sanchez J, Barach P, Johnson H, Jacobs J (eds.). Perioperative Patient Safety and Quality: Principles and Practice, Springer, 2017. ISBN 978-3-319-44010-1.

151. Subbe C, Kellet J, Barach P, et al. Crisis checklists for in-hospital emergencies: expert consensus, simulation testing and recommendations for a template determined by a multi-institutional and multi- disciplinary learning collaborative. *BMC Health Services Research* 2017;**17**:334. https://doi.org/10.1186/s12913-017-2288-y.

Enhancing medication safety during the perioperative period

11

Ephrem Abebe, MS, MPHARM, PhD[1,2], **R. Lebron Cooper, MD**[3],
Richard J. Zink, BA, MBA[2], **Poching DeLaurentis, PhD**[2],
Dan Degnan, PharmD, MS, CPPS, FASHP[1,2],
Paul Barach, B.Med.Sci, MD, MPH, Maj (ret.), AUA[4,5,6,7]

[1]*Department of Pharmacy Practice, College of Pharmacy, Purdue University, West Lafayette, IN, United States;* [2]*Regenstrief Center for Healthcare Engineering, Purdue University, West Lafayette, IN, United States;* [3]*Department of Anesthesiology, Indiana University Health Arnett Hospital, Lafayette, IN, United States;* [4]*Thomas Jefferson University, School of Medicine, Philadelphia, PA, United States;* [5]*Honorary Professor, Faculty of Medicine, The University of Queensland, Brisbane, QLD, Australia;* [6]*Honorary Professor, University of Birmingham, Birmingham, United Kingdom;* [7]*Professor, Sigmund Freud University, Vienna, Austria*

Introduction

This chapter presents an overview of medication safety hazards and mitigation strategies during the perioperative period. The goal of the chapter is to aid surgical team members to better appreciate the complexity and mitigate the risks of the medication use process. The perioperative environment is complex and marked by a high degree of safety hazards. Thankfully, this patient care setting has seen remarkable progress in patient safety and reliablity over the past few decades. Advances in perioperative care have saved countless number of lives and improved surgical patient outcomes from preventing medical gas tube misconnections to rescuing patients during crises situations. Needless to say, many of these advances are the result of painful lessons following catastrophic incidents that were linked to patient disability and/or death.

Despite advances in safety practices, the perioperative medication administration remains one of the most vulnerable for unsafe patient outcomes due to several reasons. For example, the intraoperative medication process—managed primarily by anesthesia providers—lacks key safety guardrails enjoyed by practitioners in other areas of the hospital. Medications are primarily ordered, dispensed, prepared, administered, and monitored by the same anesthesia provider, removing the potential for valuable safety checks by other clinicians such as pharmacists and nurses.[1] Additional factors that contribute to this safety vulnerability, but are not limited to, poorly designed technology and user interfaces, uncertainty of patient information, cognitively demanding tasks and a lack of appropriate support, poor teamwork, ambiguous communication,[2] inadequate work coordination, little performance feedback, and a poor unit culture.[3]

Healthcare organizations have instituted several measures to improve medication safety in the perioperative setting. Key interventions include color-coding of medication labels and containers,[4] using prefilled syringes of medications,[5] standardization of medication concentrations,[6] and deployment of safety enhancing technology such as smart infusion pumps.[7] Technologies such as point-of-care barcode systems—though widely used in other areas of the hospital—are yet to be fully leveraged during anesthesia at the point of care, including in assisting with syringe labeling and automated documentation of administered medications.[8] Even in the context of such progress and safety investments, medication errors continue to occur in the perioperative care setting and harm patients. A recent study, for example, showed that 1 in 20 medication administrations was associated with a medication error and/or adverse effect.[9]

There is a need to reexamine existing management strategies, improve current systems that remain risky, and ensure implementation of effective and reliable strategies that have been learned from analyzing perioperative adverse events.[10] Creating a culture of safety and continuous learning where speaking up is encouraged and deep reflection after practice is supported will be key and where data generated during routine care are consistently used to improve medication safety and overall patient outcomes.[11] We emphasize that medication safety is produced or degraded as a result of a complex interplay among social and technical systems—collectively referred to as a sociotechnical system—situated within the perioperative care delivery setting. We believe that this reframing of the perioperative service line will help the reader embrace a new view of medication safety hazards, enabling technologies and potential solutions.

Medication safety hazards and risk management during the perioperative period (Fig. 11.1)

The perioperative setting is a sociotechnical system with high complexity—where social (i.e., people) and technical elements interact and work together to produce individual and shared goals.[12] Each of the preoperative, intraoperative, and postoperative phases involves multiple clinical roles, care protocols, and medical technologies, including hardware and software (e.g., electronic health records (EHRs), computerized provider order entry (CPOE), and clinical decision support (CDS) systems, infusion pump systems, etc. Even though each surgical patient goes through the perioperative care process in the same order, care events may manifest quite differently due to the wide variation in their disease types and states, patient characteristics and comorbidities, provider preferences, resource availability and constraints, the inherent uncertainty in the process and given different unit, and organizational cultural environments. In particular, unexpected variations have amplified effects on subsequent procedures, all relevant services, and downstream hospital units.

To achieve reliable care and operational efficiency in this dynamic environment, each team member must be responsible for their specific tasks while working collaboratively and interdependently throughout the perioperative process. In this system, not only do the clinical actors and clinical technologies need to collaborate, interact, and follow protocols, they also need to be comfortable speaking when they see a problem and have the ability to respond appropriately and quickly to unanticipated events or situations. A high level of coordination in terms of resource allocation, physical and information workflows, communications, as well as a sustained culture of safety are essential in each steps of the clinical process in order to achieve reliable outcomes.[10]

The perioperative complex sociotechnical system has inherent challenges and increased opportunities for potential errors and harm. Several aspects of the process are key. First, a variety of medications need to be correctly prepared and appropriately stocked in the operating room (OR) for a surgical case. At times, the anesthesia provider needs to quickly and accurately administer the right medications in response to an unexpected situation. This cannot be achieved without the correct medications and dosing tools readily available. Clinicians must also follow the correct sequential steps when preparing and administering these medications. Second, patient information and clinical records, such as anesthesia notes, infusion records, and nursing documentation, need to be updated quickly and truthfully to ensure patient status and conditions are the most up-to-date and available to all surgical team members. Third, communication and coordination between and among members of the surgical care team, within and between perioperative phases, is highly shaped by implicit organizational norms and needs to be accurate and effective.[13]

While intraoperative medication use may receive the most attention and direct oversight of the anesthesia provider, the pre- and postoperative phases represent dangers to the patient and different challenges to safe medication administration.[14] This is particularly important when care responsibility is handed off across service boundaries, such as when a patient is moved out of the OR and transferred to the postanesthesia care unit (PACU).[15] Under these circumstances, multiple factors can contribute to unsafe conditions including, but not limited to, differences in drugs and dosings, and variable technology used across these settings (e.g., different narcotics, infusion pumps and dosing configurations), differences in medication concentrations, and professional norms and expectations unique to each particular clinical setting.

Communication gaps across care settings is a key contributor of unsafe medication practices.[16] For example, the ability of clinicians in the PACU and ICU to easily access and view intraoperative anesthesia records not only influences therapeutic decisions but also can have a direct impact on planning and safe medication practices.[17] Communication gaps may also be exacerbated by unanticipated external pressures, as in the case of the COVID-19 pandemic. Early in the pandemic, the sole focus on containing the infection and protecting clinical staff drove key workflow decisions across many healthcare organizations, such as in limiting clinical staff to the most essential personnel, canceling, or postponing non-urgent elective surgical procedures, and restricting family visits.[18] For example, during the immediate postoperative period, a family member may be the only person to receive education on postoperative plans and medications that need to be continued after the patient is discharged. Limited interactions with family members meant lost opportunities for education on safe and appropriate medication use, which often is the only instruction a patient may receive before a patient is discharged, and before they see an outpatient provider or a member of their surgical team during a follow-up visit.

Fig. 11.1 depicts the perioperative sociotechnical workflow system with the opportunities for medication safety advancement. The top part of the figure depicts the patient/family journey before, during, and after the surgical experience, highlighting the longitudinal care needs of the patient across the care continuum. The alignment of the perioperative work system's resources and processes (lower part of the figure) to the patient/family needs is key to achieve safe patient outcomes.[19] The timeline suggests this may not always be the case and gaps in care may develop when the patient transitions from one setting to another (e.g., from postoperative care to home discharge).[20]

Medication safety technology in the perioperative care settings

Technology plays a key role in risk reduction through a variety of technologies such as CPOE with CDS systems that may recognize dosing errors and reduce transcription errors. Other technologies include infusion pumps, automated dispensing cabinets (ADCs), and electronic documentation of medication administration and patient information. Technologies such as barcode medication administration

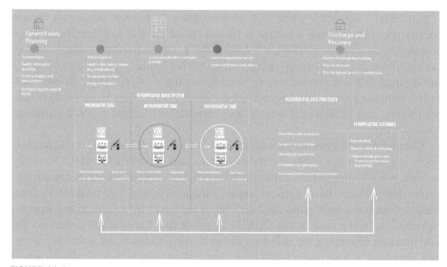

FIGURE 11.1

The perioperative sociotechnical work system[18], medication use processes, and the patient's care journey.

(BCMA) systems are rarely used at the anesthesia point of care, with current reports of their use mostly limited to research studies.[21] However, many frustrations still exist with the usability, interoperability, and implementation of these technological advances. Another concern is that these complex order entry systems and barcode technologies have been reported to add to the cognitive load on nurses and physicians and degrade their communication and may result in medication administration delays and errors.[22] The following section provides a brief overview of the most common medication safety technologies in current use.

Infusion pumps

An infusion pump is a medical device that allows clinicians to deliver controlled amounts of fluids—such as intravenous (IV) medications and nutrients—into a patient's body. Although infusion pump designs can vary by vendors, most share similar core features. The ability to program volume and a rate of medication flow allows precision in medication delivery—an advantage over traditional methods of IV medication administration. While infusion pumps have been in use since the 1960s, significant improvements in their safety mechanisms were only realized in the last two decades when "smart" infusion pumps were introduced on the market. Smart infusion pumps feature a Dose Error Reduction Software/System (DERS) that helps prevent programming errors. The DERS allows incorporation of predefined drug dose limits within which a medication can safely be administered and generate alerts when these limits are violated. Smart infusion pumps help prevent programming missteps that were common sources of serious medication errors in the pre-smart infusion pump era.

In contrast to other areas of the hospital, some of the key safety features of smart infusion pumps may be challenging to implement in the OR. For example, the hard dose limits seen elsewhere (where a provider cannot proceed with pump programming unless input settings are changed) would be impractical to deploy in the urgent and changing circumstances of intraoperative care where medications need to be rapidly titrated in response to changing patient circumstances and a desired pharmacologic effect such as when the patient's blood pressure drops precipitously. For this reason, smart infusion pump may include an "Anesthesia Mode," a pump configuration "workaround" which allows no restrictions on programming by the anesthesia provider, effectively bypassing the safety potential of the infusion pumps. This mode supersedes the pump's preprogrammed drug limits and allows the anesthesia provider to work-around the smart infusion pump's limits and potentially to cause serious adverse drug event by delivering the wrong medication dose/drug/rate of infusion.

With widespread adoption of EHR systems, the opportunity exists for greater integration and true interoperability between the pump system and other clinical technologies including BCMA and EHR. Multiple health systems in the United States are slowly undertaking this form of integration outside of the OR, and to achieve additional safety by preprogramming the infusion pump with verified medication orders directly from the EHR as well as documenting pump-delivered medications directly into the EHR. However, in 2022, only about 15% of hospitals in the United States purported to using auto-populated data in their infusion pumps.[7a] With a deeper understanding of the OR workflow and clinician's needs, these interoperability principles may be leveraged to bring an additional safety layer and add more resilience to the OR environment.

Barcoding

Barcoding is among the most commonly used safety technologies in hospitals and serves as an additional medication checkpoint feedback for the anesthesia provider and has been shown to be effective in the emergency department.[8] Machine-readable codes that constitute the barcode allow identification and tracking of products along the supply chain as well as automated documentation of tasks such as when a medication is administered to the patient. Anesthesia providers and other clinicians in the perioperative setting will recognize these barcodes in prefilled syringes, medication vials, and fluids bags used in the care of patients. During intraoperative care, barcoded syringe labels offer the opportunity to minimize errors that may result from swapping similar looking syringes that have been manually and illegibly labeled. Eliminating the need for manual labeling of syringes once medications have been drawn from their original container is also another advantage. Pairing these systems with computerized decision support systems and the EHR potentially adds another layer of defense guarding against medication errors such as those resulting from lapses in documentation of administered medications.[23] However, these systems are not commercially available.

Automated dispensing cabinets (ADC)

ADCs are decentralized medication distribution systems that enable computerized medication storage. ADCs allow ready access to medications and key supplies needed by anesthesia providers and other clinicians. The ADCs are designed to allow access control and management of medication and supply inventories by requiring user identification and input to track product use patterns. These features provide feedback or reports to the central pharmacy and supply departments to restock the cabinet when a low inventory threshold is met. ADCs also provide valuable risk management and serve as a safety check for the provider and others overseeing intraoperative medication administration.[24,25]

A user interacts with a computerized interface to remove a requested product from one of the several drawers. Within each drawer, medications and supplies are typically segregated into individual open pockets, which can all be accessed simultaneously when an authorized user opens the drawer. A user can inadvertently remove the wrong drug from these types of drawers, as there is no restriction to access any medications in the specific drawer. Other drawers allow high-risk and controlled substance medications to be accessed only from secured and locked pockets that open individually, restricting the user from inadvertently accessing other medications in the drawer.[26] Some models provide a decision support in the form of indicator lights and guide the user to the location of the requested medication. The designs of the user interface and medication compartments have both contributed to errors, suggesting opportunities for redesign and medication safety improvement.[27]

A tragic case occurred in the United States in 2017 with the use of an ADC for a patient undergoing a routine radiology procedure. In preparation for an MRI, a patient was ordered the drug "Versed" by a nurse using common order sets to alleviate anxiety associated with the scan. When accessing the medication, a nurse typed in "VE" the first two letters of the ordered drug name and ultimately accessed the drug "Vecuronium." Although the ADC quired the user about their drug choice, this query was ignored and overuled by the nurse and the ADC provided the muscle relaxant to the nurse. The drug was administered and ultimately the patient died. Multiple causes and failures were identified with the design of the ADC system, and a detailed root cause analysis found that the use of this technology without appropriate checks and balances by the provider contributed to the error and patient death.[27a] Overriding the dispensing machines was routine at this lead medical center instead of in emergent situations due to frequent malfunctions, thereby negating a critical safety measure meant to ensure administration of the proper medication to the correct patient.

Anesthesia drug carts and trays (Fig. 11.2)

The anesthesia provider makes use of carts and trays to prepare medications before they can be administered to the patient. The design, utility, and safety contributions of these tools—and the anesthesia workspace as a whole—have also been a focus of

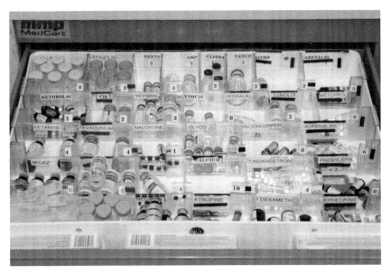

FIGURE 11.2

Standard anesthesia drug tray.

medication safety research in the perioperative setting.[28] Interventions designed using sound human factors principles include standardizing the anesthesia workspace, including the medication trays, to reduce the opportunities for errors.[29] For example, Long et al. implemented a custom-designed syringe organization device using a 3D printing technology and have observed improved usability and convenience by anesthesia providers.[30] Some anesthesia carts also feature the function of ADCs thus adding the benefits afforded by the latter. A recent randomized, open-label trial demonstrated a reduction in documentation-related medication errors following implementation of an automated anesthesia cart.[31,32]

Medication safety improvement strategies

Drawing lessons from the study of safety and hazardous conditions in high-risk industries—such as from aviation and nuclear power plants—the healthcare industry has embraced multiple safety principles, albeit to varying degree of success.[33] Notably, anesthesia and the perioperative care setting have been pioneers in this movement and have led the charge in the development and implementation of high reliability medication safety interventions.[34] These interventions aim to support clinician performance by providing common definitions, decision support, standardizing processes and products, promoting a safety culture, and a data-driven approach in which routine operational information is used to appreciate and highlight practice gaps and drive quality improvements.[35] The medication safety improvement and opportunities for safety advancement are reviewed in the following sections.

Standardizing learning about medication concentrations, labeling challenges, and anesthesia workspace designs

Much has been published on the incidence and causes of medication errors in the OR.[36–39] Researchers have consistently found, for more than three decades, that failure to read the label, "syringe swaps," inattention, pressure or haste to proceed or perform, lack of electronic (or manual) double-checks, lack of electronic hardware or software support that may aid in decision-making, and even unfamiliarity with dose or concentration are common sources of errors and lead to patient harm.[9,40,41] An additional likely cause is the historically accepted work norms of the anesthesia provider working in isolation to draw up, dilute, label, program infusion pumps, and administer all medications with little to no oversight or verification.[42–44] These practices characterize low reliable and less mature industries.[45]

Evidence-based strategies provide guidance to anesthesia providers to avoid medication errors. Jensen and colleagues developed evidence-based recommendations for minimizing IV drug administration errors.[46] The authors reviewed 98 publications and reports related to anesthesia IV drug errors and proposed potential interventions that were shown to reduce medication errors in anesthesia—these include carefully reading the label, optimizing agreed upon standards for legibility and contents of medication labels, formally organizing and standardizing drug drawers and workspaces, as well as double-checking drug doses/concentrations (with a second person or a device, such as a barcode reader). They found that a well-conducted, independent double-check could have prevented 58% of the errors reviewed, making it the single most effective medication error prevention strategy.

The Anesthesia Patient Safety Foundation (APSF) proposed in 2010 an approach to reduce medication errors.[47] They recommended that high-alert drugs should be available only in standardized concentrations, infusions should be delivered via smart pump device, and ready-to-use syringes and drug infusions have fully compliant machine-readable labels. Despite these well-reported evidence informed recommendations few hospitals have implemented the APSF recommendations.

Merry and colleagues reported a novel approach based on the principles of systems and human factors design.[48] The system includes drug trays that support a well-organized anesthesia workspace, as well as color and barcoded labeling of syringes. The same group later reported a 35% reduction in drug administration errors with their new system when compared to a conventional system but there has been no independent validation of this system.[49]

Grigg and colleagues evaluated the impact of an anesthesia medication template (AMT) that provides formal organization, standardization, and identification of syringes in the anesthesia workplace[29,50] (Fig. 11.3). Clinicians select the medications to administer and then identify the correct medication by text, shape, size, color, and location.

The authors demonstrated that AMTs could reduce syringe swaps and dosing errors by decreasing the mean number of medication errors that reached patients from 1.24 to 0.65 per 1000 anesthetics (Fig. 11.4). Surprisingly, the medication errors that

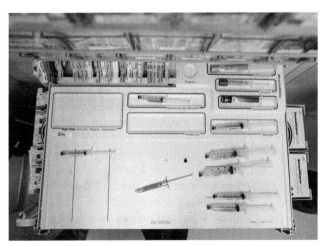

FIGURE 11.3

The anesthesia cart top template for the operating room.

With permission from Roesler A, Grigg EB, Martin LD, et al. Practice-centered design of an anesthesia medication template to reduce medication handling errors in the operating room. Int J Des. 2019;13(1):53–68.

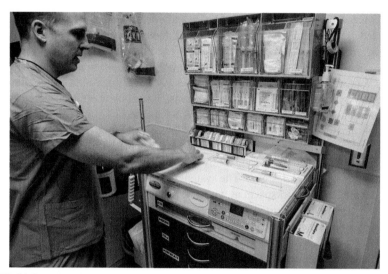

FIGURE 11.4

The AMT shown with the anesthesia cart.

With permission from Roesler A, Grigg EB, Martin LD, et al. Practice-centered design of an anesthesia medication template to reduce medication handling errors in the operating room. Int J Des. 2019;13(1):53–68.

resulted in patient harm did not change after implementation, and only 10 serious safety events were reported.

In 2018, Grigg and Roesler identified numerous weaknesses in the organizational culture in anesthesia departments that makes addressing medication errors so difficult.[42] Culture of care is known to directly and indirectly impact patient outcomes.[51] The true number of medication errors in the OR is hampered by limited self-reporting,[52] which is estimated at below 10%. Moreover, most errors go unreported or unnoticed.[53] Grigg and Roesler argued that an entrenched culture of resistance to standardization of medication concentrations/handling and resistance to arranging medications in the anesthesia workspace are important barriers to learning and improvement. Dangerous myths that undermine changing the behavior of anesthesia care providers include: "(1) Concern has been expressed in the past, for example, that color coding of syringes may contribute to syringe swaps within drug classes if it discourages providers from scrutinizing labels more closely, (2) hand-written labels are reliable in high-stress environments, and (3) pre-filled syringes have questionable safety benefits." Multiple sources in the industrial design literature suggest that the most robust way to identify hazards (in this case syringes) is to use multiple indicators in tandem. Location, color, size, and shape are all important visual cues in addition to textual information.[54]

Currently, visual or auditory alarms for bolus medications are not widely implemented,[49] limiting error detection. While medication labeling may be more standardized, with the American Society for Testing and Materials (ASTM) color-coded syringe standards and computer-generated labels being readily available, anesthesia providers still rely on the "read the label" exhortation.[4] Prefilled syringes are now available with barcoded labels, yet in the United States there is no anesthesia automated record management system that will read syringe or infusion labels and integrate them into the EHR.[5]

International anesthesia societies and safety organizations have promulgated specific recommendations for safe medication practice. In 2018, the Institute for Safe Medication Practices (ISMP) identified safety issues in the practice of anesthesia. Color-coding by drug class can be dangerous, so vials containing drugs in the same class should not be stored next to each other, and color-coding by drug class is not recommended for commercial vial caps and labels.[55] The ISMP in 2021 began implementing a medication safety assessment tool to support hospitals and other settings performing surgical procedures in their perioperative medication safety improvement efforts.[56]

An essential component of safety improvement is building a human factors-based, actionable body of knowledge about adverse drug events based on what makes the most sense to clinicians and is driven bottom-up, designed to support the work as-is, versus the perceived work of perioperative clinicians.[57] These learnings include all reportable clinical and administrative unsafe circumstances, from situations that have not yet produced an incident to serious adverse events.[57] Receiving these incidents without the system being prepared to respond can be a waste of the organization's time and resources, and can lead to more cynicism and loss of trust. Research has documented these actions main sources for medical providers' frustration regarding adverse drug reporting systems.[58]

Two strategies have been proposed to address the limited resources allocated to adverse drug incident analysis:

(i) Introduce a dynamic risk assessment and triage matrix to focus on those medication incidents that combine a high probability of recurrence (frequency) and a high harm potential (severity)[59] (Table 11.1).

Table 11.1 Error severity and probability matrix.

Risk matrix (Adapted from safety assessment code matrix)				
Severity and probability	Catastrophic	Major	Moderate	Minor
Frequent	High	High	Moderate	Low
Occasional	High	Moderate	Low	Low
Uncommon	High	Moderate	Low	Low
Remote	High	Moderate	Low	Low

Severity refers to potential severity (in the event of repetition), whereas probability is the likelihood of repetition in the future. Adapted from Bagian JP, Lee C, Gosbee J, et al. Developing and deploying a patient safety program in a large health care delivery system: you can't fix what you don't know about. Joint Comm J Qual Improv. October 2001;27(10):522-532. https://doi.org/10.1016/s1070-3241(01)27046-1.

(ii) Target-specific high-risk types of incidents[60] identified by prospective techniques such as failure modes and effects analysis (FMEA),[61] probabilistic risk assessment (PRA),[62] hazard reliability analysis (HRA),[63] and critical control point analysis.[64,65] These tools can be most beneficial for predicting clinical impact based on past anesthesia incidents and practices and can support future entrustment of clinicians instead of merely reporting of low-impact incidents that lead to little gains of patient safety.

The American Society of Health-System Pharmacists (ASHP) published an FDA-funded "Standardize 4 Safety" program in 2018, that recommended standardized concentrations for continuous IV medications as an error-reducing strategy.[6] The American Society of Anesthesiologists (ASA), building on the work of ASHP "Standardize 4 Safety" recommendations for standardized medication concentrations and the most frequently used medication concentrations in the United States found in the REMEDI database,[67] approved a position statement on the recommended standardized medication concentrations of 10 of the most common high-alert medications involved in the most significant medication errors in anesthesia practice[68] (Table 11.2). The collaborative shared efforts of ASHP, ASA, and other professional societies in supporting common definitions and drug concentration standardization should lead to a significant reduction of medication errors in anesthesia practice.

Data-informed approaches to perioperative medication safety

Data-informed approaches to improve medication safety allow clinicians to utilize data generated during the medication administration process to make evidence-based decisions for improving patient care. Using medication safety data allows organizations to develop a deep culture of continuous learning and improve their care.[69,70] Most hospitals have electronic medical records of their clinical data and medical devices such as smart infusion pumps and ADCs. A third data resource, shared patient data sets, can provide organizations with data from other hospitals for benchmarking helping to guide efforts on where to focus medication safety efforts. The Regenstrief National Center for Medical Device Informatics (REMEDI) is an example of a shared national dataset (Fig. 11.5). REMEDI was developed in 2009 by the Regenstrief Center for Healthcare Engineering, an interdisciplinary research center located at Purdue University, West Lafayette, Indiana.

The REMEDI database is used to improve intravenous medication administration practices and patient safety. The REMEDI member hospitals share four types of infusion pump data: (i) IV smart pump programming alerts, (ii) DERS-use compliance percentages, (iii) operational alarms, and (iv) drug limit libraries. The shared database allows users to conduct their own comparisons and analyses for quality improvement studies and benchmarking practices.[71] In 2020, the Institute of Safe Medication Practice (ISMP) released Guidelines for Optimizing Safe Implementation and Use of Smart Pumps.[7] These guidelines include regularly monitoring Continuous Quality Improvement (CQI) data and establishing CQI metrics. As an

Table 11.2 Top 10 high-alert medications involved in significant anesthesia-related intravenous medication errors.

Drug name	Administration	Adult Concentration(s)	Pediatric Concentration(s)
Dexmedetomidine	IV bolus	4 mcg/mL, 10 mcg/mL	2 mcg/mL, 4 mcg/mL
Dexmedetomidine	IV infusion—via pump	4 mcg/mL, 10 mcg/mL	2 mcg/mL, 4 mcg/mL
Epinephrine	IV bolus	10 mcg/mL, 32 mcg/mL[a]	1 mcg/mL, 10 mcg/mL[a]
Epinephrine	IV infusion—via pump	10 mcg/mL, 16 mcg/mL, 32 mcg/mL	10 mcg/mL, 16 mcg/mL, 32 mcg/mL
Heparin	IV bolus	1000 units/mL	10 units/mL, 100 units/mL, 1000 units/mL
Heparin	IV infusion—via pump	100 units/mL	50 units/mL, 100 units/mL
Hydromorphone	IV bolus	0.2 mg/mL	0.2 mg/mL
Hydromorphone	IV infusion—via pump	0.2 mg/mL, 0.5 mg/mL, 1 mg/mL	0.2 mg/mL, 0.5 mg/mL, 1 mg/mL
Insulin	IV bolus	1 unit/mL	1 unit/mL
Insulin	IV infusion—via pump	1 unit/mL	1 unit/mL, 0.2 units/mL
Ketamine	IV bolus	10 mg/mL, 50 mg/mL	10 mg/mL
Ketamine	IV infusion—via pump	1 mg/mL, 10 mg/mL	10 mg/mL
Lidocaine	IV bolus	10 mg/mL, 20 mg/mL	10 mg/mL, 20 mg/mL
Lidocaine	IV infusion—via pump	4 mg/mL	4 mg/mL, 8 mg/mL
Norepinephrine[b]	IV infusion—via pump	16 mcg/mL, 32 mcg/mL	16 mcg/mL, 32 mcg/mL
Phenylephrine	IV bolus	40 mcg/mL, 100 mcg/mL	40 mcg/mL, 100 mcg/mL
Phenylephrine	IV infusion—via pump	40 mcg/mL, 100 mcg/mL	40 mcg/mL, 100 mcg/mL
Remifentanil	IV bolus	25 mcg/mL, 50 mcg/mL	25 mcg/mL, 50 mcg/mL
Remifentanil	IV infusion—via pump	25 mcg/mL, 50 mcg/mL	25 mcg/mL, 50 mcg/mL

[a] *Facilities and anesthesiology groups may also consider having Epinephrine 100 mcg/mL dose available for pediatric and adult emergencies.*
[b] *Norepinephrine is rarely used via IV bolus administration. Therefore, the workgroup does not recommend an IV bolus drug concentration for norepinephrine.*

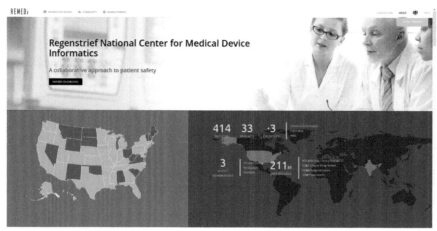

FIGURE 11.5

REMEDI—a shared dataset for medication safety.

example, one hospital used the REMEDI database to identify their highest alerting drugs. Fig. 11.6 shows one hospital's top 10 perioperative alerting drugs.

The ISMP guidelines expect DERS usage will increase across all hospital service lines, including the perioperative and procedural areas. Perioperative clinicians can

Top Alerting Drugs

Drug	Alerts
Phenylephrine	418
propofol	372
Propoven (OR)	13
remifentanil	12
Epinephrine	12
Amiodarone	11
Dexmedetomidine	10
Nitroglycerin	9
Vasopressin	7

FIGURE 11.6

REMEDI top 10 alerting drugs with number of generated alerts.

work with the pharmacy department to investigate and identify which medications may need drug library changes to better align clinical experience with the pump with the design of the library. In one case, a pharmacist went to the patient floor and talked with a nurse about administering one of the medications to better understand why a high number of alerts were being generated. This allowed the pharmacist to understand that many of these alerts were nonactionable and contributed to clinician alarm fatigue, leading to the drug library modification and to the reduction in the number of nonactionable alerts. This is important because distractions—such as those caused by alerts—in the perioperative work environment can adversely affect vigilance, situation awareness, and the ability to respond promptly to changes in the patient's condition and pose a risk to patients.[72] The result was a signification reduction in the number of false alerts generated by the medication as shown in Fig. 11.7.

The ISMP further identifies the introduction of smart pump technology (i.e., DERS) throughout the organization as a best practice.[7] The DERS usage is measured by compliance, where compliance is defined as the number of infusions given using the DERS divided by the total number of infusions given (both using DERS and without DERS). A 95% compliance or better is the ISMP target. The use of DERS is intended to reduce medication adverse events where the patient is over- or underdosed. This metric can be used to drive changes in DERS usage. As an example, a REMEDI member hospital used the compliance application to

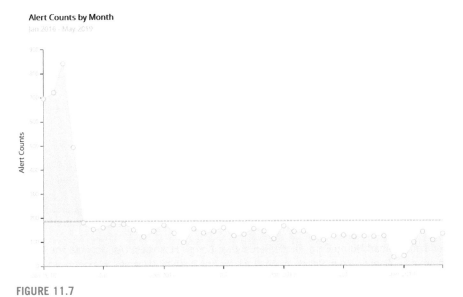

FIGURE 11.7

REMEDI alert trend for a top 10 alerting medication before and after intervention and subsequent changes in pump alerts.

benchmark their practice in compared to other hospitals and noted that their compliance rate was lower than that in the comparison hospitals (Fig. 11.8A).

The hospital pharmacist (see magenta line) seeing that other hospital pump users were doing a better job of using the smart pump features (see purple and teal lines) gave the hospital leadership confidence that they could improve their compliance rates. The hospital implemented a corrective plan resulting in improved alarm compliance moving from the 70% range to the high 90s% compliance rates (Fig. 11.8B).

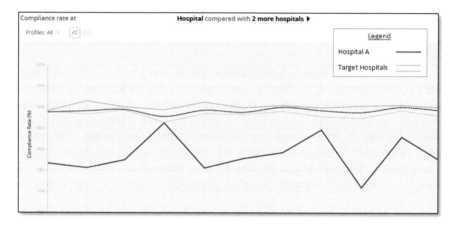

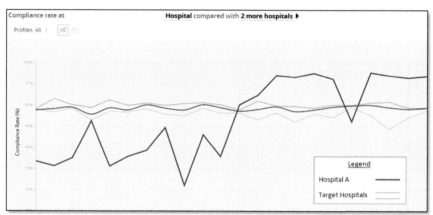

FIGURE 11.8

Comparing Smart Pump Compliance Percentage Across Hospitals. (A) Magenta line shows compliance with smart pump features for one hospital (Hospital A) compared against other two hospitals (blue and teal lines). (B) Magenta line shows compliance with smart pump features for the same hospital (Hospital A) in (A), as compared against two other hospitals (purple and teal lines) following a pharmacist-led intervention to improve pump compliance rates.

Another example of leveraging the REMEDI compliance data is to use the compliance by profile (i.e., care areas or clinical specialty) report to identify which hospital profiles need additional work to improve their reporting compliance. Fig. 11.9 shows that the Anesthesia infusion pump profile has an 86% alarm compliance.

The drug limit library in REMEDI allows hospitals to see how and which medications are used at other hospitals. Fig. 11.10 shows the concentration distribution for dexmedetomidine for adults (left) and pediatrics (right) across 111 REMEDI hospitals.

The list below identifies five reports to assist clinicians in monitoring smart pump data that are available to review on a monthly basis including:

1. Top 10 alerting drugs in the OR. Identifies which medications are generating the most false alerts (Fig. 11.4).

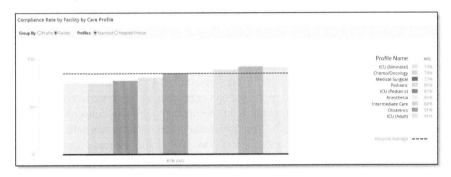

FIGURE 11.9

Smart Pump Compliance by service line profile. Bars represent individual profiles in smart infusion pump usage, which may correspond to clinical care areas where drug libraries are specifically built to accommodate the needs of particular patient care settings.

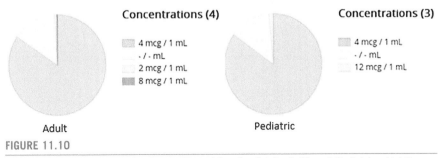

FIGURE 11.10

Concentration Distribution for Dexmedetomidine for Adults (left) and Pediatrics (right). These distributions identify room for improvement in complying with ASA Drug concentration recommendations. The "-/- mL" construct indicates a wildcard or variable concentration that is allowed for infusion.

2. REMEDI Alert trends. Identifies which drugs are generating alerts and can see how changes to the drug library reduce the number of nonactionable alerts (Fig. 11.5).
3. Compliance trend. A line graph or spark chart showing if DERS compliance is going up or down for a quarter or a year (Fig. 11.6A and B).
4. Compliance by profile. This report drills down into the OR to see how well the DERS is used (Fig. 11.7).
5. Alert details. This report identifies the details of each alert (medication, date/time, care area, programmed value, limit value, volume to be infused, etc.) and may be helpful in understanding why the alert was generated (Fig. 11.11).

A systems approach to medication safety improvement

The implementation of medication safety strategies must be guided by a systems approach that leverages concepts from disciplines ranging from clinical expertise, project management, organizational change, and human factors engineering. Human factors concerns, such as ease of use and ergonomics, need to be addressed to effectively, efficiently, and safely use new technology.[73] New technology often contains hardware and software that requires dedicated support personnel to ensure it is free of programming bugs and in working order and programmers to make changes and improvements. Although there is no excuse for failing to read medication and syringe labels, the failure to do so represents an expected "slip," more likely to occur with fatigue, distraction, or other causes of momentary lapses in concentration and failures in automatic behaviors.[74,75] The pharmaceutical industry has belatedly realized the importance of packaging medications to easily facilitate rapid identification

DRUGNAME	/	LIBRARY	PROFILE	/	THERAPY	TYPE	DATE	LIMIT	VALUE	TIMES LIMIT	UNITS	HARD/SOFT	ACTION TAKEN
propofol			Operating Room (OR) Therapy			Dose	07-14-2016 07:11:00	100	125	1.25		N/A	Pull Back
propofol			Operating Room (OR) Therapy			Dose	07-14-2016 08:41:00	100	125	1.25		N/A	Double Confirmation
propofol			Operating Room (OR) Therapy			Dose	07-14-2016 14:50:00	100	120	1.2		N/A	Double Confirmation
propofol			Operating Room (OR) Therapy			Dose	07-21-2016 09:28:00	100	150	1.5		N/A	Double Confirmation
propofol			Operating Room (OR) Therapy			Dose	07-21-2016 13:49:00	100	150	1.5		N/A	Double Confirmation
propofol			Operating Room (OR) Therapy			Dose	07-21-2016 15:00:00	100	125	1.25		N/A	Double Confirmation
propofol			Operating Room (OR) Therapy			Dose	07-22-2016 13:25:00	100	125	1.25		N/A	Double Confirmation
propofol			Operating Room (OR) Therapy			Dose	07-25-2016 07:20:00	100	150	1.5		N/A	Double Confirmation
propofol			Operating Room (OR) Therapy			Dose	07-25-2016 10:08:00	100	150	1.5		N/A	Double Confirmation
propofol			Operating Room (OR) Therapy			Dose	07-25-2016 10:18:00	100	125	1.25		N/A	Double Confirmation

FIGURE 11.11

Sample report from the REMEDI database providing details for each alert generated by a smart infusion pump.

of, and discrimination between, potent drugs used in ORs. For examples, for years, muscle relaxants such as pancuronium vials were very similar to those of heparin. Some manufacturers continue to package ephedrine in ampules similar to those of oxytocin and epinephrine. This problem also occurs with different doses of the same drug—the vials for at least three concentrations of atropine sulfate from one manufacturer are similar. This can result in inadvertent over- and underdosing of medications. Any medication drawn into a syringe for later use should be labeled immediately. Unlabeled and incorrectly labeled syringes invite errors in drug administration and dosing and should be discarded.[76]

Attention to the system factors within which a technology or care process is embedded is also crucial for success of any safety intervention. Ignoring the systems-level components can lead to patient harm. Fig. 11.12 summarizes what happens when one of these systems components is omitted. When implementing a new process, a common failure is to look at the processes as if they are isolated to a single functional area instead of across many departments. For example, the administration of medications and fluids is not entirely a nurse or anesthesiologist's task. Others in the process include the pharmacy that define dosing limits and the IT department who set up the medication order templates. In the case of smart pumps, the design of the drug library by the pharmacy must address how clinicians use the pump in the OR or the mismatch between what pharmacy and OR clinicians do can lead to clinical workarounds, false alarms, or patient harm.[76a]

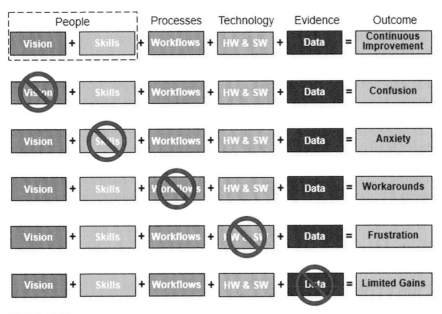

FIGURE 11.12

Key characteristics for implementing medication safety projects.

Conclusions, unmet needs, and future research directions

Perioperative medication use is a complex process associated with safety hazards that exist at the intersection of people, technologies, and organizational cultures. Unsafe conditions emerge through the acts of commission or omission of well-meaning clinicians operating in difficult and poorly designed healthcare environments. Implementation of clinical interventions that do not appreciate the realities of the sharp end, clinical work, and their context-specific workflows is likely to fail to have a significant impact on improving patient safety. There is a need to better understand the benefits of available technology and a growing awareness to the need for medical device and pharmaceutical companies to be more transparent and adopt ethical technology design guidelines.[77] Utmost attention should be paid to the context and culture of the perioperative care environment. Not taking this into consideration will likely undermine medication safety technology implementation including the willingness to report on near misses and harmful events. Continuous participation of clinicians is essential during all steps of technology design to ensure meaningful appreciation of the complex challenges and risk trade-offs, in implementing new technology.

Increasing interprofessional collaboration is key to enhance medication safety in the perioperative setting. Often, clinicians from diverse backgrounds, such as pharmacists, nurses, and physicians, will have different goals and expectations with respect to achieving safety and the means to achieve these goals. This is partly attributed to the differences in socialization and disciplinary culture, norms, and how clinicians are trained within their respective fields of study.

Creating a robust data infrastructure and systems that capture routine clinical care information that can inform practice improvements is essential for safety progress. The perioperative safety community, led by organizations such as the ASA and APSF, can develop a common framework for data elements that are captured at the institutional level and are shared across organizations through practice improvement collaboratives. This will avoid the limitations that plague common data systems involving administrative data (e.g., claims databases) as they often lack information relevant to clinicians and patients alike. This information can help answer the range of questions for research and quality improvement projects—from quantitative descriptions to complex statistical modeling, to a rich description of care-related phenomena that can reveal what the patient and family actually experience throughout their care journey. The latter approach—achieved through qualitative methods such as process maps, interviews, focus groups, observations, patient diaries, and artifact analysis—can offer rich and contextualized information that often is difficult to answer using traditional quantitative data common in epidemiological research projects.

With the growing digitization of healthcare, security and privacy of patient and clinician information will also be key considerations to progressing patient safety and cannot be overlooked. Healthcare organizations will continue to be challenged in maintaining the integrity of their data systems, from monitoring and preventing unauthorized access to patient records to dealing with enterprise-wide cyberthreats. These challenges will only escalate as new devices and technologies create additional points of vulnerability.

Finally, since the COVID-19 pandemic began, however, many indicators make it clear that healthcare safety has declined. At the height of the pandemic, in early to mid-2020, healthcare organizations' response to contain the infection and protect clinical staff may potentially have introduced communication and process breakdowns. The fact that the pandemic degraded patient safety so quickly and severely suggests that our healthcare system lacks a sufficiently resilient safety culture and infrastructure.[78] The pandemic and the breakdown it has caused presents a rare opportunity and an obligation to reevaluate healthcare safety with an eye toward building a more resilient healthcare delivery system, capable not only of achieving safer routine care but also of maintaining consistent high safety levels in times of crisis.[79,80]

References

1. Cooper L, Barach P. Sweeping it under the rug: why medication safety efforts have failed to improve care and reduce patient harm. *ASA Newsl* 2018;**82**(5):36−8.
2. Johnson JK, Barach P, Vernooij-Dassen M. Conducting a multicentre and multinational qualitative study on patient transitions. *BMJ Qual Saf* December 2012;**21**(Suppl. 1): i22−8. https://doi.org/10.1136/bmjqs-2012-001197.
3. Kohn LT, Corrigan JM, Donaldson MS, Institute of Medicine. *To err is human: building a safer health system*. National Academies Press (US); 2000.
4. Grissinger M. Color-coded syringes for anesthesia drugs—use with care. *PT* 2012;**4**: 199−201.
5. Makwana S, Basu B, Makasana Y, Dharamsi A. Prefilled syringes: an innovation in parenteral packaging. *Int J Pharm Investig* October 2011;**1**(4):200−6. https://doi.org/10.4103/2230-973x.93004.
6. ASHP. *Standardize 4 Safety Initiative*. https://www.ashp.org:443/Pharmacy Practice/ Standardize 4 Safety Initiative. [Accessed 20 November 2019].
7. ISMP. *Draft guidelines for optimizing safe implementation and use of smart infusion pumps*. 2019. https://www.ismp.org/resources/draft-guidelines-optimizing-safe-implementation-and-use-smart-infusion-pumps;
   (7a) Pedersen CA, Schneider PJ, Ganio MC, Scheckelhoff DJ. ASHP national survey of pharmacy practice in hospital settings: dispensing and administration-2020. *Am J Health Syst Pharm* June 7, 2021;**78**(12):1074−93. https://doi.org/10.1093/ajhp/zxab120. PMID: 33754638; PMCID: PMC8083667.
8. Bonkowski J, Carnes C, Melucci J, et al. Effect of barcode-assisted medication administration on emergency department medication errors. *Acad Emerg Med* August 2013; **20**(8):801−6. https://doi.org/10.1111/acem.12189.
9. Nanji KC, Patel A, Shaikh S, Seger DL, Bates DW. Evaluation of perioperative medication errors and adverse drug events. *Anesthesiology* January 2016;**124**(1):25−34. https://doi.org/10.1097/aln.0000000000000904.
10. Cassin BR, Barach PR. Making sense of root cause analysis investigations of surgery-related adverse events. *Surg Clin North Am* February 2012;**92**(1):101−15. https://doi.org/10.1016/j.suc.2011.12.008.

11. Bognar A, Barach P, Johnson JK, et al. Errors and the burden of errors: attitudes, perceptions, and the culture of safety in pediatric cardiac surgical teams. *Ann Thorac Surg* April 2008;**85**(4):1374−81. https://doi.org/10.1016/j.athoracsur.2007.11.024.

12. Entin EB, Lai F, Barach P. Training teams for the perioperative environment: a research agenda. *Surg Innovat* September 2006;**13**(3):170−8. https://doi.org/10.1177/1553350606294248.

13. Rattray NA, Flanagan ME, Militello LG, et al. "Do you know what I know?": how communication norms and recipient design shape the content and effectiveness of patient handoffs. *J Gen Intern Med* February 2019;**34**(2):264−71. https://doi.org/10.1007/s11606-018-4755-5.

14. Azocar R, Barach P. Safe anesthesia and Analgesia practice. In: Sanchez JBP, Johnson H, Jacobs J, editors. *Perioperative patient safety and quality: principles and practice.* Springer; 2017.

15. Hesselink G, Schoonhoven L, Barach P, et al. Improving patient handovers from hospital to primary care: a systematic review. *Ann Intern Med* September 18, 2012;**157**(6):417−28. https://doi.org/10.7326/0003-4819-157-6-201209180-00006.

16. Toccafondi G, Albolino S, Tartaglia R, et al. The collaborative communication model for patient handover at the interface between high-acuity and low-acuity care. *BMJ Qual Saf* December 2012;**21**(Suppl. 1):i58−66. https://doi.org/10.1136/bmjqs-2012-001178.

17. Fraind DB, Slagle JM, Tubbesing VA, Hughes SA, Weinger MB. Reengineering intravenous drug and fluid administration processes in the operating room: step one: task analysis of existing processes. *Anesthesiology* July 2002;**97**(1):139−47. https://doi.org/10.1097/00000542-200207000-00020.

18. Singhal R, Dickerson L, Sakran N, et al. Safe surgery during the COVID-19 pandemic. *Curr Obes Rep* October 28, 2021:1−12. https://doi.org/10.1007/s13679-021-00458-6.

19. Holden RJ, Carayon P, Gurses AP, et al. SEIPS 2.0: a human factors framework for studying and improving the work of healthcare professionals and patients. *Ergonomics* 2013;**56**(11):1669−86. https://doi.org/10.1080/00140139.2013.838643.

20. Groene RO, Orrego C, Sunol R, Barach P, Groene O. "It's like two worlds apart": an analysis of vulnerable patient handover practices at discharge from hospital. *BMJ Qual Saf* December 2012;**21**(Suppl. 1):i67−75. https://doi.org/10.1136/bmjqs-2012-001174.

21. Dunn L, Anderson J. Barcode medication administration implementation in the operating room. *Am J Health Syst Pharm : AJHP Off J Am Soc Health-System Pharmacists* 2019;**10**:636−7.

22. Gartner D, Zhang Y, Padman R. Cognitive workload reduction in hospital information systems : decision support for order set optimization. *Health Care Manag Sci* June 2018;**21**(2):224−43. https://doi.org/10.1007/s10729-017-9406-6.

23. Paoletti RD, Suess TM, Lesko MG, et al. Using bar-code technology and medication observation methodology for safer medication administration. *Am J Health Syst Pharm : AJHP Off J Am Soc Health-System Pharmacists* March 1, 2007;**64**(5):536−43. https://doi.org/10.2146/ajhp060140.

24. Douglas C, Desai N, Aroh DAM, et al. Automated dispensing cabinets and nurse satisfaction. *Nurs Manage* November 2017;**48**(11):21−4. https://doi.org/10.1097/01.numa.0000526064.53973.54.

25. Grissinger M. Safeguards for Using and designing automated dispensing cabinets. *PT* September 2012;**37**(9):490−530.

26. Epstein RH, Dexter F, Gratch DM, Perino M, Magrann J. Controlled substance reconciliation accuracy improvement using near real-time drug transaction capture from

automated dispensing cabinets. *Anesth Analg* June 2016;**122**(6):1841−55. https://doi.org/10.1213/ane.0000000000001289.

27. Burton SJ. Automated dispensing cabinets can help or hinder patient safety based on the implementation of safeguard strategies. *J Emerg Nurs* July 2019;**45**(4):444−9. https://doi.org/10.1016/j.jen.2019.05.001.27a . Institute for safe medication practices. www.ismp.org/resources/another-round-blame-game-paralyzing-criminal-indictment-recklessly-overrides-just-culture. Accessed July 31, 2022.

28. Leahy IC, Lavoie M, Zurakowski D, Baier AW, Brustowicz RM. Medication errors in a pediatric anesthesia setting: incidence, etiologies, and error reduction strategies. *J Clin Anesth* September 2018;**49**:107−11. https://doi.org/10.1016/j.jclinane.2018.05.011.

29. Grigg EB, Martin LD, Ross FJ, et al. Assessing the impact of the anesthesia medication template on medication errors during anesthesia: a prospective study. *Anesth Analg* May 2017;**124**(5):1617−25. https://doi.org/10.1213/ane.0000000000001823.

30. Long DR, Doney A, Bartels DL, et al. Anesthesia workspace cleanliness and safety: implementation of a novel syringe Bracket using 3D printing techniques. *Anesthesiol Res Pract* 2019;**2019**:2673781. https://doi.org/10.1155/2019/2673781.

31. Chadha R, Brull SJ. Revolutionizing medication administration safety: automated carts are here - are anesthesiologists ready? *J Clin Anesth* August 2017;**40**:105−6. https://doi.org/10.1016/j.jclinane.2017.05.003.

32. Wang Y, Du Y, Zhao Y, Ren Y, Zhang W. Automated anesthesia carts reduce drug recording errors in medication administrations - a single center study in the largest tertiary referral hospital in China. *J Clin Anesth* August 2017;**40**:11−5. https://doi.org/10.1016/j.jclinane.2017.03.051.

33. Barach P, Small SD. Reporting and preventing medical mishaps: lessons from non-medical near miss reporting systems. *BMJ* March 18, 2000;**320**(7237):759−63. https://doi.org/10.1136/bmj.320.7237.759.

34. Academies. *CoIaPMEBoHCSIoMotN. Preventing medication errors: quality chasm series.* 2006. https://www.nap.edu/read/11623. https://www.nap.edu/catalog/11623/preventing-medication-errors.

35. Nebeker JR, Barach P, Samore MH. Clarifying adverse drug events: a clinician's guide to terminology, documentation, and reporting. *Ann Intern Med* May 18, 2004;**140**(10):795−801. https://doi.org/10.7326/0003-4819-140-10-200405180-00009.

36. Llewellyn RL, Gordon PC, Wheatcroft D, et al. Drug administration errors: a prospective survey from three South African teaching hospitals. *Anaesth Intensive Care* January 2009;**37**(1):93−8. https://doi.org/10.1177/0310057x0903700105.

37. Webster CS, Merry AF, Larsson L, McGrath KA, Weller J. The frequency and nature of drug administration error during anaesthesia. *Anaesth Intensive Care* October 2001;**29**(5):494−500. https://doi.org/10.1177/0310057x0102900508.

38. Cooper JB, Newbower RS, Long CD, McPeek B. Preventable anesthesia mishaps: a study of human factors. *Anesthesiology* December 1978;**49**(6):399−406. https://doi.org/10.1097/00000542-197812000-00004.

39. Yamamoto M, Ishikawa S, Makita K. Medication errors in anesthesia: an 8-year retrospective analysis at an urban university hospital. *J Anesth* 2008;**22**(3):248−52. https://doi.org/10.1007/s00540-008-0624-4.

40. Khan FA, Hoda MQ. Drug related critical incidents. *Anaesthesia* January 2005;**60**(1):48−52. https://doi.org/10.1111/j.1365-2044.2004.04014.x.

41. Cooper L, DiGiovanni N, Schultz L, Taylor AM, Nossaman B. Influences observed on incidence and reporting of medication errors in anesthesia. *Can J Anaesth* June 2012;**59**(6):562−70. https://doi.org/10.1007/s12630-012-9696-6.

42. Grigg EB, Roesler A. Anesthesia medication handling needs a new vision. *Anesth Analg* January 2018;**126**(1):346−50. https://doi.org/10.1213/ane.0000000000002521.

43. Shultz J, Davies JM, Caird J, Chisholm S, Ruggles K, Puls R. Standardizing anesthesia medication drawers using human factors and quality assurance methods. *Can J Anaesth* May 2010;**57**(5):490−9. https://doi.org/10.1007/s12630-010-9274-8.

44. Cooper RL, Fogarty-Mack P, Kroll HR, Barach P. Medication safety in anesthesia: epidemiology, causes, and lessons learned in achieving reliable patient outcomes. *Int Anesthesiol Clin* 2019;**57**(3):78−95. https://doi.org/10.1097/aia.0000000000000232. Summer.

45. Sanchez JA, Barach PR. High reliability organizations and surgical microsystems: re-engineering surgical care. *Surg Clin No rth Am* February 2012;**92**(1):1−14. https://doi.org/10.1016/j.suc.2011.12.005.

46. Jensen LS, Merry AF, Webster CS, Weller J, Larsson L. Evidence-based strategies for preventing drug administration errors during anaesthesia. *Anaesthesia* May 2004;**59**(5):493−504. https://doi.org/10.1111/j.1365-2044.2004.03670.x.

47. Eichhorn JH. APSF Hosts Medication Safety Conference. APSF Newsletter. https://www.apsf.org/article/apsf-hosts-medication-safety-conference/.

48. Merry AF, Webster CS, Mathew DJ. A new, safety-oriented, integrated drug administration and automated anesthesia record system. *Anesth Analg* August 2001;**93**(2):385−90. https://doi.org/10.1097/00000539-200108000-00030. 3rd contents page.

49. Webster CS, Larsson L, Frampton CM, et al. Clinical assessment of a new anaesthetic drug administration system: a prospective, controlled, longitudinal incident monitoring study. *Anaesthesia* May 2010;**65**(5):490−9. https://doi.org/10.1111/j.1365-2044.2010.06325.x.

50. Roesler A, Grigg EB, Martin LD, et al. Practice-centered design of an anesthesia medication template to reduce medication handling errors in the operating room. *Int J Des* 2019;**13**(1):53−68.

51. Burbakk K, Svendsen MV, Hofoss D, Barach P, Tjomsland O. Associations between work satisfaction, engagement and 7-day patient mortality: a cross-sectional survey. *BMJ Open* 2019;**9**:e031704. https://doi.org/10.1136/bmjopen-2019-031704.

52. Orser BA, Chen RJ, Yee DA. Medication errors in anesthetic practice: a survey of 687 practitioners. *Can J Anaesth* February 2001;**48**(2):139−46. https://doi.org/10.1007/bf03019726.

53. Classen DC, Pestotnik SL, Evans RS, Burke JP. Computerized surveillance of adverse drug events in hospital patients. *JAMA* November 27, 1991;**266**(20):2847−51.

54. Ware C. *Information visualization: perception for design.* 3rd ed. Morgan Kaufmann; 2013.

55. News PP. *Medication errors 2018: the year in review.* November 20, 2019. https://www.pharmacypracticenews.com/Review-Articles/Article/10-18/Medication-Errors-2018-The-Year-in-Review/53076?sub=F09D4E1AEB1935236B7DD88EBF3511796624D-D9967A417E04A63FAD9FB86&enl=true?ses=ogst.

56. Practices IfSM. *Medication safety self assessment® for perioperative settings.* https://www.ismp.org/resources/medication-safety-self-assessmentr-perioperative-settings. [Accessed 13 March 2022].

57. Sanduende O, Villalón C, Romero G, Diaz-Cambronero O, Barach P, Arnal-Velasco D. A ten-year review of adverse medication incidents in a national incident reporting system. *Br J Anesth* 2020;**124**(2):197−205. https://doi.org/10.1016/j.bja.2019.10.013. ISSN 0007-0912.

58. Macrae C. The problem with incident reporting. *BMJ Qual Saf* February 2016;**25**(2): 71−5. https://doi.org/10.1136/bmjqs-2015-004732.

59. Battles JB, Kaplan HS, Van der Schaaf TW, Shea CE. The attributes of medical event-reporting systems: experience with a prototype medical event-reporting system for transfusion medicine. *Arch Pathol Lab Med* March 1998;**122**(3):231−8.

60. Ong MS, Magrabi F, Coiera E. Automated identification of extreme-risk events in clinical incident reports. *J Am Med Inf Assoc : JAMIA* June 2012;**19**(e1):e110−8. https://doi.org/10.1136/amiajnl-2011-000562.

61. Goodrum L, Varkey P. Prevention is better: the case of the underutilized failure mode effect analysis in patient safety. *Isr J Health Policy Res* 2017:10.

62. Wilwerding J, White A, Apostolakis G, Barach P, Fillipo B, Graham L. Modeling techniques and patient safety. In: C S US, VN D, editors. *Probabilistic safety assessment and management*. Springer; 2004.

63. Zaitseva ELV, Barach P. Healthcare system reliability analysis addressing uncertain and ambiguous data. In: *Presented at: the international conference on information and digital technologies*; 2017. https://ieeexplore.ieee.org/abstract/document/8024334.

64. Howell AM, Burns EM, Hull L, Mayer E, Sevdalis N, Darzi A. International recommendations for national patient safety incident reporting systems: an expert Delphi consensus-building process. *BMJ Qual Saf* February 2017;**26**(2):150−63. https://doi.org/10.1136/bmjqs-2015-004456.

65. Mitchell I, Schuster A, Smith K, Pronovost P, Wu A. Patient safety incident reporting: a qualitative study of thoughts and perceptions of experts 15 years after 'To Err is Human'. *BMJ Qual Saf* February 2016;**25**(2):92−9. https://doi.org/10.1136/bmjqs-2015-004405.

66. Bagian JP, Lee C, Gosbee J, et al. Developing and deploying a patient safety program in a large health care delivery system: you can't fix what you don't know about. *Joint Comm J Qual Improv* October 2001;**27**(10):522−32. https://doi.org/10.1016/s1070-3241(01) 27046-1.

67. Purdue University. *REMEDI: Regenstrief National Center for Medical Device Informatics*. https://catalyzecare.org/remedi. [Accessed 20 November 2019].

68. Anesthesiologists ASA Statement on Drug Concentration Standardization. https://www.asahq.org/standards-and-guidelines/statement-on-drug-concentration-standardization?&ct=7b64574c0d8d684c2c413f78310d3fba4afa142bf49f0e3cc7115c2bc60bdea167ba7-d31096ed36d6ec2cde0f0dd2621dd2a0e2436396457b6c7a1916d03e66b. [Accessed 21 November 2019].

69. Classen DC, Metzger J. Improving medication safety: the measurement conundrum and where to start. *Int J Qual Health Care : Journal of the International Society for Quality in Health Care/ISQua* December 2003;**15**(Suppl. 1):i41−7. https://doi.org/10.1093/intqhc/mzg083.

70. Kleinman L, Barach P. Towards a learning system for pediatric outcomes: Harvesting meaning from evidence. *Prog Pediatr Cardiol* 2018;**49**:20−6.

71. Purdue University. *Regenstrief Center for Healthcare Engineering (RCHE)*. https://www.purdue.edu/discoverypark/rche/centers/remedi/remedi-overview.php. [Accessed 15 December 2019].

72. Weinger MB, Herndon OW, Gaba DM. The effect of electronic record keeping and transesophageal echocardiography on task distribution, workload, and vigilance during cardiac anesthesia. *Anesthesiology* July 1997;**87**(1):144−55. https://doi.org/10.1097/00000542-199707000-00019. discussion 29A-30A.

73. Barach P, Van Zundert A. The crucial role of human factors engineering in the future of safe perioperative care and resilient providers. *ESA Newsletter* 2019;**76**:1–5.

74. Rasmussen J. *Information processing and human machine interaction*. Elsevier; 1986.

75. Reason J. A preliminary classification of mistakes. In: Rasumussen J, Duncan K, Lelpat J, editors. *Technology and human error*. Wiley; 1987. p. 15–22.

76. Sones S, Barach P. Medication safety. In: Sanchez J, Barach P, Johnson H, Jacobs J, editors. *Perioperative patient safety and quality: principles and practice*. Springer; 2017.

76a Solet J, Barach P. Managing alarm fatigue in cardiac care. *Prog Pediatr Cardiol* 2012; **33**:85–90.

77. Kim YW, Barach P, Melzer A. The Seoul declaration: a manifesto for ethical medical technology. *Minim Invasive Ther Allied Technol* April 2019;**28**(2):69–72. https://doi.org/10.1080/13645706.2019.1596956.

78. Lee F, Schreiber M, Cardo D, Srinivasan A. Health care safety during the pandemic and beyond — building a system that ensures resilience. *N Engl J Med* 2022;**386**:609–11. https://doi.org/10.1056/NEJMp2118285.

79. Dal Mas F, Cobianchi L, Piccolo D, Barach P. Knowledge translation during the COVID-19 pandemic. In: Lepeley MT, Morales O, Essens P, Beutell NJ, Majluf N, editors. *Human centered organizational culture global dimensions*. Routledge; 2021. p. 139–50. https://doi.org/10.4324/9781003092025-11-14.

80. Barach P, Rivkind A, Israeli A, Berdugo M, Richter ED. Emergency preparedness and response in Israel during the Gulf war. *Ann Emerg Med* 1998;**32**(2):224–33.

Surgical site and other acquired perioperative infections

12

Sanda A. Tan, MD, PhD, FACS, FASCRS [1,2], **Juan A. Sanchez, MD, MPA, FACS** [3]

[1]*Program Director in General Surgery Residency, UCF/HCA Florida West Hospital, Pensacola, FL, United States;* [2]*Professor, University of Central Florida, College of Medicine, Orlando, FL, United States;* [3]*Group Vice President for Graduate Medical Education, HCA Healthcare, Nashville, TN, United States*

Introduction

When a patient awakens from anesthesia after surgery, they usually look at their wound site to see how big the incisional bandage is. Usually, the patient and their family are relieved to hear that the operation was a success and believe the whole ordeal is over, even though patients are generally informed before surgery that unexpected events, including infections, can develop during their recovery, even after discharge. Such healthcare-associated infections (HAIs) are a considerable burden to the patient and the healthcare delivery system. These events alter a patient's expected course delaying full recovery and increasing the risk of undesirable outcomes such as death and disability. In this chapter, we describe HAIs with a focus on surgical site infections (SSIs) and outline the methods that help reduce their occurrence.

HAIs can be acquired within any healthcare setting, even in medical offices, laboratories, and ambulatory sites. However, the perioperative setting presents a particularly high-risk environment given the metabolic derangements and damage resulting from the surgical manipulation of tissues, alteration of tissue perfusion, and other transient disruptions of homeostasis. HAIs jeopardize surgical outcomes and increase a patient's length of stay, morbidity, and mortality resulting in billions of dollars in additional healthcare costs.[1] There are multiple opportunities along the health delivery process where healthcare teams can intervene to reduce HAI and improve the outcomes. All interprofessional healthcare team members have a role to play in infection prevention. For a surgical case, practices can be instituted before, during, and after surgery to reduce the risks of infections.

Increasingly, the rates of postsurgical infections at a hospital are accessible by the general public, and, often, detailed data are available for individual procedures and surgeons. These and other types of clinical quality data, such as patient mortality and patient satisfaction, may be used to determine payment for services and for accreditation decisions. Guidelines reflecting best practices to reduce infections have been established, and healthcare agencies promote and monitor the implementation of such practices. For example, the Centers for Medicare and Medicaid Services (CMS)[2] tracks the rates of major complications after common surgical procedures (https://www.cms.gov/Medicare/Quality-Initiatives-Patient-Assessment-Instruments/QualityMeasures). In the United States, validated national standards of care and treatment processes, or Core Quality Measures, reflect the quality of care a hospital provides and allow stakeholders in the healthcare system to assess and compare provider organizations to reduce complications and improve patient outcomes. Compliance with Core Measures demonstrates the commitment of healthcare organizations to achieve optimal outcomes.

Definition of healthcare-associated infections

Common HAIs associated with perioperative care include postoperative pneumonia (including VAP), catheter-related bloodstream infection (CRBSI), catheter-associated urinary tract infections (CAUTIs), *Clostridium difficile* infections (CDIs), and SSIs, discussed below. In all cases, strict handwashing between patients and appropriate prophylactic antibiotics help decrease the transfer of microorganisms to patients. To be considered an HAI, the infection must occur after 48 h of initial admission, and the identification of the infection should not be present at the time of admission. VAP is determined to be an acquired condition if it occurs 48–72 h after endotracheal intubation.[1] Table 12.1 outlines the criteria for an infection to qualify as HAI.

Table 12.1 Criteria required for HAI classification.

CAUTI	• Catheter in place for >48 h or removed the day before event date • Presence of one symptom or sign of UTI • Positive urine culture
CRBSI	• Positive blood culture as the culture from catheter tip or culture of same organism in at least two blood samples • Laboratory confirmed bloodstream infection with central line within 48 h
Pneumonia	• VAP more than 48–72 h after intubation • Pneumonia that occurs in a nonhospitalized patient with extensive healthcare contact • Appropriate clinical, radiographical, and histopathological signs and symptoms
CDI	• Presence of an unexplained new episode of 3 or more loose stool within 24 h and/or • Stool test positive for presence of *Clostridium difficile* or its toxin or colonoscopic or histopathologic finding demonstrating pseudomembranous colitis

CAUTIs, *catheter-associated urinary tract infections;* CDI, Clostridium difficile *infection;* CRBSI, *catheter-related bloodstream infection;* HAI, *healthcare-associated infection;* UTI, *urinary tract infection;* VAP, *ventilator-associated pneumonia.*

Surgical site infections

SSIs are infections at or near surgical incisions within 30 days of an operative procedure and account for 15% of all nosocomial infections.[3] They are the leading type of HAIs occurring between 2% and 5% of patients having surgery and are associated with a 2- to 11-fold increase in mortality.[4] They increase the cost of healthcare by $20,842 per admission leading to over a billion dollars yearly in direct expenditures and nearly another billion in readmission costs. The Centers for Disease Control (CDC) of the United States estimated that over 110,000 SSIs are associated with inpatient surgeries annually, accounting for 20% of all HAIs, resulting in an estimated cost of $3.3 billion. Rates of SSIs appear to be decreasing modestly due to the considerable focus on eliminating preventable patient harm by provider organizations (https://www.cdc.gov/nhsn/pdfs/pscmanual/9pscssicurrent.pdf).

The surveillance period for SSIs begins on the day of surgery and lasts either 30 or 90 days, depending on the type of surgery. The CDC defines two major SSI categories: **incisional** and **organ space** infections (Table 12.2). Incisional SSIs can be

Table 12.2 Surgical site infection (SSI) classification system.

	Superficial incisional SSI	Deep space SSI	Organ/ space SSI
Time after procedure	Within 30 days	Within 30–90 days	Within 30 –90 days
Layer of involvement	Skin and subcutaneous tissue	Deep soft tissue—fascial and muscle layer	Body space deeper than fascial/ muscle layer
And at least one of	• Purulent drainage from the incision • Culture from wound or abscess • Wound deliberately opened and culture and patient has at least one of the following signs: Localized pain or tenderness; localized swelling, erythema, or heat • Diagnosis of SSI by a physician	• Purulent drainage • Deep incision spontaneously dehisces or deliberately opened and cultured or noncultured and has at least symptom of fever, localized pain, or tenderness • Abscess or infection involving deep incision	• Purulent drainage from a drain • Cultured organism • Evidence of abscess or infection
Not including	• Cellulitis • Stitch abscess • Localized stab wound or pin site infection		

*Adapted from CDC guidelines, Berrfos-Torres SI et al. Centers for disease control and prevention guideline for the prevention of surgical site infection, 2017. Jama Surgery 2017;**152**(8):784—91. https:// doi.org/10.1001/jamasurg.2017.0904.*

"superficial" involving only skin and subcutaneous tissue, and "deep," involving underlying soft tissues such as fascia or muscle.

Evidence-based practices to prevent SSI

Many perioperative strategies may be able to reduce the risk of infection substantially. In the following section, we identify several factors that help reduce SSIs.

Preoperation

Surgical procedures can inflict significant stress on the body. Strategies to optimize nutritional status and lower perioperative risk are described in Chapter 8, Prehabilitation and Enhanced Recovery After Surgery. In general, the most common factors that can increase the risk of infection are smoking, diabetes, obesity, and coincident remote site infections or colonization with virulent strains such as Methicillin-resistant *Staphylococcus aureus* (MRSA). Cigarette smoking is a leading cause of morbidity and may negatively impact wound healing and the body's immunologic response to injury. Studies show that smoking cessation for as little as 4 weeks before surgery significantly reduces incisional wound infection.[5−7] In addition, frailty can predispose patients to life-threatening infectious complications.[8]

The association between SSI and diabetes remains controversial. However, several studies show a positive correlation between elevated perioperative blood glucose levels and increased SSI rates. Similarly, obesity has been linked to higher rates of SSI. This may be connected to an increased risk of diabetes, suboptimal physical conditioning, and other factors associated with obese patients. Moreover, a more extensive layer of adipose tissue with limited blood supply through which the incision has to be carried, along with the use of electrocautery, can result in fat necrosis leading to wound infection.[9−11]

Nasal colonization of *S. aureus*, found in approximately 10%−30% of the general population, constitutes a risk factor for SSIs.[12] Preoperative strategies to reduce risk include selectively screening all patients for MRSA and treating identified carriers. Alternatively, all patients undergoing surgery may undergo treatment of suspected colonization immediately prior to surgery.[13,14] The efficacy of intranasal mupirocin for decolonization and SSI prevention has been demonstrated in several clinical studies, particularly in patients undergoing cardiothoracic and orthopedic surgeries. However, concern about increasing mupirocin resistance and treatment failures has resulted in the exploration of other nasal decolonization agents including chlorhexidine and povidone-iodine compounds. In a meta-analysis report by Tang et al. conducted on 20 relevant randomized controlled trials published between 1996 and 2019 involving 10,526 patients, nasal decolonization of *S. aureus* using chlorhexidine was associated with a reduction in SSIs in patients undergoing surgery.[15] Although additional studies are needed to understand the impact of preoperative nasal decolonization, most preoperative protocols include a strategy to address nasal colonization.

The effectiveness of showering or bathing with antiseptic soap to reduce skin contamination before surgery in reducing SSI has not convincingly been proven although it remains a part of most preoperative protocols.[13,16,17] Removal of hair over surgical areas has been traditionally done with the idea that hair may be a reservoir of infectious agents and that skin antisepsis can be better accomplished. However, routine preoperative hair removal has not decreased the incidence of SSIs. In cases where excessive hair may interfere with wound closure, clipping is the preferred method. Clipping has been shown to have lower SSI rates when compared to shaving, which may result in abrasion of the epidermis and folliculitis.[18]

Intraoperative considerations

Once in the operating room, many precautions must be taken to reduce the exposure of the operative field to endogenous and environmental pathogens. Besides meticulous maintenance of a sterile environment and practicing aseptic methods, other factors have been correlated with the risk of SSI. The entire healthcare team should be aware of the following associations: the length of procedure, copious use of subcutaneous electrocautery, excessive blood loss, and hypothermia. The longer the surgery, the longer the operative field is exposed to circulating pathogens and exposed tissue that remains in a state of hypothermia.[19] Excessive electrocautery damages tissues and limits blood flow to the subcutaneous tissue. Obese patients are more susceptible to this effect, leading to local hypoxia increasing their chances of infection. Excessive blood loss and hypothermia can also exacerbate hypoxia near the wound area and should be continuously monitored. Maintaining normothermia and optimizing oxygenation is especially important in cases where large areas are exposed such as in an exploratory laparotomy.

Besides preparing the patient for surgery, the surgical team must maintain a sterile environment and use aseptic techniques to avoid inoculating the sterile field. All team members have a role in ensuring that the operative environment remains as clean and sterile as possible. This includes proper hand scrubbing by the surgeons and all staff who assist in the surgical field, assistance with donning gowns and gloves to the surgical team, use of barrier methods on the incision wound, meticulous surgical techniques which minimize bleeding and tissue trauma, and a reduction of the number of personnel that flow through the operating room. These are mainstay concepts underlying intraoperative infection prevention strategies. Unfortunately, foot traffic is common, resulting in unnecessarily opening and closing doors in the OR room. The presence of individuals should be limited to essential personnel only. Frequent traffic compromises the negative pressure in the OR suite and increasing the chances of introducing contaminants.

Careful hand and forearm scrubbing by the surgical team using a surgical antiseptic before gowning has been the mainstay of surgical practice for many years. Perforations of surgical gloves occur more frequently than recognized and can lead to the transfer of organisms to the surgical site. Double gloving is the most effective method that protects the healthcare worker and reduces SSIs, particularly with an indicator inner pair that visibly alerts the user that the outer glove is compromised.[20] This practice also may reduce the risk of an accidental needle stick injury to the user and minimize exposure to bodily fluids from a patient.

Patients should be given appropriate prophylactic antibiotics tailored to the scheduled surgery dosed according to weight and redosing as appropriate for lengthy procedures. This is determined by the type of microflora that is most commonly associated with the specific type of surgery. The benefits of parenteral antimicrobial prophylaxis in reducing SSIs are unclear in comparison to the unintended risk of antibiotics.[21] However, the administration of appropriate antimicrobial agents, when indicated, before skin incision only and no additional doses after the surgery, perhaps even in clean-contaminated cases, is considered optimal. Hospital antibiotic stewardship programs and infection control and prevention teams should be available for consultation to determine what is the most appropriate prophylaxis in a given case.

Patients undergoing a wide variety of surgical procedures should participate in bundled practices or clinical guidelines to reduce SSIs. These tools include the use of a separate closing tray in certain types of cases such as colon resections. Such trays include new instruments, drapes, electrocautery, suction, sponges, and other materials which may have been contaminated during the course of the procedures. The use of approved intraoperative wound protectors may also be of value. However, intraoperative irrigation of deep subcutaneous tissue with iodophor aqueous solution in contaminated or dirty procedures is not generally recommended. Despite the precautions taken, SSIs may not be completely eliminated, given the complex interaction between host and infectious agents.

A meta-analysis by Zywot et al. showed a significant reduction in SSIs following colon and rectal surgery after implementing such bundled practices.[22] Their meta-analysis consisted of 35 studies involving 17,557 patients. Their results indicated that using separate closure trays reduced the incidence of SSIs from 58.6% to 33.1%. The practice also requires all scrubbed personnel to change into new gowns and gloves. Preclosure glove change alone showed a decrease from 56.9% to 28.5%. Closing trays are set up and covered z-drape on a separate surgical table and remain untouched until the abdominal fascia is ready to be closed. Fig. 12.1 shows a typical closing table. Dirty gowns and gloves are doffed, and OR staff will assist in donning new ones. Previously used instruments are isolated. A separate count is recorded for the closing table to prevent contamination during the initial stages of the surgical procedure. The closing tray should have instruments that will be needed for the entire wound closure. In cases needing the maturation of an ostomy, the required instruments can be included with the closing tray instruments.

Other adjunctive measures include the maintenance of normoglycemia, normothermia, tissue oxygenation, and minimizing blood transfusion intraoperatively which are important considerations in reducing the occurrence of SSI.

Maintaining blood glucose levels under 200 mg/dL intraoperatively regardless of whether or not the patient has diabetes is a desirable goal to minimize SSI risk. Additionally, control of blood glucose postoperatively is associated with a reduction in SSI rates.[23] A study involving 462 patients showed that tight glycemic control

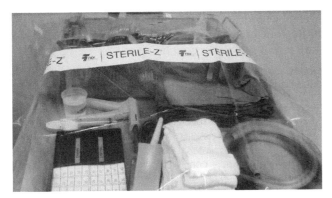

FIGURE 12.1

Picture of a typical closing tray with separate set of instruments, drapes, cautery, suction and sharp container under sterile drape.

with a target HbA1C below 6.5 reduces SSIs from 14.6% to 5.7% after implementation of the program. Increased oxygen delivery to tissues in patients undergoing general anesthesia with endotracheal intubation and after extubation in the immediate postoperative period is an important goal of perioperative management.

Many studies have described the potential association between blood transfusions and an increased risk of postoperative SSI in a dose-related fashion.[24] While it is unclear whether this is a causal relationship, methods to lessen perioperative blood loss and optimize blood conservation strategies are always warranted.

Wound classification and management

Given the strong correlation between wound classification (Table 12.3) and the incidence of SSIs, accurate documentation of the wound class and other intraoperative findings is essential in alerting the care team to patients at risk for postoperative complications. Infections that are present at the time of surgery (PATOS) should be documented carefully but do not eliminate the need for close SSI surveillance in the postoperative period. An organ space infection that develops postoperatively may not meet the definition of an SSI under certain situations when an infection was found at the time of surgery. For example, a PATOS exclusion may be applicable if an intra-abdominal abscess is found intraoperatively and a deep or organ space infection occurs. However, even in these cases, SSIs involving the skin incision are generally seen as acquired and not subject to the PATOS exclusion. As such, obtaining cultures and carefully reporting the findings in the operative note are important steps.

The wound classification is determined by the most contaminated procedure if there are multiple incision sites, such as with a colostomy take-down surgery. In this example, the old colostomy site is considered dirty or infected. In the event that more than one incision becomes infected, the SSI is categorized at the site where the deepest tissue level occurs.

Table 12.3 Wound classification (CDC)[25]: The wound classification is determined at the time of surgery by individuals directly involved with the procedure, such as the surgeon or circulating nurse.

Wound class	Wound definition	Description
I	Clean	An uninfected wound with no inflammation is encountered The respiratory, alimentary, genital, or uninfected urinary tract is entered
II	Clean-contaminated	Respiratory, alimentary, genital, or urinary tract is entered under controlled conditions and without unusual contamination No evidence of infection or major break in sterile technique is encountered
III	Contaminated	Open, fresh, accidental wounds Operation with major breaks in sterile technique including gross spillage from the gastrointestinal tract, and incision in which acute or no purulent inflammation is encountered
IV	Dirty/infected	Old traumatic wounds with retained devitalized tissue and those that involve existing clinical infection of perforated viscera. Organisms causing postoperative infection were present in the operative field before the operation

Recently, negative pressure incisional wound vac systems (NPIWVSs) are available to prevent or reduce the extent of SSIs. In clean-contaminated cases, such as colon and rectal surgeries in which SSI rates can be as high as 25%, NPIWVS therapy has reduced the incidence of SSIs. Willy et al. have reviewed the literature between the years 2000 and 2015.[26] Most of these studies support the use of NPIWVS, especially in patients with a body mass index over 30 kg/m^2, and those who use tobacco, are diabetic, or have undergone a lengthy surgical procedure.

Discharge considerations

Appropriate discharge planning and comprehensive patient education are critical elements in improving surgical outcomes and reducing infectious complications. Discharge instructions tailored to each patient should include how to identify early signs of infections, how to keep the wound clean, and information about dressings, drains, and ostomy care when appropriate. Home health nursing visits may be necessary to assist patients who may need a higher level of care after discharge.

Other healthcare-associated infections

Postoperative pneumonia and VAP

Pneumonia is the most frequently encountered HAI in the hospital (CDC). Risk factors include extreme age, underlying respiratory conditions such as chronic obstructive pulmonary disease (COPD), acute respiratory distress syndrome (ARDS), impaired consciousness, aspiration, and mechanical ventilation. Duration of mechanical ventilation is one of the highest risk factor for development of postoperative pneumonia. Avoiding intubation and mechanical ventilation altogether, whenever possible, is the most effective way to reduce postoperative pneumonia.

When postoperative mechanical ventilation is necessary, measures to minimize the intubation period such as sedation breaks, daily extubation assessment, early mobilization, and use of secretion suctioning may reduce risk. Additionally, oral hygiene care (OHC) and gastric decontamination have also been shown to reduce VAP risks. In a Cochran Review, OHC, including chlorhexidine mouthwash or gel, reduced the risk of VAP in critically ill patients from 26% to 18% although mortality, duration of mechanical ventilation, and length of stay in ICU were not impacted. In this review, OHC, including oral antiseptics and tooth brushing, may be more effective than antiseptics alone.[27]

Plowman et al.[28] have recently shown a high frequency of tracheal aspiration and an increased prevalence of swallowing impairment in adults following cardiac surgery. These may result in aspiration and pneumonia, increasing morbidity and mortality. Early detection using laryngoscopic monitoring for vocal cord impairment, and identifying vocal fold injury following extubation may minimize the risk of aspiration.[21] In nonintubated patients, early mobilization, incentive spirometry, and sitting up in a chair for oral intake to reduce aspiration have decreased the incidence of pneumonia. Many of these measures can be continued after discharge from the hospital to help reduce the incidence of readmission.

Catheter-associated urinary tract infections

CAUTIs are the second most common HAIs after pneumonia in hospitalized patients (CDC). They are caused by indwelling urinary catheters or instrumentation of the urinary tract. Advanced age, female sex (likely due to the shorter urethra), malnutrition, diabetes mellitus, renal insufficiency, ureteral stents, and inappropriate management of catheter draining systems, including reflux of urine from collecting bags, all predispose patients to urinary infections. In the surgical patient, CAUTIs are commonly encountered in complex and critically ill patients where the necessity to monitor urine output closely is essential.

Many CAUTIs are asymptomatic and not associated with urosepsis. A catheter in the urinary bladder increases the risk of bacteriuria by 5% each day.[29] The microflora of CAUTI is mainly associated with perineal and colonic organisms but may originate from other sources, including the hands of healthcare workers during placement or manipulation of indwelling catheters. Host proteins and microbial exoglycocalyx matrix result in a biofilm along the catheter's surfaces, creating a reservoir that may be responsible for urinary bacterial and fungal contamination.

Minimizing or eliminating the use of indwelling catheters whenever possible and removing them as soon as possible are essential in preventing these infections. In selected patients, intermittent bladder catheterization may minimize the risk. In males, external collection devices can reduce the risk of CAUTIs. Strict aseptic insertion techniques and ensuring that the drainage system is properly functioning and below the level of the patient at all times are essential. Decision-making tools, appropriateness criteria, and nurse-driven protocols to remove catheters when no longer necessary have dramatically reduced CAUTI rates. Other approaches such as bladder scanning can reduce the need for urinary catheters. Additionally, antimicrobial-coated catheters may reduce the incidence of infection, although their efficacy has not been defined.

Catheter-related bloodstream infections

Bloodstream infections from intravascular catheters can result from improper sterility during insertion. They also correlate with the number of days an intravascular catheter usage remains in place. Measures have been developed, particularly for critically ill patients, to help eliminate these infections. Proper skin preparation, the meticulous use of aseptic technique during insertion, the use of barrier precautions, the systematic use of antibiotics, and the removal of unnecessary catheters are crucial elements of infection prevention. Protocols used at many institutions, including weekly dressing changes employing aseptic techniques and daily visual inspection of puncture sites for early signs of infection, have shown improvement in reducing the CRBSI rate. The use of antimicrobial-impregnated materials in catheters and other devices, as well as the use of chlorhexidine during dressing changes, has also shown promise. The frequent manipulation of catheters and inattention to sterile protocols during medication administration increase colonization and must be avoided. Femoral central venous catheters are more challenging to manage aseptically compared to other insertion sites such as subclavian and jugular catheters and should be discouraged. The daily and careful assessment of all intravascular insertion sites and early removal once they are no longer needed are paramount to prevention. In severe sepsis, endocarditis, suppurative thrombophlebitis, or persistent infection, long-term catheters should be removed as soon as possible. If no other intravenous access is available, removal should occur as early as possible after antimicrobial therapy.[30,31]

Clostridium difficile infections

With the widespread use of antibiotics, CDIs have become a significant cause of morbidity, accounting for over 70% of gastrointestinal illnesses.[32,33] An emerging problem in many hospitals, CDI has the potential to cause severe disease, prolong hospitalization, and may result in death in surgical patients. Risk factors for acquiring CDIs postoperatively include advanced age, obesity, diabetes, other gastrointestinal diseases such as inflammatory bowel disease, and chronic immunosuppression. Reducing CDIs involves strategies to minimize transmission between patients by establishing strict contact precautions, using personal protective equipment, and ensuring proper handwashing between each patient encounter. Additionally, frequently cleaning with a bleach solution decreases CDI transmission. Good handwashing with water and soap is necessary since sanitizing solutions containing alcohol do not effectively kill the virus. Environmental disinfection and cleaning must be conducted to control transmission of *C. difficile* to other patients. Limiting certain antibiotics such as clindamycin and fluoroquinolones that promote CDI is also important.[34]

Reducing infectious complications requires an interprofessional approach

The primary strategy for eliminating HAIs is to prevent the transmission of infectious agents to patients from the environment in which care is delivered, particularly from vectors such as healthcare personnel. Each perioperative team member plays a crucial role by strictly adhering to infection prevention protocols. Diligent handwashing and strictly following established processes by all care team members requires an organizational culture in which the care team shares the psychological safety to point out deviations from protocols in achieving continuous improvement. Infection prevention requires extensive education so that all healthcare workers reliably use proper aseptic techniques when interfacing with the surgical patient, such as when performing invasive procedures, changing wound dressings, and securing catheters. Facility managers, environmental services personnel, and administrators also play a vital role in reducing infection by ensuring that all patient care areas across a facility are clean to reduce the risk of environmental contamination. Additionally, given the rise in antibiotic-resistant organisms, hospital infection control and prevention committees are critical to ensuring that antibiotics are used appropriately. These committees should include a broad scope of healthcare professionals, including pharmacists and infection control epidemiologists to improve healthcare outcomes.

Conclusion

This chapter addresses common HAIs, mostly preventable events, which cause significant morbidity in postoperative patients, and drive unnecessary healthcare costs. We have discussed definitions of HAI including SSI, and approaches to help reduce their occurrence. While a goal of eliminating all acquired infections may be challenging, particularly in complex and severely ill patients, methods to prevent these infections have been proven to be successful. Many surgical teams have achieved outstanding and sustained success by implementing the practices and protocols described here. The need for accurate documentation, a strong safety culture, and continuous improvement guided by careful data analysis are essential to achieve reductions in infection rates.

Surgical care is a team sport. Outstanding surgical outcomes result from the coordinated actions of many committed professionals whose contributions are essential during a patient's perioperative journey. Each individual has an important role in eliminating acquired conditions such as SSIs. As such, a holistic understanding of the risks to patients from the healthcare environment is critical. A sustained effort to minimize deviations from best practices is vital to achieving optimal results.

References

1. Ellner SJ, Umer A. In: Sanchez JA, Barach P, Johnson JK, Jacobs JP, editors. *Healthcare-associated infections in surgical practice in surgical patient care. Improving safety, quality and value*. Baltimore: Springer; 2017. p. 449−60.
2. CMS Quality Measures. https://www.cms.gov/Medicare/Quality-Initiatives-Patient-Assessment-Instruments/QualityMeasures. Accessed August/2/2022.
3. Watanabe M, Suzuki H, Nomura S, Maejima K, Chihara N, Komine O, et al. Risks factors for surgical site infections in emergency colorectal surgery: a retrospecitve analysis. *Surg Infect (Larchmt)* 2014;**15**(3):256−61. https://doi.org/10.1089/sur.2012.154. 24810804.
4. Mazzeffi M, Galvagno S, Rock C. Prevention of healthcare-associated infections in intensive care unit patients. *Anesthesiology* 2021;**135**:1122−31. https://doi.org/10.1097/ALN.0000000000004017. 34731244.
5. Thomsen T, Villebro N, Moller AM. Interventions for preoperative smoking cessation. *Cochrane Database Syst Rev* 2014;**3**:CD002294. https://doi.org/10.1002/14651858.CD002294.pub4.
6. Nolan MB, Martin DP, Thompson R, Schroeder DR, Hanson AC, Warner DO. Association between smoking status, preoperative exhaled carbon monoxide levels, and postoperative surgical site infection in patients undergoing elective surgery. *JAMA Surg* May 1, 2017;**152**(5):476−83. https://doi.org/10.1001/jamasurg.2016.5704. PMID: 28199450.
7. Turan A, Mascha EJ, Roberman D, Turner PL, You J, Kurz A, Seller DI, Saager L. Smoking and perioperative outcomes. *Anesthesiology* April 2011;**114**(4):837−46. https://doi.org/10.1097/ALN.0b013e318210f560. PMID: 21372682.
8. Meng Y, Zhao P, Yong R. Modified frailty index independently predicts postoperative pulmonary infection in elderly patients undergoing radical gastrectomy for gastric cancer. *Cancer Manag Res* December 11, 2021;**13**:9117−26. https://doi.org/10.2147/CMAR.S336023. PMID: 34924772; PMCID: PMC8675092. National Healthcare Safety Network on Surgical Site Infection Event (SSI), https://www.cdc.gov/nhsn/pdfs/pscmanual/9pscssicurrent.pdf. [Accessed 2 August 2022].
9. Thelwall S, Harrington P, Sheridan E, Lamagni T. Impact of obesity on the risk of wound infection following surgery: results from a nationwide prospective multicentre cohort study in England. *Clin Microbiol Infect* November 2015;**21**(11):1008.e1−8. https://doi.org/10.1016/j.cmi.2015.07.003. Epub 2015 Jul 18. PMID: 26197212.
10. Tongyoo A, Chatthamrak P, Sriussadaporn E, Limpavitayaporn P, Mingmalairak C. Risk assessment of abdominal wall thickness measured on pre-operative computerized tomography for incisional surgical site infection after abdominal surgery. *J Med Assoc Thai* July 2015;**98**(7):677−83. PMID: 26267990.
11. Chang Y, Murphy K, Yackzan D, Thomas S, Kay D, Davenport D, Evers BM, Bhakta AS. Abdominal wall thickness is a predictor for surgical site infections in patients undergoing colorectal operations. *Am Surg* 2021. Jul;**87**(7):1155−62. https://doi.org/10.1177/0003134820956932. Epub 2020 Dec 19. PMID: 33345564.

12. Sakr A, Brégeon F, Rolain JM, Blin O. *Staphylococcus aureus* nasal decolonization strategies: a review. *Expert Rev Anti Infect Ther* May 2019;**17**(5):327–40. https://doi.org/10.1080/14787210.2019.1604220. Epub 2019 Apr 23. PMID: 31012332.

13. Edmiston Jr CE, Leaper DJ, Barnes S, Johnson HB, Barnden M, Paulson M, Wolfe JL, Truitt K. Revisiting perioperative hair removal practices. *AORN J* May 2019;**109**(5): 583–96. https://doi.org/10.1002/aorn.12662. PMID: 31025350.

14. Humphreys H, Becker K, Dohmen PM, Petrosillo N, Spencer M, van Rijen M, Wechsler-Fordos A, Pujol M, Dubouix A, Garau J. *Staphylococcus aureus* and surgical site infections: benefits of screening and decolonization before surgery. *J Hosp Infect* November 2016;**94**(3):295–304. https://doi.org/10.1016/j.jhin.2016.06.011. PMID: 27424948.

15. Tang J, Hui J, Ma J, Mingquan C. Nasal decoloniztion of *Staphylococcus aureus* and the risk of surgical site infection after surgery: a meta-analysis. *Ann Clin Microbiol Antimicrob* July 30, 2020;**19**(1):33. https://doi.org/10.1186/s12941-020-00376-w. PMID: 32731866.

16. Kamel C, McGahan L, Polisena J, Mierzwinski-Urban M, Embil JM. Preoperative skin antiseptic preparations for preventing surgical site infecions: a systematic review. *Infect Control Hosp Epidemiol* June 2012;**33**(6):608–17. https://doi.org/10.1086/665723. Epub 2012 Apr 16. PMID: 22561717.

17. Webster J, Osbone S. Preoperative bathing or showering with skin antiseptics to prevent surgical site infection. *Cochran Database Syst Rev* 2012;**9**:CD004985.

18. Global Guidelines for the Prevention of Surgical Site Infection. *Web Appendix 7, Summary of a systematic review on the effectiveness and optimal method of hair removal.* Geneva: World Health Organization; 2018. Available from: https://www.ncbi.nlm.nih.gov/books/NBK536407/.

19. Leaper D, Ousey K. Evidence update on prevention of surgical site infection. *Curr Opin Infect Dis* April 2015;**28**(2):158–63. https://doi.org/10.1097/QCO.0000000000000144. PMID: 25672267.

20. Tanner J, Parkinson H. Double gloving to reduce surgical cross-infection. *Cochrane Database Syst Rev* July 19, 2006;**2006**(3):CD003087. https://doi.org/10.1002/14651858.CD003087.pub2. PMID: 16855997; PMCID: PMC7173754.

21. Plowman EK, Chheda N, Anderson A, York JD, DiBase L, Vasilopoulos E, Arnaoutakis G, Beaver T, Marin T, Bateh T, Jeng E. Vocal fold mobility impairment after cardiovascular surgery: incidence, risk factors and sequela. *Ann Thorac Surg* 2021 July; **112**(1):53–60.

22. Zywot A, Lau CSM, Fletcher HS, Paul S. Bundles prevent surgical site infections after colorectal surgery: meta-analysis and systemic review. *J Gastrointest Surg* November 2017;**21**(11):1915–30. https://doi.org/10.1007/s11605-017-3465-3.

23. Hopkins L, Brown-Broderick J, Hearn J, Malcolm J, chan J, Hicks-Boucher W, De Sousa F, Walker MC, Gagne S. Implementation of a referral to discharge glycemic control initiative for reduction of surgical site infections in gynecologic oncology patients. *Gynecol Oncol* August 2017;**146**(2):228–33. https://doi.org/10.1016/j.ygyno.2017.05.021. Epub 2017 May 20.

24. Yuan Y, Zhang Y, Shen L, Xu L, Huang Y. Perioperative allogeneic red blood cell transfusion and wound infections: an observational study. *Anesth Analg* November 2020; **131**(5):1573–81.

25. Berrfos-Torres SI, et al. Centers for disease control and prevention guideline for the prevention of surgical site infection, 2017. *Jama Surgery* 2017;**152**(8):784–91. https://doi.org/10.1001/jamasurg.2017.0904.

26. Willy C, Agarwal A, Andersen CA, De Santis G, Gabriel A, Grauhan O, Guerrra OM, Lipsky BA, Malas MB, Mathiesen LL, Singh DP, Reddy VS. Closed incision negative pressure therapy: international multidisciplinary consensus recommendations. *Int Wound J* April 2017;**14**(2):385−98. https://doi.org/10.1111/iwj.12612. Epub 2016 May 12.

27. Zhao T, Wu X, Zang Q, Li C, Worthington HV, Hua F. Oral hygiene care for critically ill patients do prevent ventilator-associated pneumonia. *Cochrane Database Syst Rev* 2020. https://doi.org/10.1002/14651858.CD008367.pub4.

28. Plowman EK, Anderson A, York JD, DiBiase L, Vasilopoulos T, Arnaoutakis G, Beaver T, Martin M, Jeng E. Dysphagia after cardiac surgery: prevalence, risk factors, and associated outcomes. *J Thorac Cardiovasc Surg* 2021 Mar 3;**S0022−5223**(21). https://doi.org/10.1016/j.jtcvs.2021.02.087. 00405-0.

29. Lobdell KW, Stamou S, Sanchez JA. Hospital-acquired infections. *Surg Clin North Am* February 2012;**92**(1):65−77. https://doi.org/10.1016/j.suc.2011.11.003. Epub 2011 Dec 5. PMID: 22269261.

30. Rupp ME, Karnatak R. *Infect Dis Clin North Am* December 2018;**32**(4):765−87. https://doi.org/10.1016/j.idc.2018.06.002. Epub 2018 Sep 18. PMID: 30241718.

31. Buetti N, Marschall J, Drees M, Fakih MG, Hadaway L, Maragakis LL, et al. Strategies to prevent central line-associated bloodstream infections in acute-care hospitals: 2022 update. *Infect Control Hosp Epidemiol* 2022;**43**(5):1−17. https://doi.org/10.1017/ice.2022.87. 35437133.

32. Bond SE, Boutlis CS, Yeo WW, Pratt WAB, Orr ME, Miyakis S. The burden of healthcare-associated *Clostridium difficile* infection in a non-metropolitan setting. *J Hosp Infect* April 2017;**95**(4):387−93. https://doi.org/10.1016/j.jhin.2016.12.009. Epub 2016 Dec 18. PMID: 27131640.

33. Chai J, Lee CH. Management of primary and recurrent *Clostridium difficile* infection: an update. *Antibiotics (Basel)* June 30, 2018;**7**(3):54. https://doi.org/10.3390/antibiotics7030054. PMID: 29966323.

34. Surawicz CM, Brandt LJ, Binion DG, Ananthakrishnan AN, Curry SR, Gilligan PH, McFarland LV, Mellow M, Zuckerbraun BS. Guidelines for diagnosis, treatment, and prevention of *Clostridium difficile* infections. quiz 499 *Am J Gastroenterol* April 2013;**108**(4):478−98. https://doi.org/10.1038/ajg.2013.4. Epub 2013 Feb 26. PMID: 23439232.

Further reading

1. Reichman DE and Greenberg JA. Reducing surgical site infections. A review. Rev Obstet Gynecol. 2009 Fall;2(4):212−21. PMID: 20111657.

Occupational well-being, resilience, burnout, and job satisfaction of surgical teams

13

Vera Meeusen, PhD, CHM, MA, RN, FACPAN, AFACHSM [1],
Stephen Paul Gatt, MD, FANZCA, FRCA, FACHSM, FCICM, AFRCMA, et alii, et eundem [2,3]**, Paul Barach, B.Med.Sci., MD, MPH, Maj (ret.), AUA** [4,5,6]**,
André Van Zundert, MD, PhD, FRCA, EDRA, FANZCA** [7]

[1]*Clinical Nurse Consultant, Princess Alexandra Hospital, Brisbane, QLD, Australia;* [2]*Professor of Anesthesiology & Reanimation, University of Udayana, Denpasar, Bali, Indonesia;* [3]*Associate Professor, University of New South Wales, Sydney, NSW, Australia;* [4]*Professor, Thomas Jefferson School of Medicine, Philadelphia, PA, United States;* [5]*Professor, Sigmund Freud University, Vienna, Austria;* [6]*Honorary Professor, School of Medicine, The University of Queensland, Brisbane, QLD, Australia;* [7]*Professor & Chair Anaesthesiology, Royal Brisbane and Women's Hospital & The University of Queensland, Faculty of Medicine, Brisbane, QLD, Australia*

Perioperative teams

A well-functioning perioperative surgical team is central to achieving the quadruple aim.[1,2] Superior outcomes can only occur when surgical team members are well and engaged in the process of improved patient outcomes. Surgical high-performance results from a relatively permanent or persistent change of behavior or behavior potential resulting from instruction, training, and practice (intentional learning) or experience (incidental learning).[3] The overall "health" of the surgical team is determined when there is trust, respect, collaboration, psychological safety,[4] and a willingness for mutual support among the members of the group. While team output is determined by the sum of its component parts, there are key knowledge, skills and attributes which guarantee or contribute to the overall wellness within the surgical environment.[5] While much can be done to improve and optimize the performance of each surgical team, there are many innate traits and behaviors of individual members which can reduce tension and stress within a team.[6] Resilience, motivation, and work satisfaction, all of which can be measured and improved, are key elements to the success of the group. Group resilience can be measured using ethnographic and qualitative methods and is a great asset for all surgical teams to possess. Individual plasticity, ability to learn, change and mental 'resilience' are at least as useful as hard work, superior work skills, and stamina in producing exceptional results in a joyful milieu.[7]

Handbook of Perioperative and Procedural Patient Safety. https://doi.org/10.1016/B978-0-323-66179-9.00016-6

Work climate

Hospitals are complex social—cultural organizations defined by their operational volatility, uncertainty, complexity, ambiguity, and interdependency. A strong casual link between the organization of care and patient outcomes has been found in several studies.[8,9] Complex organizations rely on authentic inputs and interactions while they deliver an array of clinical services.[10] Numerous initiatives have been promoted to enhance the quality of the patient's journey when in hospital and after their discharge, and yet at least one in three postsurgical patients suffers adverse events.[11] The impact of organizational culture on quality, reporting of data, and safety in nonmedical organizations is well documented.[12] A positive work climate can result in highly engaged teams and increased job satisfaction. Work climate refers to the perceptions of individuals on how well the organization is realizing their full potential and enabling their ability to comfortably speak up.[13] Monitoring staff perceptions of their work environment and their organizational culture is used by managers to discover what is deemed meaningful and makes organizational sense to employees.[14] Leggat et al. have consistently demonstrated a positive relationship between high-performance workplaces and organizational outcomes also applies to patient outcomes in healthcare organizations.[15]

Hackman and Oldham[16] determined that the opportunity for team growth emerges as an important determinant of employee job satisfaction. Jobs with a high motivating potential often offered additional opportunities for learning. Empowering employees to expand their potential and positive work climate has been demonstrated to enhance job satisfaction, health, retention and can mitigate against burnout.[17] Maslach posited that burnout is particularly relevant for medical professions where the gaps between demands and resources often leads to exhaustion.[18] Burnout exists in all occupations but is more prevalent in medicine, and "people work" fields, such as police work, social work, nursing, and teaching professionals.[19—21]

Kristof et al.[22] introduced the term "Fit for the Job" defined as a match of perceptions between personal competence and well-being versus work environment and organisational requirements. The level of being "fit for the job" influences job satisfaction, organizational commitment, turnover intention, well-being, and performance.[23] In practice, it is important to create the right work climate by providing the essential job resources that effectively buffer the negative aspects of the job and stimulate staff motivation.[24,25] Motivational models introduced by Maslow, Herzberg, Hackman and Oldham, and Karasek and Bakker, the founders of most modern motivation theories, demonstrate that five work context factors are considered important (demands and resources) in understanding staff burnout:

- Job demands: physical and/or mental effort;
- Decision latitude or job control: acquired knowledge and skills enabling decision-making;
- Social support, the important factor determining employees' resilience;

- Physical/environmental risk factors; and
- Job insecurity: labor market requirements for particular skills and possibilities targeting future career development.

Identifying and anticipating the demands of clinicians is crucial in order to better apply resources effectively and prevent negative outcomes. Job 'resources' constitute the physical, organizational, and social aspects of the job that help in achieving work goals, reducing job demands, and stimulating personal growth, learning, and development.[25,26]

The power of motivation

Motivation or 'the eagerness to do something' can vary in (a) level or intensity; or (b) type—(1) extrinsic type is stimulated by an incentive (reward or command); or (2) intrinsic type which is inherently geared toward personal interest or in line with personal goals. The theories pertaining to what motivates individuals are myriad and have benefited from much research attention both about the motivation factors (what motivates people) and the motivation processes (how behavior is influenced by the motivation factors).

There are different theories as to how intrinsic and extrinsic factors can influence behavior especially in medicine where providers and medical students are highly motivated and self-driven.[27] Neuroscientific analysis of the neural reward mechanisms shows that the prediction error of the perceptual connotations of objects is the mechanism that underlies reward.[28] A positive and unexpected 'error in reward prediction' in the timing and quality of an event causes a release of the neuromodulator dopamine, a neurotransmitter which activates or modulates global brain status. Dopaminergic neurons in the substantia nigra and ventral tegmental areas, are activated by rewards, especially when the reward is not anticipated, or is mediated by reward-dependent behavior. From a neuroscientific perspective, it is not the motivation factor itself, which is important, but the unexpected prediction of rewards.

Expectations, especially when they are wrong, can influence behavior: e.g., an event that ultimately is less negative than expected results in fewer negative emotions.[29] The emotional mismatch between expectation and an ensuing event outcome can influence job satisfaction. The physiological process of dopamine release is the cause of intrinsically rewarding states or their subjective feelings.[30]

In economics, the study of how people use resources and respond to incentives, an effective motivator is money, stated succinctly as 'everything has its price.' The strong relationship between reward and performance is reflected in the principal—agent theory. Individuals are persuaded to work harder when monetary incentive rises. The 'principal' uses rewards and commands in order to raise performance of the 'agent.' The principal assumes that the agent only does work for which they get paid. Intrinsic motivation is of no importance; only extrinsic motivation is relevant. From the point of view of the principal—agent theory, financial rewards for nurses and physicians can increase productivity. Psychologists tend to emphasize the behavioral motives emanating from within the person. The empirical psychology of the 1940s–60s enshrined two dominant behavioral theories:

- Behavior motivated by rewards, i.e., extrinsically motivated activities where the reward is the activity itself and
- Behavior motivated by physiological drive, i.e., intrinsic motivated activities satisfying personal psychological needs.

DeCharms introduced intrinsic motivation or 'work moral' in 1968, now a firmly established concept in psychology.[31] Establishing high-level intrinsic motivation results from experiencing satisfaction of needs of competence and autonomy. Choice and opportunity for self-direction enhance intrinsic motivation by creating a greater sense of autonomy and personal caustation. Threats, deadlines, directives, and competitive pressure undermine intrinsic motivation because people experience these variables as 'controlling'.[32,33] Maintenance of autonomy, rather than control, is essential. Personality and culture influence needs and desires and, thereby, affect intrinsic motivation.[34] The content and context of tasks of physicians can increase intrinsic motivation if they are relevant and consistent with their needs, wants, or desires. Intrinsic motivation is essential to cognitive and social development and represents a key part of vitality[35,36] which is an essential part of work engagement[37]. Vitality has to do with energy, feeling strong and fit, and the experience of success, happiness, or joy.

In some circumstances in which surgical team members are burned-out, an intervention leads to higher performance without interfering with intrinsic motivation; in other cases, interventions can lead to such a sharp drop of intrinsic motivation that productivity does not change or even decreases. Intrinsic motivation can vary and is not always of similar importance.[38,39] The feeling of self-esteem is fostered, and the person feels that he is given more freedom to act, thus enhancing their self-determination and increasing job satisfaction[40,41] triggering positive emotions.[42,43] Subjective perceptions become the pervading determinant with the same intervention being perceived by one person as controlling and supportive by another.[38,39,44] Psychological reactions are often more intense when individuals are confronted with strict commands because at least there is a choice with a monetary reward; one can refuse the reward and not be forced.

In a continuum from no motivation, neither extrinsic nor intrinsic, to pure intrinsic motivation, we recognize six levels of extrinsic motivation that depend on the degree of clinician autonomy[36]:

- No motivation: lack of any intention to complete the task from feelings of noncompetence or nonbelief in the desired outcome;
- External regulation: principal–agent theory where the task is performed to satisfy an external demand or reward;
- Introjected regulation: pressure is applied through feelings of guilt, anxiety, pride, or ego but where self-esteem is still present;

- Identification: regulation becomes personalized because control is identified as of personal importance;
- Integrated regulation: regulations are fully assimilated with individual values and needs producing an integrated autonomous form of extrinsic motivation with behavior motivated by integrated regulation for its instrumental value (outcome); and
- Pure intrinsic motivation for self-enjoyment.

Good performance induced by intrinsic motivation is not necessarily the only way to get work done, but the advantages of intrinsic work motivation[39] are as follows:

- Enhanced mental and physical health;
- Higher learning capacity;
- Better resolution of cognitively difficult tasks; and
- Reduced need for supervision.

The disadvantages of intrinsic work motivation are as follows:

- A tendency toward one wrong word or action can produce anger and resentment in highly inner motivated people;
- Overreaction and overzealousness, sometimes to the point of rule breaking, in those with extreme moral standards; and
- Self-centeredness to the detriment of society or the hospital.

Measuring motivation focuses on assessing work attitudes, feelings, and experience. Seminal studies at the Hawthorne plant of the Western Electric Company between 1924 and 1932 analyzed work restriction norms, productivity, leadership, and social relations and found that environmental changes, positive or negative, had the same effect on work performance.[45] Increased productivity was due to increased attention focus and social relations with improved interpersonal social relations being the main motivation factors.

In 1943, Maslow introduced the Needs Hierarchy Theory where the individual's ultimate goal is self-actualization (Fig. 13.1). The hierarchical motivational structure has five needs: physiological, safety, love, esteem, and self-actualization. When the needs of the lowest level are satisfied, new and higher needs will arise and behavior is then driven by the needs that are not satisfied. The first four needs are deficit needs and motivation will become less once they are met. The top level, self-actualization, is a growth need and is continually felt and will become stronger once initiated. Individual progress can be disrupted due to failure to meet lower needs but also can fluctuate due to external circumstances.

Herzberg during the late 1950s, interviewed 200 engineers and accountants who worked in Pittsburgh's industry looking for factors leading to satisfaction or dissatisfaction. He developed two lists of factors. The first set, he called 'motivators,' were task related and caused positive job attitudes because they satisfy the worker's need for self-actualization: recognition, achievement, the possibility of growth,

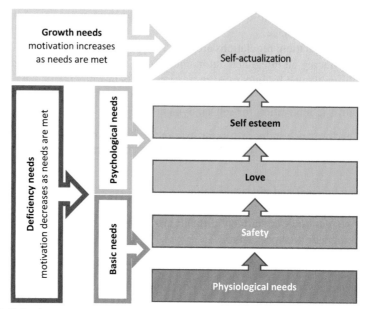

FIGURE 13.1 Hierarchy of needs according to Maslow.

The hierarchical motivational structure has five needs: Physiological, safety, love, esteem, and self-actualization. When the needs of the lowest level are satisfied, new and higher needs will arise and behavior is then driven by the needs that are not satisfied. The first four needs are deficit needs and motivation will become less once they are met. The top level, self-actualization, is a growth need and is continually felt and will become stronger once initiated. Individual progress can be disrupted due to failure to meet lower needs but also can fluctuate due to external circumstances.

advancement, responsibility, and the work imperative itself. Motivators always promote action over time producing long-running attitudes and satisfaction. Motivators create greater job satisfaction; however, the absence of motivators does not cause dissatisfaction but a lack of satisfaction. The second set, he called 'hygiene' factors, were not directly related to the job itself but to the work conditions (i.e., salary, interpersonal relations with supervisor, subordinates and peers, technical supervision, company policy, and administration), factors of personal life, status, and job security. Hygiene factors cause temporary action, and the presence of these factors causes no satisfaction and their absence can cause great dissatisfaction.[46,47] Herzberg stressed the need for management to pay close attention to both sets of factors (Fig. 13.2).

Hackman and Oldham developed the job characteristics model in 1980 that structures work in order to achieve high internal motivation, job satisfaction, and effectiveness by integrating job characteristics with employee well-being (Fig. 13.3). Internal motivation requires three basic conditions, the so-called 'critical psychological states.' If one of these conditions is missing, intrinsic motivation will

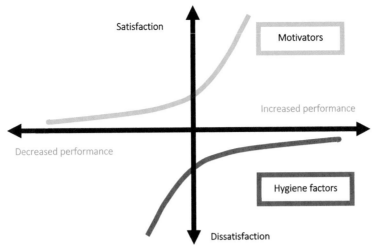

FIGURE 13.2 Herzberg's two-factor theory.

The first set of 'motivators' are task related and cause positive job attitudes because they satisfy the worker's need for self-actualization. Motivators create greater job satisfaction; absence of motivators does not cause dissatisfaction but a lack of satisfaction. The second set of 'hygiene' factors are not directly related to the job itself but to work conditions, factors of personal life, status, and job security. The presence of these factors causes no satisfaction. However, their absence can cause great dissatisfaction.

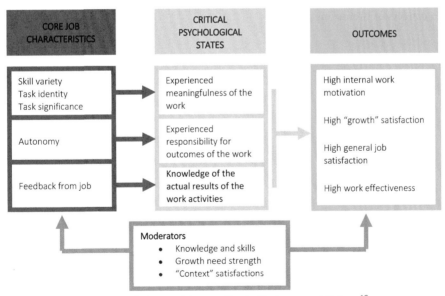

FIGURE 13.3 Job characteristics model according to Hackman and Oldham[16].

The job characteristics model (JC-model) structures work in order to achieve high internal motivation, job satisfaction, and effectiveness by integrating job characteristics with employee well-being. Internal motivation requires the so-called 'critical psychological states.' If one of these conditions is missing, intrinsic motivation will not occur. The psychological states are facilitated by 'core' job characteristics: Centered around meaningfulness, autonomy, feedback, support, and communication. Jobs with high intrinsic motivation potential provide the best performance by meeting personal needs and talents.

not occur; the stronger these factors are, the higher the intrinsic motivation. These psychological states are facilitated by a series of 'core' job characteristics: centered around meaningfulness, autonomy, feedback, support, and communication. Jobs with high intrinsic motivation potential provide the best performance by meeting the personal needs and talents of workers. Those with enough knowledge and skills receive satisfaction from doing well (and vice versa). Secondly, jobs with high motivating potential often offer additional opportunities for learning and growth. The appreciation of challenging work is not universal. Surgical team members with strong growth needs experience high intrinsic motivation when performing complex tasks.[48] The extent to which individuals are satisfied with extrinsic motivation factors (pay, job security, supervision, and coworkers) can influence the extent of positive reactions to new challenges and enrichment opportunities.

Warr's 'Vitamins Model'[49] argued that the relationship between job characteristics and mental health outcomes (well-being) is analogous to the nonlinear effects that vitamins have on physical health as suggested by Hackman and Oldham (Fig. 13.4). An absence of job characteristics impairs mental health. As job characteristics increase, a beneficial effect on mental health is experienced; furthermore, beyond a certain level, further increase of job characteristics may either produce a constant or plateau effect (analogously to water-soluble vitamins C and E overtreatment where excess vitamin intake is excreted with little benefit) or even could impair mental health (analogously to dangers of overdosing on fat-soluble vitamins A and D).

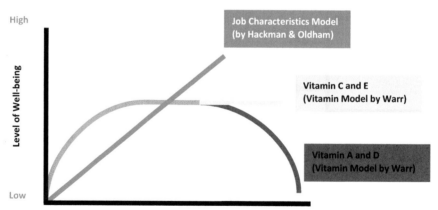

FIGURE 13.4 Relationship between job characteristics according to Hackman and Oldham[16] and Warr[49].

The relationship between job characteristics and mental health outcomes (well-being) is analogous to the nonlinear effects that vitamins have on physical health and not linear as suggested by Hackman and Oldham. An absence of job characteristics impairs mental health. As job characteristics increase, a beneficial effect on mental health is experienced; beyond a certain level, further increase of job characteristics may either produce a constant or plateau effect (in analogy to overdose of water soluble vitamins C and E) or impair mental health (in analogy to increased administration of vitamins A and D).

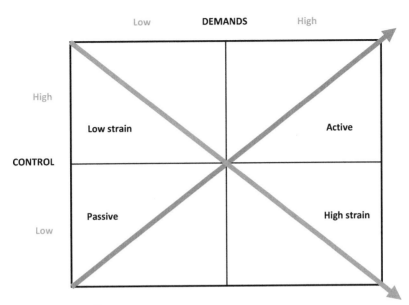

FIGURE 13.5 Karasek's[50] 'Job Demands—Control' model of workload and work-related stress.

This model explains how a control factor can buffer the impact of physical, psychological, social, and organizational job demands (strain) on stress levels. The control factor is defined as 'decision latitude.' Jobs with high demands (strain) and low decision-making authority have increased levels of stress. Low-demanding jobs are usually low in decision latitude making them routine, repetitive, and nonchallenging with low intrinsic motivation.

Karasek's[50] 'Job Demands—Control' model (Fig. 13.5) explains how a control factor can buffer the impact of physical, psychological, social and organizational job demands on stress levels. The control factor was defined as 'decision latitude,' i.e., the freedom to decide how to organize and perform assigned tasks. Jobs with high demands (strain) and low decision-making authority, such as surgeons in training, have increased levels of stress. Low-demanding jobs are usually low in decision latitude making them routine, repetitive, and nonchallenging with low intrinsic motivation. High-demanding jobs with high control (or many deadlines) with high decision latitude are not experienced as stressful and provide intrinsic motivation by life-long growth and development. Unfortunately, the model did not include individual characteristics and focused only on negative outcome variables (e.g., burnout, sickness, mental strain).

The Job Demand—Resources (JD-R) Model[51] includes integrated resources such as coping, social support, and self-efficiency and argues that strain is an imbalance between demands and the available resources to cope with the demand.[51] The JD-R model includes negative and positive variables for understanding individual's well-being. Personal and workplace resources are physical, psychological, social, and organizational factors that contribute to work goals and stimulate growth and development. The demand—resource imbalance can cause energy depletion and health-related issues. An abundance of resources increases work engagement and performance excellence. High demands with insufficient rewards cause a reciprocity deficit that increases the stress and negative emotions. Individual surgeons can try to recover from this imbalance by either reducing demands and/or maximizing rewards (e.g., money, esteem, job security, and career opportunities).

The importance of job satisfaction in perioperative team members

Job satisfaction, work attitudes, and organizational behavior influence organizational outcomes including job turnover.[17] Job satisfaction is usually defined as a (negative or positive) judgment regarding one's job situation[43] and is related to personality, job characteristics, situational, and genetic determinants.[52,53] Negative working conditions have an impact on both the work environment and persona and eventually impact life satisfaction.[24,54] Poor job satisfaction can result in lower productivity and higher rates of absenteeism, burnout, and job turnover.[55] The extent to which personal desires and needs match job characteristics determines the overall level of perceived job satisfaction.[43]

Job satisfaction is described as an attitude with two components: affective and cognitive. Cognitive job satisfaction is a personal judgment or perception of the job based on an evaluation of a job's concrete features such as pay levels, job characteristics, and career mobility. These concrete features are evaluated by employees who measure their perceptions against standards like values and needs. The degree of similarity between perceptions and standards (values and needs) determines the level of cognitive job satisfaction.[43]

Lynn et al., in 2009, developed and validated the Satisfaction in Nursing Scale that is comprised of four factors: workload and barriers, intrinsic rewards and satisfiers, administrative support, and collegiality.[56] The Affective Events Theory of Weis and Cropanzano[43] describes the influence of emotions on the affective component of job satisfaction. Work incidents, positive and negative, trigger emotions that alter affective job satisfaction: positive emotions increase job satisfaction: but, conversely, negative emotions decrease satisfaction. Triggered by incidents and driven by emotions, affective job satisfaction fluctuates throughout the working day. The intensity of the emotion depends on the level of importance and context of the specific event for that specific individual. Improving the work environment can be achieved by stimulating positive events with positive emotions and thus creating a sense of empowerment and self-regard that can lead to a better perceived sense of self and better patient outcomes.[57] A high frequency of net positive emotions gives a higher level of job satisfaction than intense, but less frequent, positive emotions.[42] Emotional support, acknowledgment, and communication are found to be important attributes that can increase positive emotions and job satisfaction among anesthesia clinicians.[58−60]

Role of personality

Certain personality traits may have a protective effect for healthcare providers against the negative consequences of work stress and burnout by using effective and well-adjusted coping mechanisms.[36,47,61] Personality traits shape the perceptions of work ethic and environment.[62] If these perceptions cause a stressful reaction, a negative impact on health and job satisfaction can be expected.[63−65] The relationships between personality and job satisfaction vary among studies (3.5%−25%) and depends on the used personality dimensions: positive and negative affectivity, Big Five,[66−68] the latter recognizing the following five dimensions:

- Conscientiousness (efficiency vs. easy going);
- Extroversion (outgoing vs. reserved);
- Openness to experience (incentive vs. consistent);
- Agreeableness (compassionate vs. detached); and
- Neuroticism (sensitive vs. confident).[69,70]

Personality also plays a critical role in affecting individual behavior at work, emotional reactions to work, and the predisposition to experience positive or negative emotions. McManus, Keeling and Sress found that physicians with high levels of stress can show higher levels of neuroticism.[63] In particular, physicians reporting more emotional exhaustion also had higher neuroticism levels, as well as being more introverted, while those with higher levels of depersonalization report lower levels of agreeableness. Overall, the career satisfaction of nurses and physicians are related to lower levels of neuroticism. The personality trait "extrovert" or "easy going" was related to higher job satisfaction scores among nurses.[67] Lue and colleagues measured the personality characteristics of physicians with high levels of burnout and found high levels of neuroticism, negative affectivity, and disengagement.[71] In summary, the literature indicates that neuroticism, low agreeableness, introversion, and negative affectivity are the main personality traits associated with burnout.

Senior workers tend to outperform younger employees in activities that require good interpersonal relationships, attention to detail, and meeting deadlines. They are more modest, conventional, careful in interactions, sympathetic, and helpful.[72,73] This expected evolution of personality dimensions is likely due to the accumulation of life events (experience) and somewhat free from social constraints causing people to be able to act in certain ways. In the work environment, these differences are noticeable in various ways in which junior surgeons and medical students, for example, have higher burnout rates than seasoned clinicians.[74]

Burnout and physical health

Clinical work can be stressful. Clinicians are repeatedly confronted with changing patient needs, fatigue, constant stress, high work volume, and work constraints compounded by productivity demands from other clinicians and hierarchical supervisors, poorly suited technology for task, unexpected morbidity or mortality, and malpractice claims arising from bad outcomes (sometimes) despite optimal care resulting in stress, burnout, and diminished job satisfaction.[75,76] Active disclosure eases clinicians conscience and this moral weight can be heavy depending on the clinician and the type and outcome of the event. Some clinicians, have even called clinicians who have been involved in patient harm 'the second victim'.[77] Other clinicians have admitted that they have felt better after disclosing an adverse event to a patient.[78]

External pressures—bringing up a family, societal demands, interpersonal relationships, extramural community leadership duties, financial pressures, teaching and research provisions, administrative duties, and time pressures from multiple competing tasks—all add to the mayhem of everyday life. Burnout among surgical team members is a negative, chronic, work-related state that is primarily characterized by emotional exhaustion, feelings of being overextended and depleted, depersonalization (indifferent attitude toward one's service or care), and negligible professional accomplishments.[55,79] In 2019, the World Health Organization added burnout to the International Classification of Diseases.

Burnout levels among surgical professionals can be as high as 50%. Surgeons, proceduralists, nurses, and allied health components are all affected to varying degrees.[53] Increasing stress levels are multifactorial, but stressors include high caseload, practice setting, unrewarding career, lack of autonomy, personal problems interfering with work, decreased clinical productivity, difficulty in funding research endeavors, diminution in reimbursement, rising debt, difficulty balancing personal and work life, inability to cope with patients' suffering and death, and a lack of administrative support.[80,81] This negativity can influence medical students as early as their second year when they are exposed, with limited training in patient safety and risk management, to the chaotic and unsafe clinical environments and management decisions that are seen as counter to their values (also called moral injury).[82,83] The negative impact of burnout on healthcare professionals' empathy and inability to alleviate the suffering of patients can decrease personal satisfaction and increase their burnout and compassion fatigue.[84] This, so called, 'cost of caring' can be measured by the Professional Quality of Life Protocols. Adapting Maslow's hierarchy of needs as a framework for surgical resident wellness has been shown to be very effective.[85]

Burnout is a response to long-standing stress at work sometimes associated with psychosomatic illness—muscular strains and injuries, cardiovascular disease, fibromyalgia, repetitive strain injury, and drug or alcohol abuse, sometimes culminating in suicide or self-harm.[61,86–88] In several studies, the incidence of psychosomatic symptoms among anesthesia staff was found to be substantially higher than among the general public.[41,86,89−91] Contributing factors included working night shifts, low social support, on-call−related stress caused by sleep deprivation and physical fatigue, lack of respect and trust from colleagues, and lack of autonomy (e.g., work pace and participation).[92] The consequences of stress are minimized by superior emotional intelligence skills that equip clinicians with more adaptive coping strategies.[93]

Clinicians could greatly benefit from recognizing the early warning symptoms of increased stress: anxiety, difficulty concentrating, feeling moody or tearful, overwhelmed or out-of-control, headaches, upset stomach and indigestion, high blood pressure, low self-esteem, lack of confidence, withdrawal, irritability, and failing personal and/or work relationships.[94,95]

Burnout often occurs among younger (age < 30 years) and less experienced clinicians, possibly due to 'reality shock' or 'early career burnout,' caused by a lack of job experience or by facing harsh realities of the operating theater suite coupled with pressures to raise and support young children.[55] However, others found that older employees experience higher sickness absence probably due to insufficient recovery time inducing physical and emotional exhaustion .[90,96] Short-term sickness absence is often considered as a type of coping behavior used in situations where a longer recovery period is needed as, for example, in cases of heightened stress.[61,97] The Hackman and Oldham's Job Characteristics Model states that job satisfaction reflects the coping capabilities of a person's competencies to work in their profession without developing stress. Based on this, it is suggested that the level of job satisfaction is a good predictor for long-term or repetitive sickness absence.[98] Burnout, psychosomatic symptoms, and sickness absence are negatively associated with job satisfaction.[90] Limited evidence is available thus far for effective strategies to prevent or decrease stress levels.[99] A physician's wellness hierarchy is effective when designed to prioritize interventions at the systems level.[100] Some studies demonstrate positive results with mindfulness and resilience training to increase surgical resident and faculty resilience and align personal and organizational goals with values by allocating specific and meaningful activities to professionals.[101−104] As burnout is a workplace-related issue, self-care may help in coping with burnout, but not preventing it. Employers are responsible to limit the causes of burnout and their accountability is insufficient when only self-care tools (mindfulness, yoga, etc.) are offered.[105] Maslach indicated the main causes of burnout are unfair treatment at work, unmanageable workload, unreasonable time pressure, lack of role clarity, communication over, and lack of support from managers as confirmed by the Gallup institute.[18,106]

Managing burnout starts with measuring burnout using the Maslach Burnout Inventory. Based on this data, effective interventions can be made at an organizational and pesonal levels.[107] Focusing on causes at an organizational and individual level, together with self-care, can facilitate healthcare professionals to recover from burnout.[108]

Fatigue and medical errors

Fatigue, a general term that describes physical and/or mental weariness, can affect personal and work life and contribute to burnout. Fatigue decreases performance and harms patients.[109] Errors increase after a 12 hour work shift, when more than 40 hours per week and during even modest overtime. It causes lapses of attention and memory, decreases the ability to detect and react to subtle changes in patient's vital signs, decreases speed and quality of intubations, causes a higher incidence of dural punctures with epidural anesthesia, and slows down information processing and abilities to manage unexpected situations.[110] Acute, and acute on chronic, fatigue contributes to communication difficulties probably caused by increased irritability.[111,112] These authors[113] found that fatigue levels of nurse anesthetists were comparable to people suffering from multiple sclerosis and twice as high as a healthy control group. Effective risk management strategies to reduce fatigue are multifactorial.[114,115] Firstly, healthcare providers should be educated on the inherent dangers of sleep deprivation, the risks associated with it, and the insidious impact on their and their team's performance. Clinicians need to consider their well-being by limiting their working hours, preventing disruption of sleep cycles, limiting alcohol and substance abuse, and eating and drinking in a sensible manner.[116–118]

Sustainable employability and its impact on occupational wellness and joy at work

Sustainable employability has become a new model to describe the employees and employers demands and resources for long-term and healthy careers. It consists of three dimensions: work ability, employability, and vitality.[119,120] Work ability is the physical, mental, and social ability to work and is also referred to as the 'House of Work Ability'.[121,122] The 'ground floor' of wellness includes the physical, mental, and social functional abilities of employees and their health/wellness state. The first floor represents the qualifications and competences. The second floor is about motivation, norms and values of employees. The third floor includes the physical and mental demands of work, working conditions, social environment, management and situational leadership. Friends, family, and society are the community in which the house is located and can influence the impact of the work to create a state of wellness.

Employability is necessary for career success and has five dimensions: balance (compromise between employers' interests and employees' own interests), anticipation and optimization (preparing for changes in order to optimize career outcomes), corporate sense (participating as members of an integrated team and anticipating the organizational culture and needs such as committee participation), personal flexibility (adapting to changes occurring in the work environment and clinical work schedules), and occupational expertise (the extent to which individuals are in possession of domain-specific knowledge and skills).[123] Studies about factors that influence sustainable employability focus not only on training and mobility but also on the health and safety measures that result from interventions at the individual, team, and organizational levels.

At an individual level this means employees should have the right knowledge, skills, and attitudinal competences and expertise to perform the work as part of a learning organization (life-long learning).[124] Possibilities to increase knowledge and skills are by job rotation and cross training, a form of informal learning. In this respect, self-efficacy (conviction of own abilities) is important as it increases the motivation for further development and the focus on employability,[125,126] creating more interest in career opportunities and increased career success.[127]

A healthcare organization can support and create the possibilities for development by offering job enrichment, job enlargement, job rotation, horizontal, and vertical flows in the organization. Further stimulation of employees' development can be established by offering continuing education, training, career opportunities and advice, with an explicit learning budget.[128] Furthermore, support from the supervisor can influence the employees' self-efficiency and job satisfaction.[129] Sustainable employability should be part of organizational governance and should involve employability policies that focus on improving life-long learning, policies that focus on factors that affect health (physical and mental), and an overall awareness of age-related needs and resources based on the workload and experiences of the employee (e.g., content of work, adapting work conditions, flexible work hours). Fig. 13.6 summarizes the range of interventions that employers and employees should consider to "break the paths" associated with burnout and help to improve job satisfaction, employee loyalty, and joy.

This chapter focuses on the incredibly important and growing awareness of addressing and optimizing the occupational well-being and joy of surgical team members given the reported large increase in burnout during the COVID-19 pandemic.[130] Growing evidence supports the importance of boosting joy at work and thus impacting staff engagement and productivity, as a means to improve the quality of care and experiences for staff and patients.

Successful interventions to enhance job satisfaction and mitigate against staff burnout should take into account the broad range of causes and should incorporate a variety of different therapeutic and integrated tools. Reducing stress is only one aspect of improving the working conditions of surgical team members and may not be sufficient to diminish the growing rates of burnout rate among surgical providers that have been exasperated by during the COVID-19 pandemic.[131] It is clear that the training in coping strategies, interpersonal skills to increase social support, management of negative emotions, improvement of communication skills, discussion of specific professional high-stress situations, and use of relaxation techniques should be considered.[132] Successful interventions during the COVID-19 pandemic undertaken at the institutional level have included adequate personal protective equipment (PPE) and a refresher training on proper PPE usage helped to mitigate the stress levels.[133] Workflows were established for managing infected patients in

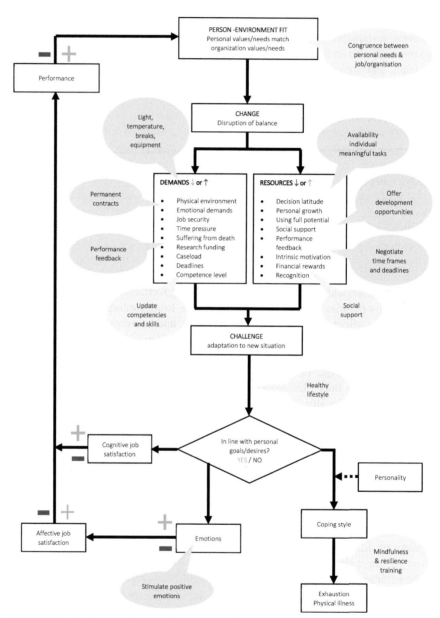

FIGURE 13.6 Mechanisms involved in burnout mitigation and acning job satisfaction.

Yellow balloons represent interventions initiated by the employer, while *blue* balloons represent interventions initiated by the employee.

different scenarios, and full-dress rehearsals were conducted to familiarize everyone with the various protocols. Staff members were sent daily e-mail updates on the progress of the pandemic.[134] Directives were updated regularly by the hospital management to keep up with the changing disease burden. Staff were also provided with resources for managing stress, such as confidential access to mental health professionals. Despite this, burnout rates and moral injuries did increase during the COVID-19 pandemic -strong cognitive and emotional response to events that violate somebody's moral or ethical code[135] Growing evidence suggests that moral injury increased during COVID-19 due to shortage of PPE, fear of catching COVID-19, breech in trust, short staffing, etc.[105,135,136] New generations of physicians and nurses should begin individual prevention training early in their careers in order to develop the skillsets and personal coping systems to provide effective inoculation against situations that may make them more prone to burnout.[137] A renewed focus on the importance of psychological safety, truth-telling, and nurturing teams all contribute to more trust, truth-telling and less likelihood of burnout and employee turnover.[138]

The roadmap for future research must include developing and sustaining team wellness and committing to serious and continuous team training that is structured, implemented, and evaluated to optimize patient safety in the perioperative setting.[139] These resilience strategies, as well demonstrated in other high-stress fields such as aviation and nuclear power, need to be adaptive and creative—not prescriptive. We must expand our understanding of the factors that drive burnout by using deep ethnographic social science methods and be informed by extensive research from occupational psychology and organizational learning. This approach explores how ideas such as job crafting—the process of actively engaging workers in codesigning their scope of work and providing them with structural job resources while minimizing negative job demands—may move us even further toward achieving a true reduction in resident and surgical team member burnout using targeted stressor countermeasures to improve training and well-being.[140] Involvement of all stakeholders, including policymakers, individual institutions, faculty, and residents, is imperative to making real and sustainable changes. The national and international dialogue on addressing the epidemic of burnout in the field of surgery and anesthesia must continue, inviting trainees and healthcare professionals at all levels to help codesign the surgical training ecosystem of the future and moving from burnout to wellness.

References

1. Gin N, Courneya P. Working to achieve the quadruple aim. *Perm J* 2020;**24**:20.046. https://doi.org/10.7812/TPP/20.046.
2. Wang A, Ahmed R, Ray J, Hughes P, Eric McCoy E, Marc A, Auerbach A, Barach P. Supporting the quadruple aim using simulation and human factors during COVID-19 care. *Am J Med Qual* 2021 March–April 01;**36**(2):73–83. https://doi.org/10.1097/01.JMQ.0000735432.16289.d2. PMID: 33830094; PMCID: PMC8030878.

3. Cosman P, Pramudith S, Barach P. Building surgical expertise through the science of continuous learning and training. In: Sanchez J, Barach P, Johnson H, Jacobs J, editors. *Perioperative patient safety and quality: principles and practice.* Springer; 2017, ISBN 978-3-319-44010-1.

4. Rosenbaum L. Cursed by knowledge—building a culture of psychological safety. *N Engl J Med* 2019;**380**(8). https://doi.org/10.1056/NEJMms1813429.

5. Salas E, Baker D, King H, Battles J, Barach P. On teams, organizations and safety. *Jt Comm J Qual Saf* 2006;**32**:109—12.

6. Barach P, Weinger M. Trauma team performance. In: Wilson WC, Grande CM, Hoyt DB, editors. *Trauma: emergency resuscitation and perioperative anesthesia management*, vol 1. New York: Marcel Dekker, Inc.; 2007. p. 101—13. ISBN: 10-0-8247-2916-6.

7. Schraagen JM, Schouten A, Smit M, van der Beek D, Van de Ven J, Barach P. Improving methods for studying teamwork in cardiac surgery. *Qual Saf Health Care* 2010;**19**:1—6. https://doi.org/10.1136/qshc.2009.040105.

8. Mitchell PH, Shortell SM. Adverse outcomes and variations in organization of care delivery. *Med Care* 1997;**35**(11):NS19—32.

9. Kohn LT, Corrigan JM, Donaldson M. *To err is human: building a safer health system.* Washington, DC: National Academy Press; 1999.

10. Brubakk K, et al. Associations between work satisfaction, engagement, and 7-day patient mortality; a cross-sectional survey. *BMJ Open* 2019;**9**:e031704. https://doi.org/10.1136/bmjopen-2019-031704.

11. Nepogodiev D, Martin J, Biccard B, Makupe A, Bhangu A. A global burden of postoperative death. *Lancet* 2019;**393**:401.

12. Singer JJ, Gaba DM, Geppert JJ, Sinaiko AD, Howard SK, Park KC. The culture of safety: results of an organization-wide survey in 15 California hospitals. *Qual Saf Health Care* 2003;**12**:112—8.

13. Bognar A, Barach P, Johnson J, Duncan R, Woods D, Holl J, Birnbach D, Bacha E. Errors and the burden of errors: attitudes, perceptions and the culture of safety in pediatric cardiac surgical teams. *Ann Thorac Surg* 2008;**4**:1374—81.

14. Barach P, Phelps P G. Clinical sensemaking: a systematic approach to reduce the impact of normalised deviance in the medical profession. *J R Soc Med* 2013;**106**(10):387—90.

15. Leggat S, Karimi L, Bartram T. A path analysis study of factors influencing hospital staff perceptions of quality of care factors associated with patient satisfaction and patient experience. *BMC Health Serv Res* 2017;**17**:739. https://doi.org/10.1186/s12913-017-2718-x.

16. Hackman JR, Oldham GR. *Work redesign.* Reading, MA: Addison-Wesley Publishing Company; 1980.

17. Meeusen V, Brown-Mahoney C, Van Dam K, van Zundert A, Knape J. Understanding nurse anaesthetists' intention to leave their job: how burnout and job satisfaction mediate the impact of personality and workplace characteristics. *Health Care Manag Rev* 2011;**36**(2):155—63.

18. Maslach C. Understanding burnout: definitional issues in analyzing a complex phenomenon. In: Paine WS, editor. *Job stress and burnout*; 1982. p. 29—40. Beverly Hills, CA.

19. Shanafelt TD, Bradley KA, Wipf JE, Back AL. Burnout and self-reported patient care in an internal medicine residency program. *Ann Intern Med* 2002;**136**(5):358—67.

20. Shanafelt TD, Balch CM, Bechamps GJ, et al. Burnout and career satisfaction among American surgeons. *Ann Surg* 2009;**250**(3):463−71.
21. Shanafelt TD, Balch CM, Dyrbye L, et al. Special report: suicidal ideation among American surgeons. *Arch Surg* 2011;**146**(1):54−62.
22. Kristof-Brown AL, Zimmerman RD, Johnson EC. Consequences of individuals'fit at work: a meta-analysis of person−job, person−organisation, person−group, and person−supervisor fit. *Person Psychol* 2005;**58**(2):281−342.
23. Kristof AL. Person-organization fit: an integrative review of its conceptualizations, measurement, and implications. *Person Psychol* 1996;**49**(1):1−49.
24. Demerouti E, Bakker AB, Nachreiner F, Schaufeli WB. A model of burnout and life satisfaction amongst nurses. *J Adv Nurs* August 2000;**32**(2):454−64. https://doi.org/10.1046/j.1365-2648.2000.01496.x. PMID: 10964195.
25. Bakker AB, Demerouti E, Euwema MC. Job resources buffer the impact of job demands on burnout. *J Occup Health Psychol* 2005;**10**:170−80.
26. Balch CM, Freischlag JA, Shanafelt TD. Stress and burnout among surgeons: understanding and managing the syndrome and avoiding the adverse consequences. *Arch Surg* 2009;**144**(4):371−6.
27. Brazeau CM, et al. Relationships between medical student burnout, empathy, and professionalism climate. *Acad Med* 2010;**85**(10 Suppl. l):S33−6.
28. Marr AJ. *Intrinsic/extrinsic motivation: the phony controversy.* 2008. www.drmezmer.com/.
29. Wilson TD, Gilbert DT. Affective forecasting. *Adv Exp Soc Psychol* 2003;**35**:346−411.
30. Hollerman JR, Schultz W. Dopamine neurons report an error in the temporal prediction of reward during learning. *Nat Neurosci* 1998;**1**(4):304−9.
31. DeCharms R. *Personal causation.* New York, NY: Academic Press; 1968.
32. Deci EL, Ryan RM. *Intrinsic motivation and self-determination in human behavior.* New York: Plenum; 1985.
33. Deci EL, Koestner R, Ryan RM. A meta-analytic review of experiments examining the effects of extrinsic rewards on intrinsic motivation. *Psychol Bull* 1999;**125**:627−68.
34. Eisenberger R, Pierce WD, Cameron J. Effects of reward on intrinsic motivation−negative, neutral and positive. *Psychol Bull* 1999;**125**(6):677−91.
35. Rathunde K, Csikszentmihalyi M. Undivided interest and the growth of talent: a longitudinal study of adolescents. *J Youth Adolesc* 1993;**22**(4):385−405.
36. Ryan RM, Deci EL. Intrinsic and extrinsic motivations: classic definitions and new directions. *Contemp Educ Psychol* 2000;**25**:54−67.
37. Bakker A, Hakanen J, Demerouti E, Xanthopoulou D. Job resources boost work engagement particularly when job demands are high. *J Educ Psychol* 2007;**99**:274−84.
38. Frey BS. On the relationship between intrinsic and extrinsic work motivation. *Int J Ind Organ* 1997;**15**:427−39.
39. Frey BS. *Not just for the money. An economic theory of personal motivation.* Cheltenham: Edward Elgar Publishing; 1997.
40. Flin R, Yule S, McKenzie L, Paterson-Brown S, Maran N. *Attitudes to teamwork and safety in the operating theatre.* 2006. www.thesurgeon.net/site/CMD=ORA/ArticleID/= 42d3a112-2e7b-4931-9b90-e5.
41. Kluger MT, Townend K, Laidlaw T. Job satisfaction, stress and burnout in Australian specialist anaesthetists. *Anaesthesia* 2003;**58**:339−45.
42. Fisher CD. Mood and emotions while working: missing pieces of job satisfaction? *J Organ Behav* 2000;**21**:185−202. http://www.jstor.org/stable/3100305.

43. Weiss HM, Cropanzano R. Effective Events Theory: a theoretical discussion on the structure, causes and consequences of affective experiences at work. In: Staw B, Cummings L, editors. *Research in organizational behaviour*, vol 18. Greenwich, CT: JAI Press; 1996. p. 1−74.

44. Spector PE. Behaviour in organizations as a function of employee's locus of control. *Psychol Bull* 1982;**91**:482−97.

45. Mullins LJ. *Management and organisational behaviour*. 5th ed. Harlow: Financial Times Prentice Hall; 2005.

46. Tietjen MA, Myers RM. Motivation and job satisfaction. *Manag Decis* 1998;**36**: 226−31.

47. Ramadanov N. Teamwork in a surgical department. In: Firstenberg MS, Stawicki SP, editors. *Teamwork in healthcare*. London: IntechOpen; 2020. https://doi.org/10.5772/intechopen.93698 [cited 2022 Mar 14]. Available from: https://www.intechopen.com/chapters/73280.

48. Warr PB. Decision latitude, job demands, and employee well-being. *Work Stress* 1990; **4**(4):285−94. https://doi.org/10.1080/02678379008256991.

49. Karasek JRA. Job demands, job decision latitude, and mental strain: implications for job redesign. *Adm Sci Q* 1979:285−308.

50. Agho AO, Mueller CW, Price JL. Determinants of employee job satisfaction: an empirical test of a casual model. *Hum Relat* 1993;**46**:1007−27.

51. Elmore LC, et al. National survey of burnout among US general surgery residents. *J Am Coll Surg* 2016;**223**(3):440−51.

52. Judge TA, Locke EA, Durham CC, Kluger AN. Dispositional effects on job and life satisfaction: the role of core evaluations. *J Appl Psychol* February 1998;**83**(1):17−34. https://doi.org/10.1037/0021-9010.83.1.17. PMID: 9494439.

53. Maslach C, Schaufeli WB, Leiter MP. Job burnout. *Annu Rev Psychol* 2001;**52**: 397−422.

54. Lynn MR, Morgan JC, Moore KA. Development and testing of the satisfaction in nursing scale. *Nurs Res* 2009;**58**(3):166−74.

55. Bruback K, Barach P, Tjomsland O. Hospital work environments affect the patient safety climate: a longitudinal follow-up using a logistic regression analysis model. *PLoS One* 2021;**16**(10):e0258471. https://doi.org/10.1371/journal.pone.0258471.

56. Lederer W, Kinzl F, Trefalt E, Traweger C, Benzer A. Significance of working conditions on burnout in anesthetists. *Acta Anaesthesiol Scand* 2006;**50**:58−63.

57. Michinov E, Olivier-Chiron E, Rusch E, Chiron B. Influence of transactive memory on perceived performance, job satisfaction and identification in anaesthesia teams. *Br J Anaesth* 2008;**100**(3):327−32.

58. Meeusen V, van Dam K, van Zundert A, Knape J. The influence of emotions on events and job satisfaction amongst Dutch nurse anaesthetists. *Int Nurs Rev* 2010;**57**:85−91.

59. Houtman I, Kornitzer M, De Smet P, Koyuncu R, De Backer G, Pelfrene E, Romon M, Boulenguez C, Ferrario M, Origgi G, Sans S, Perez I, Wilhelmsen L, Rosengren A, Isacsson S, Östergren P. The job stress, absenteeism and coronary heart disease European cooperative study (the JACE-study)-design of a multicenter prospective study. *Eur J Publ Health* 1999;**9**:52−7.

60. Friedberg MW, et al. Factors affecting physician professional satisfaction and their implications for patient care, health systems, and health policy. *RAND Health Q* 2014;**3**(4).

61. McManus IC, Keeling A, Paice E. *Stress, burnout and doctors' attitudes to work are determined by personality and learning style: a twelve year longitudinal study of U.K. medical graduates.* 2004. http://www.biomedcentral.com/1741-7015/2/29.

62. Unden AL. Social support at work and its relationship to absenteeism. *Work Stress* 1996;**10**:46−61.

63. Dusschoten-de Maat C. *Mensen maken het verschil.* Assen: Koninklijke Van Gorcum BV; 2004.

64. Watson D, Suls J, Haig J. Global self-esteem in relation to structural models of personality and affectivity. *J Pers Soc Psychol* 2002;**83**:185−97.

65. Meeusen V, Brown-Mahoney C, Van Dam K, van Zundert A, Knape J. Personality dimensions and their relationship to job satisfaction amongst Dutch nurse anaesthetists. *J Nurs Manag* 2010;**18**:573−81.

66. Connolly JJ, Viswesvaran C. The role of affectivity in job satisfaction: a meta-analysis. *Pers Indiv Differ* 2000;**29**:265−81.

67. McCrea RR, Costa PT. Reinterpreting the Myers-Briggs type indicator from the perspective of the five-factor model of personality. *J Pers* 1989;**57**:17−40.

68. Warr P, Miles A, Platts C. Age and personality in the British population between 16 and 64 years. *J Occup Organ Psychol* 2001;**74**:165−99.

69. Lue BH, Chen HJ, Wang CW, Cheng Y, Chen MC. Stress, personal characteristics and burnout among first postgraduate year residents: a nationwide study in Taiwan. *Med Teach* 2010;**32**(5):400−7.

70. Warr P. Age and work behaviour: physical attributes, cognitive abilities, knowledge, personality traits and motives. *Int Rev Ind Organ Psychol* 2001;**16**:1−36.

71. Gambles M, Wilkinson SM, Dissanayake C. What are you like? A personality profile of cancer and palliative care nurses in the United Kingdom. *Cancer Nurs* 2003;**26**: 97−104.

72. Dyrbye LN, Thomas MR, Shanafelt TD. Systematic review of depression, anxiety, and other indicators of psychological distress among US and Canadian medical students. *Acad Med* 2006;**81**(4):354−73.

73. Balch CM, et al. Distress and career satisfaction among 14 surgical specialties, comparing academic and private practice settings. *Ann Surg* 2011;**254**(4):558−68.

74. Tawfik DS, Profit J, Morgenthaler TI, et al. Physician burnout, well-being, and work unit safety grades in relationship to reported medical errors. *Mayo Clin Proc* 2018; **93**(11):1571−80.

75. Wu A. Medical error: the second victim. The doctor who makes the mistake needs help too. *Br Med J* 2000;**320**:726−7.

76. Cantor M, Barach P, Derse A, Maklan C, Woody G, Fox E. Disclosing adverse events to patients. *Jt Comm J Qual Saf* 2005;**31**:5−12.

77. World Health Organization. *Burn-out an "occupational phenomenon": international classification of diseases.* 2019. https://www.who.int/mental_health/evidence/burnout/en/.

78. Arora M, Diwan AD, Harris IA. Burnout in orthopaedic surgeons: a review. *ANZ J Surg* 2013;**83**(7−8):512−5. https://onlinelibrary.wiley.com/doi/full/10.1111/ans.12292.

79. Dimou FM, Eckelbarger D, Riall TS. Surgeon burnout: a systematic review. *J Am Coll Surg* June 2016;**222**(6):1230−9. https://doi.org/10.1016/j.jamcollsurg.2016.03.022. Epub 2016 Mar 25. PMID: 27106639; PMCID: PMC4884544.

80. Mayer D, Gunderson A, Klemen D, Barach P. Designing a patient safety undergraduate medical curriculum: the telluride interdisciplinary invitational roundtable experience. *Teach Learn Med* 2009;**21**(1):52−8.

81. Vohra P, Daugherty C, Mohr J, Wen M, Barach P. Housestaff and medical student attitudes towards adverse medical events. *JCAHO J Qual Saf* 2007;**33**:467−76.

82. Stamm BH. *The concise ProQOL manual.* 2nd ed. Pocatello, ID: ProQOL.org; 2010.

83. Hale AJ, Ricotta DN, Freed J, Smith CC, Huang GC. Adapting Maslow's hierarchy of needs as a framework for resident wellness. *Teach Learn Med* 2019;**31**(1):109−18.

84. Jackson SH. The role of stress in anaesthetists' health and well-being. *Acta Anaesthesiol Scand* 1999;**43**:583−602.

85. Melamed S, Shirom A, Toker S, Berlinger S, Shapira I. Burnout and risk of cardiovascular disease: evidence, possible causal paths, and promising research directions. *Psychol Bull* 2006;**132**:327−53.

86. Hawton K, Malmberg A, Simkin S. Suicide in doctors: a psychological autopsy study. *J Psychosom Res* 2004;**57**:1−4.

87. Meretoja OA. We should work less at night. *Acta Anaesthesiol Scand* 2009;**53**:277−9.

88. Meeusen V, Brown-Mahoney C, Van Dam K, van Zundert A, Knape J. Burnout, psychosomatic symptoms and job satisfaction among Dutch nurse anaesthetists: a survey. *Acta Anaesthesiol Scand* 2010;**54**:616−21.

89. Morais A, Maia P, Azevedo A, Amaral C, Tavares J. Stress and burnout among Portuguese anaesthesiologists. *Eur J Anaesthesiol* 2006;**23**:433−9.

90. Nurok M, Lee Y, Ma Y, Kirwan A, Wynia M, Segal S. Are surgeons and anesthesiologists lying to each other or gaming the system? A national random sample survey about "truth-telling practices" in the perioperative setting in the United States. *Patient Saf Surg* 2015;**9**:34. https://doi.org/10.1186/s13037-015-0080-7. Published online 2015 Nov 10.

91. Montes-Berges B, Augusto JM. Exploring the relationship between perceived emotional intelligence, coping, social support and mental health in nursing students. *J Psychiatr Ment Health Nurs* 2007;**14**:163−71.

92. Civil Aviation Safety Authority. Human performance. In: *Safety behaviours: human factors: resource guide for pilots.* 2nd ed. 2019.

93. Daniels AH, DePasse JM, Kamal RN. Orthopaedic surgeon burnout: diagnosis, treatment, and prevention. *J Am Acad Orthop Surg* April 2016;**24**(4):213−9. https://doi.org/10.5435/JAAOS-D-15-00148. PMID: 26885712.

94. Andrea H, Beurskens AJHM, Metsemakers JFM, Van Amelsvoort LGPM, Van den Brandt PA, Van Schayck CP. Health problems and psychosocial work environment as predictors of long-term sickness absence in employees who visited the occupational physician and/or general practitioner in relation to work: a prospective study. *Occup Environ Med* 2003;**60**:295−300.

95. Hardy GE, Woods D, Wall TD. The impact of psychological distress on absence from work. *J Appl Psychol* 2003;**88**:306−14.

96. Cropanzano R, Rupp DE, Byrne ZT. The relationship of emotional exhaustion to work attitudes, job performance, and organizational citizenship behaviors. *J Appl Psychol* 2003;**88**:160−9.

97. West CP, Dyrbye LN, Erwin PJ, Shanafelt TD. Interventions to prevent and reduce physician burnout: a systematic review and meta-analysis. *Lancet* 2016;**388**(10057):2272−81.

98. Shapiro DE, Duquette C, Abbott LM, Babineau T, Pearl A, Haidet P. Beyond burnout: a physician wellness hierarchy designed to prioritize interventions at the systems level. *Am J Med* 2019;**132**(5):556–63.

99. Rothenberger DA. Physician burnout and well-being: a systematic review and framework for action. *Dis Colon Rectum* 2017;**60**(6):567–76.

100. Lebares CC, Guvva EV, Ascher NL, O'Sullivan PS, Harris HW, Epel ES. Burnout and stress among US surgery residents: psychological distress and resilience. *J Am Coll Surg* 2018;**226**(1):80–90.

101. Van Wulfften Palthe OD, Neuhaus V, Janssen SJ, Guitton TG, Ring D. Among musculoskeletal surgeons, job dissatisfaction is associated with burnout. *Clin Orthop Relat Res* August 2016;**474**(8):1857–63. https://doi.org/10.1007/s11999-016-4848-6. Epub 2016 Apr 25. PMID: 27113597; PMCID: PMC4925415.

102. Salles A, Liebert CA, Esquivel M, Greco RS, Henry R, Mueller C. Perceived value of a program to promote surgical resident well-being. *J Surg Educ* 2017;**74**(6):921–7.

103. Song YK, Mantri S, Lawson JM, Berger EJ, Koenig HG. Morally injurious experiences and emotions of health care professionals during the COVID-19 pandemic before vaccine availability. *JAMA Netw Open* 2021;**4**(11):e2136150. https://doi.org/10.1001/jamanetworkopen.2021.36150.

104. Wigert B, Agrawal S. Employee burnout, part 1: the five main causes. In: *How to prevent employee burnout*. Washington, DC: The Gallup Institute; 2022.

105. Moss J. Rethinking burnout: when self care is not the cure. *Am J Health Promot* 2020;**34**(5):565–8. https://doi.org/10.1177/0890117120920488b.

106. Almén N. A cognitive behavioral model proposing that clinical burnout may maintain itself. *Int J Environ Res Publ Health* 2021;**18**(7):3446. 26.

107. Landrigan CP, Rothschild JM, Cronin JW, Kaushal R, Burdick E, Katz JT, et al. Effect of reducing interns' work hours on serious medical errors in intensive care units. *N Engl J Med* 2004;**351**:1838–48.

108. Gander PH, Merry A, Millar MM, Weller J. Hours of work and fatigue related error: a survey of New Zealand anaesthetists. *Anaesth Intensive Care* 2000;**28**:178–83.

109. Harrison Y1, Horne JA. The impact of sleep deprivation on decision making: a review. *J Exp Psychol Appl* 2000;**6**(3):236–49.

110. Rogers AE1, Hwang WT, Scott LD, Aiken LH, Dinges DF. The working hours of hospital staff nurses and patient safety. *Health Aff (Millwood)* 2004 July–August;**23**(4):202–12.

111. Meeusen V, Van Zundert A, Hoekman J. High fatigue levels in Dutch nurse anaesthetists. *AANA J (Am Assoc Nurse Anesth)* 2014;**82**(3):227–30.

112. Air Line Pilots Association International. *ALPA White Paper: fatigue risk management systems: addressing fatigue within a just safety culture*. June 2008. Available at: www.alpa.org/-/media/ALPA/Files/pdfs/news-events/white-papers/white-paper-fatigue-risk-management-systems.pdf?la=en. [Accessed December 2019].

113. Wong LR, Flynn-Evans E, Ruskin KJ. Fatigue risk management: the impact of anesthesiology residents' work schedules on job performance and a review of potential countermeasures. *Anesth Analg* 2018;**126**(4):1340–8.

114. Graves K, Simmons D. Reexamining fatigue: implications for nursing practice. *Crit Care Nurs Q* 2009 April–June;**32**(2):112–5. https://doi.org/10.1097/01.CNQ.0000348198.16788.df.

115. Williamson A, Friswell R. *Survey of pilot fatigue for Australian commercial pilots*. Australia: UNSW Fatigue Survey Report; 2017.

116. Sinha A, Singh A, Tewari A. The fatigued anesthesiologist: a threat to patient safety? *J Anaesthesiol Clin Pharmacol* 2013;**29**(2):151−9. https://doi.org/10.4103/0970-9185.111657.

117. Van der Klink JJL, Burdorf A, Schaufeli WB, Van der Wilt GJ, Zijlstra FRH, Brouwer S, Bültmann U. Duurzame inzetbaarheid bij oudere werknemers, werk als waarde. *Gedrag Organ* 2011;**4**(24).

118. Van Vuuren T, Caniëls MCJ, Semeijn JH. Duurzame inzetbaarheid en een leven lang leren. *Gedrag Organ* 2011;**4**:356−73.

119. Gould R, Ilmarinen J, Järvisalo J, Koskinen S. *Dimensions of work ability: results of the health 2000 survey.* Helsinki: Finnish Centre of Pensions (ETK), The Social Insurance Institution (KELA), National Public Health Institute (KTL), and Finnish Institute of Occupational Health (FIOH); 2008.

120. Ilmarinen J, Tuomi K, Seitsamo J. New dimensions of work ability. *Int Congr Ser* 2005; **1280**:3−7.

121. Van der Heijde CM, Van der Heijden BIJM. In: Costa G, Goedhard WJA, Ilmarinen J, editors. *The development and psychometric evaluation of a multi-dimensional measurement instrument of employability—and the impact of aging*; 2005.

122. Ramaswamy R, Barach P. Towards a learning system for enhanced recovery after surgery (ERAS): embedding implementation and learning evaluation. In: *Enhanced recovery after surgery—a complete guide to optimizing outcomes.* Olle Ljungqvist, Rich Urman and Nader Francis; 2020. p. 361−72. Ch. 39, ISBN 978-3-030-33443-7.

123. Hazelzet AM, Paagman H, El Marini S. Werknemers motiveren voor scholing. Het belang van een 'evidence based' aanpak. *Opleiding & Ontwikkeling* 2008;**10**.

124. Nauta A, Dessing R, Kooiman T. Carrière met kikkersprongen: met succes werken aan inzetbaarheid. *Gids Pers* 2008;**87**(10).

125. Bandura A. *Self-efficacy: the exercise of control.* New York: W.H. Freeman; 1997.

126. Schoppers M. *A study on sustainable employability of employees at 'Company X'.* The Netherlands: University of Twente; April 2014.

127. Meeusen V, Brown-Mahoney C, Van Dam K, Van Zundert A, Knape J. Discriminating work context factors in the working environment of Dutch nurse anaesthetists. *Acta Anaesthesiol Belg* 2008;**59**:1−7.

128. Barach P, Fisher S, Adams A, Burstein G, Brophy P, Kuo D, Lipshultz S. Disruption of healthcare: will the COVID pandemic worsen non-COVID outcomes and disease outbreaks? *Pediatr Cardiol* 2020. https://doi.org/10.1016/j.ppedcard.2020.101254.

129. Houdmont J, Daliya P, Theophilidou E, Adiamah A, Hassard J, Lobo DN, East Midlands Surgical Academic Network (EMSAN) Burnout Study Group. Burnout among surgeons in the UK during the COVID-19 pandemic: a cohort study. *World J Surg* 2022;**46**:1−9. https://doi.org/10.1007/s00268-021-06351-6.

130. Kabir T, Tan AYH, Koh FHX, Chew M-H. Burnout and professional fulfilment among surgeons during the COVID-19 pandemic. *Br J Surg* 2021:e3−5. https://doi.org/10.1093/bjs/znaa001.

131. Chew MH, Chau KC, Koh FH, Ng A, Ng SP, Ng SF, Tan MG, Ong SGK, Teo LM, Ong BC. Safe operating room protocols during the COVID-19 pandemic. *Br J Surg* August 2020;**107**(9):e292−3. https://doi.org/10.1002/bjs.11721. Epub 2020 Jun 7. PMID: 32506427; PMCID: PMC7300865.

132. Williamson V, Murphy D, Phelps A, Forbes D, Greenberg N. Moral injury: the effect on mental health and implications for treatment. *Lancet Psychiatry* 2021;**8**(6):453−5.

133. Auerbach MA, Abulebda K, Bona AM, Falvo L, Hughes PG, Wagner M, Barach PR, Ahmed RA. A national US survey of Pediatric Emergency Departments coronavirus pandemic preparedness. *Pediatr Emerg Care* January 1, 2021;**37**(1):48−53.

134. Luton OW, James OP, Mellor K, Eley C, Hopkins L, Robinson DBT, Lebares CC, Powell AGMT, Lewis WG, Egan RJ. Enhanced stress-resilience training for surgical trainees. *BJS Open* July 6, 2021;**5**(4):zrab054. https://doi.org/10.1093/bjsopen/zrab054. PMID: 34323917; PMCID: PMC8320339.

135. Edmondson A. Psychological safety and learning behavior in work teams. *Adm Sci Q* 1999;**44**(2):350−83. https://doi.org/10.2307/2666999.

136. Baker DP, Salas E, King H, Battles J, Barach P. The role of teamwork in the professional education of physicians: current status and assessment recommendations. *Jt Comm J Qual Patient Saf* April 2005;**31**(4):185−202. https://doi.org/10.1016/s1553-7250(05)31025-7. PMID: 15913126.

137. Robinson DBT, Luton O, Mellor K, James OP, Hopkins L, Powell AG, Hemington-Gorse S, Harries RL, Egan RJ, Lewis WG. Trainee perspective of the causes of stress and burnout in surgical training: a qualitative study from Wales. *BMJ Open* 2021;**11**:e045150. https://doi.org/10.1136/bmjopen-2020-045150. PMID 34341033.

138. Wickström G, Bendix T. The "Hawthorne effect"—what did the original Hawthorne studies actually show? *Scand J Work Environ Health* 2000;**26**(4):363−7. https://doi.org/10.5271/sjweh.555.

139. Bakker AB, Demerouti E. The job demands-resources model: state of the art. *J Manag Psychol* 2007;**22**(3):309−28.

140. Hughes AM, Doos D, Ahmed R, Pham T, Barach P. How can personal protective equipment be best used and reused: a closer look at donning and doffing procedures. *Disaster Med Public Health Prep* 2022;**26**:1−8. https://doi.org/10.1017/dmp.2022.209. PMID: 36155649.

Redesigning the operating room for safety

14

Marius Fassbinder, MD [1], **James H. Abernathy, III, MD, MPH** [2]

[1]*Assistant Professor, Department of Anesthesiology, George Washington University, Washington, DC, United States;* [2]*Interim Executive Vice Chair, ACCM, Chief, Division of Cardiac Anesthesiology, Core Faculty, Armstrong Institute of Patient Safety, Department of Anesthesiology & Critical Care Medicine, Johns Hopkins University, Baltimore, MD, United States*

Why design matters?

We have been designing hospital operating rooms (ORs) for nearly 300 years. One of the first such spaces was designed with seats so that observers at St Thomas Hospital in 1751 could watch and learn.[1] Consequently, even today, ORs are often referred to as operating theaters.

Prior to the establishment of ORs, surgical procedures took place on hospital wards, patient homes, or in doctors' consulting rooms. As medicine discovered important concepts such as antisepsis, and surgical techniques advanced, specifically designed rooms became a necessity. The size, layout, and design of these rooms have changed enormously over time to accommodate for the ongoing evolution in surgical practice and medicine.[1] Today, ORs are expected to facilitate an increasingly diverse variety of procedures. However, there is relatively little understanding about the impact of design on human error, and evidence showing effects of OR design on surgical outcomes is scarce. Given the rising complexity of surgical procedures and the introduction of robotic and hybrid procedures, these complex interactions between humans and machines become even more important. Understanding how design impacts errors will allow healthcare architects to create safer spaces for an ever-complex procedural environment. One type of error is described as a flow disruption, which is defined as an obstruction of the ideal workflow. Importantly, these flow disruptions have been linked to adverse patient events.[2,3] It stands to reason that if through optimizing the built environment we can reduce flow disruptions, then we can improve patient and provider outcomes.[4–7]

Is there an optimal OR design?

Little empiric evidence exists on the optimal layout and design of the hospital OR. It is imperative that design, size, and layout not lag behind surgical advances, a task difficult to achieve when hospital structures are built to last for decades while surgical changes occur more rapidly. The optimal OR environment is free from physical

Handbook of Perioperative and Procedural Patient Safety. https://doi.org/10.1016/B978-0-323-66179-9.00010-5

231

hazards to patients and workers; optimizes personnel flow; minimizes adverse events; provides optimal conditions for sterility, communication, concentration, efficiency, and comfort; prevents stress; and incorporates best practices to reduce environmental contamination. Key principles can be generalized as: standardize the position of the head of the table and the handedness of the room, provide adequate space for staff and equipment to move around, establish and maintain a line of sight for personnel to the patient at all times, and use technology to help workflow.[8,9] Many experts highlight these key points, but few studies provide a link to better outcomes. The following sections will take a closer look at studies and the importance of the physical space and ergonomics.[10]

Components of an OR

Layout

When a new OR is being designed, its layout will be influenced by its anticipated use balanced against available space and the cost of construction. Optimal layout in the OR should be guided toward facilitating personnel flow while maintaining patient and workers safety. Evidence exists that the layout of an OR can influence movement patterns as well as flow disruptions.[11,12] These disruptions in workflow during a surgical procedure have been linked to higher levels of stress, a higher perceived workload for surgical staff, increased surgery duration, and negative patient outcomes.[3,13–17] In one study, OR layout was the most frequent cause of flow disruptions.[12]

Key factors in the overall layout of ORs need to be divided into static factors such as overall size, storage cabinets, doors, access to gas and electrical supply, ventilation versus variable factors such as the placement of surgical and anesthesia equipment based on the anticipated surgery, the patient position, and the number of personnel.

Existing literature on the relationship between architectural layout and healthcare outcomes has primarily focused on understanding the dynamics of movement patterns at the unit level such as across surgical suites, across the hospital, or within units such as the general medical or surgical units and outpatient clinics.[18–24] Little work has focused on the movement patterns within small-scaled rooms, such as the OR. However, when developing the optimal layout, it is important to focus on the contribution of spatial adjacencies to work patterns and flow disruptions at a microsystems level. Architectural diagrams aimed at monitoring movement and interactions of OR personnel have been developed to help diagnose and address potential system design issues and to facilitate workflow within the operating unit. In order to analyze working patterns and flow within the OR, Ahmad et al. categorized the OR into eight different zones[11]:

1. Console zone
2. CN zone
3. Anesthesiology zone
4. Sterile zone
5. Supply zone 1
6. Supply zone 2
7. Transit zone 1
8. Transit zone 2

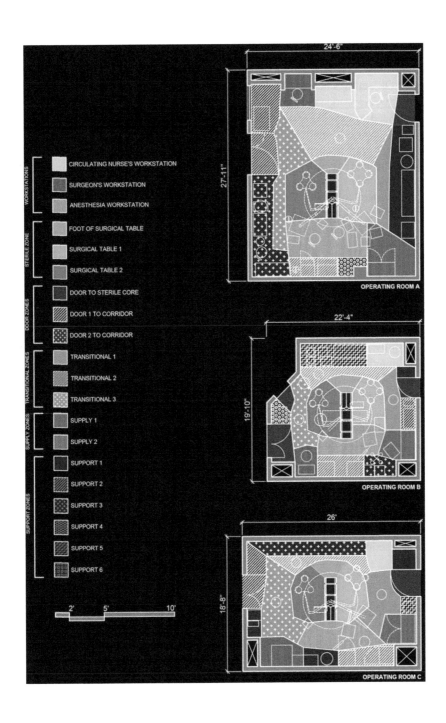

WORKSTATIONS
- CIRCULATING NURSE'S WORKSTATION
- SURGEON'S WORKSTATION
- ANESTHESIA WORKSTATION

STERILE ZONE
- FOOT OF SURGICAL TABLE
- SURGICAL TABLE 1
- SURGICAL TABLE 2

DOOR ZONES
- DOOR TO STERILE CORE
- DOOR 1 TO CORRIDOR
- DOOR 2 TO CORRIDOR

TRANSITIONAL ZONES
- TRANSITIONAL 1
- TRANSITIONAL 2
- TRANSITIONAL 3

SUPPLY ZONES
- SUPPLY 1
- SUPPLY 2

SUPPORT ZONES
- SUPPORT 1
- SUPPORT 2
- SUPPORT 3
- SUPPORT 4
- SUPPORT 5
- SUPPORT 6

2' 5' 10'

OPERATING ROOM A — 24'-6" × 27'-11"

OPERATING ROOM B — 22'-4" × 19'-10"

OPERATING ROOM C — 26' × 18'-8"

Floor plans of different operating rooms with assigned zones {Bayramzadeh: 2018hv}.

Circulatory nurse (CN) movement analysis during surgical procedures in different OR settings helped identify the need for adjacency between these specific zones. The CNs workstation serves as the central hub for CN activities. Due to the frequent need to provide additional equipment, direct proximity between the CNs workstation and the supply zone where key supplies are located is recommended. Indirect adjacency between the CNs workstation and the areas surrounding the surgical table is also suggested. This allows for a timely response while maintaining a safe distance from the sterile zone, thus avoiding contaminating the area. Unsuitable adjacencies need to be avoided to prevent the number of zones through which a CN travels. During video analysis by human factors engineers, transitional zones, those areas where two zones interface, were identified as high-risk zones for flow disruptions as they need to accommodate both equipment and personnel travel.[24] These findings provide scientific evidence to support certain principles[25]:

1. The importance principle: components and equipment that are vital to the achievement of a procedure or task should be placed in convenient locations
2. The frequency of use principle: components and equipment that are frequently used during the completion of a procedure or task should be located in close proximity and be easily accessible
3. The function principle: components, equipment, or information/displays that serve the same function or are commonly used together to make decisions or complete a task should be placed in similar locations or close to one another
4. The sequence of use principle: during completion of a procedure or task, certain tools and technology may be consistently used in a set sequence or order and should therefore be arranged in a manner to facilitate this process

It is important to note that the location of various equipment and other OR components may interfere with communication between nurses, anesthesia providers, and surgeons. Therefore, research (Realizing Improved Patient Care Through Human-Centered Design in the Operating Room RIPCHD.OR, AHRQ HS24380) is ongoing evaluating the optimal architectural layout based on human and equipment interactions in the OR.

Size

The optimal size for an OR varies based on the procedure. While the size for transplant ORs can sometimes exceed 75qm^2 (800 square feet), the common recommendation for cardiovascular ORs is around 55qm^2.[26]

Intuitively, one would think the bigger the better in order to reduce the amount of clutter and improving overall organization. Maybe, bigger rooms create storage space to accommodate all of the necessary equipment within the room. However, large ORs may decrease efficiency on various levels. While congestion may be prevented in certain spaces by the increase in size, areas such as the anesthesia workstation will still be affected by unavoidable equipment and personnel density. Increased space inadvertently leads to higher travel time to retrieve equipment from storage rooms. This creates potential for increasing flow disruptions and could increase surgical risks. Another problem could arise from difficulties in locating equipment. Increased OR size also correlates with decreased speech intelligibility. In one analysis, 40 ORs of varying size were assessed for acoustics. It was found that the increasing size correlated with impaired speech intelligibility, while increasing amounts of OR contents improved the acoustics.[27] The available evidence suggests that while an OR should be able to accommodate the necessary equipment and supplies, there may be a point at which increased size can itself be a cause of surgical errors.[26]

Noise

Effective communication is a critical precondition of effective teamwork and high-reliability performance in high-risk and high-consequence environments such as the OR. Noise levels in ORs can be deafening, however, and significantly impair communication. Sometimes, noise in the OR can reach levels up to 80 dB and higher, a level corresponding to the passing of a freight train at 15 m distance. Measured noise levels sometimes exceed both Occupational Safety and Health Administration and National Institute for Occupational Safety and Health standards.[28,29] At this level, surgical performance can be impaired.[30–32]

In the OR, auditory distractions most commonly stem from equipment alarms, OR traffic, conversations, and sometimes music.

Equipment-related alarms as a frequent cause for noise pollution need to be addressed. It was previously found that up to 90% of alarms generated during cardiac surgery are false positives or have no therapeutic effect, desensitizing staff to true alarms.[33] Research is needed for the development of more sensitive and specific alarm systems. The use of advanced algorithms and an improved systems design could help limit alarms generated by machinery.[34] The optimal placement of large equipment can further help in the reduction of noise.[27] Furthermore, standards should be developed across manufacturers that allow for differentiation among high alert alarms and simple attention requiring noises.

Efforts need to be made to reduce overall OR traffic, both from a noise and flow disruption perspective.[35] Strategies to reduce traffic include: preoperative briefings incorporating a discussion about equipment needed during the case can limit traffic.[36,37] Extraneous conversations should be limited as they contribute to the noise in the OR and distract members of the team. Conversations about nonsurgery-related topics were associated with significantly higher sound levels.[32]

Research findings about music in the OR remain controversial. Music can be relaxing to providers and reduce overall stress.[38] However, this can be compounded by the fact that a team consisting of nurses, surgeons, and anesthesiologists share different opinions on the optimal choice for music. What is relaxing to one of the team members can induce stress in the other.[39]

It has been suggested to address noise pollution in the OR via the "sterile cockpit" approach.[40] Yet, different members of the team share different cognitive workloads at different times during the case—making this suggestion impractical and impossible to implement. Structured and scripted conversations, while awkward, if used during key portions of the case can reduce noise clutter and improve communication.[41]

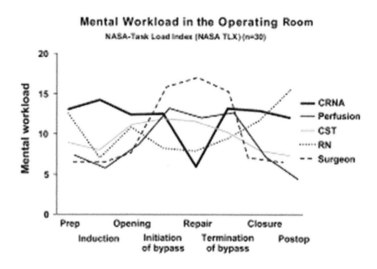

Cognitive workload measures during cardiac surgical procedures: (CRNA 1⁄4 certified registered nurse anesthetist; CST 1⁄4 certified surgical technologist; Postop 1⁄4 postoperative period; Prep 1⁄4 surgical preparation; RN 1⁄4 registered nurse). (Reprinted from Wadhera RK, Parker SH, Burkhart HM et al. Is the "sterile cockpit" concept applicable to cardiovascular surgery critical intervals or critical events? The impact of protocol-driven communication during cardiopulmonary bypass. The Journal of Thoracic and Cardiovascular Surgery. 2010;139:312–9, with permission from Elsevier).

Airflow and doors

Heating, ventilation, and air conditioning systems are crucial components in the OR with direct effects on infection rates.[42] Airflow must be carefully designed to maintain positive pressure in order to move contaminants away from the surgical field. Several different modes of OR ventilation exist (laminar airflow, ultraclean laminar airflow, and mobile zoned/exponential laminar airflow), with no clear evidence suggesting the benefit of one over another.[43–46] Nonetheless, having an effective system in place is important, since 80%—90% of bacterial contaminants in the OR stem from the ambient air.[47] Simultaneously, it remains critical that infection control and the prevention of surgical site infections include the prevention of hypothermia in the patient. Decreases in patient temperature have a clear, direct relationship to the incidence of surgical wound infections.[48]

Airflow within the OR is affected by the opening and closing of doors. The ability to enter and leave an OR is crucial but is important to limit traffic. Ample evidence exists between the amount of door openings and traffic and the risk for bacterial contamination of the OR.[49–53] Further, traffic through the OR can be a distractor to the team.[7]

The most common reasons for door openings during cases include retrieval of equipment and supplies, information issues, communication between surgeons or other clinical personnel not involved in the case, staff breaks, and shift changes. With proper design of rooms, equipment, and procedures, 60% of overall OR traffic can be prevented. The distribution and frequency of door opening times appear to be independent from the type of surgery and room layout, but it was found that during incision and closure times, significantly less traffic occurred.[54]

Despite multiple indicators pointing toward limiting door opening, no study to date could find beneficial results with limiting door access.[55] Nonetheless, taking all research findings into account, doors should be positioned away from the sterile field. Unnecessary traffic should be limited through preoperative discussion, improved communication strategies via phone, or electronic medical records. Design and layout should focus on positioning doors in a way to limit shortcuts and therefore decrease incentives to cross an OR when the workforce is not immediately taking part of the surgical case.

Equipment

Technological advancements and the introduction and distribution of laparoscopic and robotic surgery have led to an enormous influx of equipment to the OR. Equipment and machines can improve and save lives by rendering otherwise impossible procedures possible (i.e., procedures involving cardiac arrest and the use of the cardiopulmonary bypass machine (CBP)). The use of this equipment can be complicated, however, and often, new equipment occupies significant space leading to spatial congestion and subsequent obstruction of workflow. The overall increasing number of wires, tubes, and cables that go to and from the patient as well as between equipment and personnel have been identified as a significant cause of workplace injury and workflow disruptions.[56,57] Often times referred to as spaghetti syndrome, wires and cables are a frequent cause of slips, trips, and falls in the OR.[58] To address this problem use the ceiling space and the installation of ceiling-mounted booms to provide gas flow to the anesthesia machine or electricity for surgical equipment.[56] The introduction of color-coding for cables and wire arrangement in unique patterns on the ceiling for easier identification can be added.[9] Rubber mats can be used to cover exposed cables and wires on the floor to further decrease the chance of a fall. One organizational strategy may be to use the operating table as the central hub for electrical power, gases, and light sources.[9] The incorporation of wireless technology into the OR could further facilitate this process.

Given that traffic is a problem and there are many obstacles to movement in modern ORs, careful thought should occur as to the ideal placement of equipment workstations. Workstations between team members and the patient can hinder communication and obstruct the line of sight toward the patient. This can lead to poor coordination and communication between team members and subsequently disrupt flow. A systematic analysis of the design and usability of CBP machines recognized the human–machine interface as a particularly high-risk locale for error occurrence. Multiple problems with the overall positioning of the machine, controls, displays, alarms, shape, and workplace design were identified, highlighting the need to incorporate usability and ergonomics insight into the development of OR equipment.[59] Misuse, poor maintenance, design flaws, and the inherent risk of using a device have increased the risk to potentially causing harm.[60] Equipment-related problems are estimated to be the cause for >10% of flow disruptions during cardiac surgery procedures.[25,37,61,62] Equipment malfunction appears to be one of the major factors in flow disruptions, poor training, or lack of certification in the use of the device and poorly designed alarm systems add to the problem.[60] Technological advancements are implemented with incremental changes to the machines we work with. Attention is principally given to mechanical efficiency and biocompatibility, with little awareness of the impact of design changes on the human user.[59] Thankfully, this is slowly changing.

Concerning the optimal arrangement of OR equipment, one needs to consider that the same OR often needs to be used by different surgeons for different types of procedures. However, while maintaining a certain degree of flexibility for the positioning of a variety of equipment, it is important to note that flexibility and variability may not always be beneficial. One argument for standardization is that fewer errors and near misses occur when providers work in a familiar environment, and that the same location of cleaning supplies, the information monitor, and booms improve overall workflow.[56,62]

Ability to clean

A hallmark of a successful operation is one that is free from infection.[63] A comprehensive program to decrease surgical site infections must therefore include an assessment of the potential sources of contamination, including the OR environment.[64]

Since the advent of antisepsis, initiated by Lister in 1867, OR design has been heavily influenced by the need to eliminate infection.[65] The overall space and equipment available are considered major contributors to the cleanliness of the OR. Cleaning efforts should not only focus on shiny floors, but instead be broadened to equipment and high touch surfaces such as the anesthesia workstation.[66] It is recommended to use materials that can easily be wiped or washed and to eliminate corners that could collect debris. For decontamination of hard to reach surfaces such as undersurfaces of tables, the use of ultraviolet light has been suggested.[67−69] Automated ultraviolet radiation devices have been also shown to reduce the number of *Clostridium difficile* spores as well as *Enterococcus* and *Staphylococcus aureus* colony-forming units present in the OR.[70]

Future directions
How should we approach design?
With the increasing variety of surgical procedures and the growing use of advanced equipment and technology in the OR (i.e., robotic surgery, hybrid cardiovascular procedures), adequate OR design is likely to be a key component for success. Human factors engineering has been increasingly studying the interactions between the OR environment and personnel and there is an ongoing need for further study and improvement. Use of 3D video modeling to optimize layout prior to construction has been suggested in the past to facilitate this complicated process.[71] Direct observation and the analysis of personnel movement is a very important component, as it can help find solutions for the work as done.

Not all space is the same (retrofit, different sizes, different buildings, ambulatory, large academic medical centers)
While there is a growing need to concentrate efforts on developing optimal working conditions through optimal design, one needs to acknowledge that not all recommendations can be applied to all the environments. Optimal design and layout need to take into consideration existing constraints in existing size, function, financial budget, and the human factors (culture) component. Research in patient safety in the OR has shown that fewer near misses arise when providers work in a familiar environment.[62] It remains challenging to export successful interventions from one hospital location to different locations within the same hospital. It may be even more challenging to transfer findings to external hospitals, whether it is on a local, regional, or international level. Overall hospital culture likely plays an important role.[8]

Perfect design remains elusive. Slowly, with the help of talented groups of investigators like the RIPCHD.OR research group, we are gathering data about how the built environment can enhance staff experiences and improve patient outcomes.

References
1. Essex-Lopresti M. Operating theatre design. *Lancet* 1999;**353**:1007−10. https://doi.org/10.1016/S0140-6736(98)11356-9.
2. de Leval MR, Carthey J, Wright DJ, Farewell VT, Reason JT. Human factors and cardiac surgery: a multicenter study. *J Thorac Cardiovasc Surg* 2000;**119**:661−72. https://doi.org/10.1016/S0022-5223(00)70006-7.

3. Wiegmann DA, ElBardissi AW, Dearani JA, Daly RC, Sundt III TM. Disruptions in surgical flow and their relationship to surgical errors: an exploratory investigation. *Surgery* 2007;**142**:658−65. https://doi.org/10.1016/j.surg.2007.07.034.

4. Reijnen MMPJ, Zeebregts CJ, Meijerink WJHJ. Future of operating rooms. *Surg Technol Int* 2005;**14**:21−7.

5. McDermott MW. Neurosurgical suite of the future. I. *Neuroimaging Clin N Am* 2001;**11**:575−9.

6. Journal SBA. Distractions and interruptions in the OR: evidence for practice. Wiley Online Library; 2007.

7. Healey AN, Sevdalis N, Vincent CA. Measuring intra-operative interference from distraction and interruption observed in the operating theatre. *Ergonomics* 2007. https://doi.org/10.1080/00140130600568899.

8. Killen AR. Operating room redesign: building safety through a culture of teamwork. *Nat Rev Urol* 2008;**5**(4):171. https://doi.org/10.1038/ncpuro1097.

9. Ofek E, Pizov R, Bitterman N. From a radial operating theatre to a self-contained operating table. *Anaesthesia* 2006;**61**:548−52. https://doi.org/10.1111/j.1365-2044.2006.04622.x.

10. Matern U, Koneczny S. Safety, hazards and ergonomics in the operating room. Surg Endosc 2007;21:1965−1969. doi:10.1007/s00464-007-9396-4.

11. Ahmad N, Hussein AA, Cavuoto L, Sharif M, Allers JC, Hinata N, et al. Ambulatory movements, team dynamics and interactions during robot-assisted surgery. *BJU Int* 2016;**118**:132−9. https://doi.org/10.1111/bju.13426.

12. Palmer G, of JATJ. Realizing improved patient care through human-centered operating room design: human factors methodology for observing flow disruptions in the .... AnesthesiologyPubsAsahqorg; 2013.

13. Wheelock A, Suliman A, Wharton R, Babu ED, Hull L, Vincent C, et al. The impact of operating room distractions on stress, workload, and teamwork. *Ann Surg* 2015;**261**:1079−84. https://doi.org/10.1097/SLA.0000000000001051.

14. Weigl M, Antoniadis S, Chiapponi C, Bruns C, Sevdalis N. The impact of intra-operative interruptions on surgeons' perceived workload: an observational study in elective general and orthopedic surgery. *Surg Endosc* 2015;**29**:145−53. https://doi.org/10.1007/s00464-014-3668-6.

15. Gillespie BM, Chaboyer W, Fairweather N. Factors that influence the expected length of operation: results of a prospective study. *BMJ Qual Saf* 2012;**21**:3−12. https://doi.org/10.1136/bmjqs-2011-000169.

16. Zheng B, Martinec DV, Cassera MA, Swanström LL. A quantitative study of disruption in the operating room during laparoscopic antireflux surgery. *Surg Endosc* 2008;**22**:2171−7. https://doi.org/10.1007/s00464-008-0017-7.

17. Catchpole KR, Giddings AEB, de Leval MR, Peek GJ, Godden PJ, Utley M, et al. Identification of systems failures in successful paediatric cardiac surgery. *Ergonomics* 2007. https://doi.org/10.1080/00140130600568865.

18. Freihoefer K, Kaiser L, Vonasek D, Bayramzadeh S. Setting the stage: a comparative analysis of an onstage/offstage and a linear clinic modules. *Herd* 2018;**11**:89−103. https://doi.org/10.1177/1937586717729348.

19. Hurst K. UK ward design: patient dependency, nursing workload, staffing and quality—an observational study. *Int J Nurs Stud* 2008;**45**:370−81. https://doi.org/10.1016/j.ijnurstu.2006.09.007.

20. Lorenz WE, Bicher M, Wurzer GX. Adjacency in hospital planning. *IFAC-PapersOnLine* 2015;**48**:862−7. https://doi.org/10.1016/j.ifacol.2015.05.118.

21. Reiling JG, Knutzen BL, Wallen TK, McCullough S, Miller R, Chernos S. Enhancing the traditional hospital design process: a focus on patient safety. *Joint Comm J Qual Saf* 2004;**30**:115−24. https://doi.org/10.1016/S1549-3741(04)30013-4.

22. Zadeh RS, Shepley MM, Waggener LT. Rethinking efficiency in acute care nursing units: analyzing nursing unit layouts for improved spatial flow. *Herd* 2012;**6**:39−65. https://doi.org/10.1177/193758671200600103.

23. Zhao Y, Mourshed M, Wright J. *Factors influencing the design of spatial layouts in healthcare buildings*. 2009.

24. Bayramzadeh S, Joseph A, San D, Khoshkenar A, Taaffe K, Jafarifiroozabadi R, et al. The impact of operating room layout on circulating nurse's work patterns and flow disruptions: a behavioral mapping study. *Herd* 2018;**11**:124−38. https://doi.org/10.1177/1937586717751124.

25. ElBardissi AW, Sundt TM. Human factors and operating room safety. *Surg Clin North Am* 2012;**92**:21−35. https://doi.org/10.1016/j.suc.2011.11.007.

26. Heinke TL, Catchpole KM, Abernathy JH. *Designing for safety: the importance of the physical space*. 2017. p. 1−4. https://doi.org/10.1007/s40140-017-0223-8.

27. McNeer RR, Bennett CL, Horn DB, Dudaryk R. Factors affecting acoustics and speech intelligibility in the operating room: size matters. *Anesth Analg* 2017;**124**:1978−85. https://doi.org/10.1213/ANE.0000000000002118.

28. Fritsch MH, Chacko CE, Patterson EB. Operating room sound level hazards for patients and physicians. *Otol Neurotol* 2010;**31**:715−21. https://doi.org/10.1097/MAO.0b013e3181d8d717.

29. Hodge B, Thompson JF. Noise pollution in the operating theatre. *Lancet* 1990;**335**:891−4. https://doi.org/10.1016/0140-6736(90)90486-O.

30. Moorthy K, Munz Y, Adams S, Pandey V, Darzi A. A human factors analysis of technical and team skills among surgical trainees during procedural simulations in a simulated operating theatre. *Ann Surg* 2005;**242**:631−9. https://doi.org/10.1097/01.sla.0000186298.79308.a8.

31. Momtahan K, Hétu R, Tansley B. Audibility and identification of auditory alarms in the operating room and intensive care unit. *Ergonomics* 2007;**36**:1159−76. https://doi.org/10.1080/00140139308967986.

32. Kurmann A, Peter M, Tschan F, Mühlemann K, Candinas D, Beldi G. Adverse effect of noise in the operating theatre on surgical-site infection. *Br J Surg* 2011;**98**:1021−5. https://doi.org/10.1002/bjs.7496.

33. Imhoff M, Kuhls S, Gather U, Fried R. Smart alarms from medical devices in the OR and ICU. *Best Pract Res Clin Anaesthesiol* 2009;**23**:39−50. https://doi.org/10.1016/j.bpa.2008.07.008.

34. Kruger GH, Tremper KK. Advanced integrated real-time clinical displays. *Anesthesiol Clin* 2011:1−18. https://doi.org/10.1016/j.anclin.2011.05.004.

35. Joseph A, Khoshkenar A, Taaffe KM, Catchpole K, Machry H, Bayramzadeh S. Minor flow disruptions, traffic-related factors and their effect on major flow disruptions in the operating room. *BMJ Qual Saf* 2018. https://doi.org/10.1136/bmjqs-2018-007957. bmjqs−2018−007957−8.

36. Henrickson SE, Wadhera RK, ElBardissi AW, Wiegmann DA, Sundt TM. Development and pilot evaluation of a preoperative briefing protocol for cardiovascular surgery. *J Am Coll Surg* 2009;**208**:1115−23. https://doi.org/10.1016/j.jamcollsurg.2009.01.037.

37. Wahr JA, Prager RL, Abernathy III JH, Martinez EA, Salas E, Seifert PC, et al. Patient safety in the cardiac operating room: human factors and teamwork. *Circulation* 2013; **128**:1139−69. https://doi.org/10.1161/CIR.0b013e3182a38efa.

38. Wong SW, Smith R, Crowe P. Optimizing the operating theatre environment. *ANZ J Surg* 2010;**80**:917−24. https://doi.org/10.1111/j.1445-2197.2010.05526.x.

39. Hawksworth C, Asbury AJ, Millar K. Music in theatre: not so harmonious. *Anaesthesia* 1997;**52**:79−83. https://doi.org/10.1111/j.1365-2044.1997.t01-1-012-az012.x.

40. Rosinski DJ. Sterile cockpit or not: it's all about team and effective communication. *J Thorac Cardiovasc Surg* 2010;**140**:10−1. https://doi.org/10.1016/j.jtcvs.2010.03.016.

41. Wadhera RK, Parker SH, Burkhart HM, Greason KL, Neal JR, Levenick KM, et al. Is the "sterile cockpit" concept applicable to cardiovascular surgery critical intervals or critical events? The impact of protocol-driven communication during cardiopulmonary bypass. *J Thorac Cardiovasc Surg* 2010;**139**:312−9. https://doi.org/10.1016/j.jtcvs.2009.10.048.

42. Yavuz SS, Bicer Y, Yapici N, Kalaca S, Aydin OO, Camur G, et al. Analysis of risk factors for sternal surgical site infection emphasizing the appropriate ventilation of the operating theaters. *Infect Control Hosp Epidemiol* 2006;**27**:958−63. https://doi.org/10.1086/506399.

43. Friberg B, Friberg S, Burman LG. Correlation between surface and air counts of particles carrying aerobic bacteria in operating rooms with turbulent ventilation: an experimental study. *J Hosp Infect* 1999;**42**:61−8. https://doi.org/10.1053/jhin.1998.0542.

44. Friberg B, Lindgren M, Karlsson C, Bergström A, Friberg S. Mobile zoned/exponential LAF screen: a new concept in ultra-clean air technology for additional operating room ventilation. *J Hosp Infect* 2002;**50**:286−92. https://doi.org/10.1053/jhin.2001.1164.

45. Friberg B, Friberg S, Ostensson R, Burman LG. Surgical area contamination−comparable bacterial counts using disposable head and mask and helmet aspirator system, but dramatic increase upon omission of head-gear: an experimental study in horizontal laminar air-flow. *J Hosp Infect* 2001;**47**:110−5. https://doi.org/10.1053/jhin.2000.0909.

46. Friberg S, Ardnor B, Lundholm R, Friberg B. The addition of a mobile ultra-clean exponential laminar airflow screen to conventional operating room ventilation reduces bacterial contamination to operating box levels. *J Hosp Infect* 2003;**55**:92−7.

47. Howorth FH. Prevention of airborne infection in operating rooms. *J Med Eng Technol* 1987;**11**:263−6.

48. Kurz A, Sessler DI, Lenhardt R. *Perioperative normothermia to reduce the incidence of surgical-wound infection and shorten hospitalization.* 2009. https://doi.org/10.1056/NEJM199605093341901.

49. Scaltriti S, Cencetti S, Rovesti S, Marchesi I, Bargellini A, Borella P. Risk factors for particulate and microbial contamination of air in operating theatres. *J Hosp Infect* 2007;**66**:320−6. https://doi.org/10.1016/j.jhin.2007.05.019.

50. Andersson AE, Bergh I, Karlsson J, Eriksson BI, Nilsson K. Traffic flow in the operating room: an explorative and descriptive study on air quality during orthopedic trauma implant surgery. *Am J Infect Control* 2012;**40**:750−5. https://doi.org/10.1016/j.ajic.2011.09.015.

51. Villafruela JM, San José JF, Castro F, Zarzuelo A. Airflow patterns through a sliding door during opening and foot traffic in operating rooms. *Build Environ* 2016;**109**:190−8. https://doi.org/10.1016/j.buildenv.2016.09.025.

52. Mousavi ES, Grosskopf KR. Airflow patterns due to door motion and pressurization in hospital isolation rooms. *Sci Technol Built Environ* 2016. https://doi.org/10.1080/23744731.2016.1155959.

53. Teter J, Guajardo I, Al-Rammah T, Rosson G, Perl TM, Manahan M. Assessment of operating room airflow using air particle counts and direct observation of door openings. *Am J Infect Control* 2017;**45**:477−82. https://doi.org/10.1016/j.ajic.2016.12.018.

54. Mousavi ES, Jafarifiroozabadi R, Bayramzadeh S, Joseph A, San D. An observational study of door motion in operating rooms. *Build Environ* 2018;**144**:502−7. https://doi.org/10.1016/j.buildenv.2018.08.052.

55. Bohl MA, Clark JC, Oppenlander ME, Chapple K, Budde A, Lei T, et al. The barrow randomized operating room traffic (BRITE) trial: an observational study on the effect of operating room traffic on infection rates. *Neurosurgery* 2016;**63**(Suppl. 1):91−5. https://doi.org/10.1227/NEU.0000000000001295.

56. Brogmus G, Leone W, Butler L, Hernandez E. Best practices in OR suite layout and equipment choices to reduce slips, trips, and falls. *AORN J* 2007;**86**:384−94. https://doi.org/10.1016/j.aorn.2007.06.003. quiz395−8.

57. Weerakkody RA, Cheshire NJ, Riga C, Lear R, Hamady MS, Moorthy K, et al. Surgical technology and operating-room safety failures: a systematic review of quantitative studies. *BMJ Qual Saf* 2013;**22**:710−8. https://doi.org/10.1136/bmjqs-2012-001778.

58. Cesarano FL, Piergeorge AR. The Spaghetti Syndrome. A new clinical entity. *Crit Care Med* 1979;**7**:182−3.

59. Wiegmann D, Suther T, Neal J, Parker SH, Sundt TM. A human factors analysis of cardiopulmonary bypass machines. *J Extra Corpor Technol* 2009;**41**:57−63.

60. Martinez EA, Thompson DA, Errett NA, Kim GR, Bauer L, Lubomski LH, et al. Review article: high stakes and high risk: a focused qualitative review of hazards during cardiac surgery. *Anesth Analg* 2011;**112**:1061−74. https://doi.org/10.1213/ANE.0b013e31820bfe8e.

61. Savoldelli GL, Thieblemont J, Clergue F, Waeber J-L, Forster A, Garnerin P. Incidence and impact of distracting events during induction of general anaesthesia for urgent surgical cases. *Eur J Anaesthesiol* 2009:1−13. https://doi.org/10.1097/EJA.0b013e328333de09.

62. Christian CK, Gustafson ML, Roth EM, Sheridan TB, Gandhi TK, Dwyer K, et al. A prospective study of patient safety in the operating room. *Surgery* 2006;**139**:159−73. https://doi.org/10.1016/j.surg.2005.07.037.

63. Jenney AW, Harrington GA, Russo PL, Spelman DW. Cost of surgical site infections following coronary artery bypass surgery. *ANZ J Surg* 2001;**71**:662−4.

64. Wahr JA, Abernathy JHI. Environmental hygiene in the operating room: cleanliness, godliness, and reality. *Int Anesthesiol Clin* 2013;**51**:93−104. https://doi.org/10.1097/AIA.0b013e31827da44b.

65. Lister BJ. *The classic: on the antiseptic principle in the practice of surgery. 1867*, vol 468. Springer-Verlag; 2010. https://doi.org/10.1007/s11999-010-1320-x.

66. Guh A, Carling P. *Options for evaluating environmental cleaning*. 2010.

67. Ritter MA, Olberding EM, Malinzak RA. Ultraviolet lighting during orthopaedic surgery and the rate of infection. *JBJS* 2007;**89**:1935. https://doi.org/10.2106/JBJS.F.01037.

68. Taylor GJ, Chandler L. Ultraviolet light in the orthopaedic operating theatre. *Br J Theatre Nurs* 1997;**6**:10−4.

69. Taylor GJS, Bannister GC, Leeming JP. Wound disinfection with ultraviolet radiation. *J Hosp Infect* 1995;**30**:85−93. https://doi.org/10.1016/0195-6701(95)90148-5.
70. Nerandzic MM, Cadnum JL, Pultz MJ, Donskey CJ. Evaluation of an automated ultraviolet radiation device for decontamination of Clostridium difficile and other healthcare-associated pathogens in hospital rooms. *BMC Infect Dis* 2010;**10**:197. https://doi.org/10.1186/1471-2334-10-197.
71. Watkins N, Kobelja M, Peavey E, Thomas S, Lyon J. An evaluation of operating room safety and efficiency: pilot utilization of a structured focus group format and three-dimensional video mock-up to inform design decision. *Herd* 2011;**5**:6−22.

A perioperative safety and quality change management model and case study: Muda Health

15

Paul Barach, B.Med.Sci, MD, MPH, Maj (ret.), AUA [1,2], Hal Wiggin, PhD [3], Paul Risner, JD [8], Julie Johnson, MSPH, PhD [4], Dave Patrishkoff, MA [5], Shankar Kurra, MD, MBA [6], Becky Southern, RN [9], Edward Popovich, PhD [7]

[1]*College of Population Health, Thomas Jefferson University, Philadelphia, PA, United States;* [2]*Sigmund Frued University, Vienna, Austria;* [3]*Dr Koran C Patel College of Osteopathic Medicine, Health Informatics Department, Nova Southeastern University, Fort Lauderdale, FL, United States;* [4]*Department of Surgery, Feinberg School of Medicine, Northwestern University, Chicago, IL, United States;* [5]*Dr Patel College of Osteopathic Medicine, Nova Southeastern University, Fort Lauderdale, FL, United States;* [6]*Sentara Virginia Beach General, Virginia Beach, VA, United States;* [7]*Dr Koran C Patel, College of Osteopathic Medicine, Nova Southeastern University, Fort Lauderdale, FL, United States;* [8]*President, Paul E. Risner, P.A;* [9]*Caldwell Butler Associates*

Every system is perfectly designed to get the results it gets.

— **Paul Batalden, M.D.**

Introduction

The surgical space is a high-risk environment where hazards lurk around every corner and for every patient. The patients who come to surgery are generally among the sickest and at more advanced stages of disease. The very act of treatment involves risky interventions that are often considerably invasive with vigorous and unpredictable physiologic responses. The level of complexity, both in task-oriented and cognitive demands, results in a dynamic, unforgiving environment that can magnify the consequences of even small lapses and errors and undermine patient safety.

The lifeblood of a hospital's revenue cycle is having well-orchestrated perioperative services as these services typically generate around 60% of overall hospital revenue. The operating room (OR) is one of the most complex and challenging areas, and value streams with multiple inputs and outputs (Fig. 15.1). Due to the revenue impact of perioperative services, hospital leadership desires to ensure that perioperative services are well managed by achieving constant readiness, improving

Handbook of Perioperative and Procedural Patient Safety. https://doi.org/10.1016/B978-0-323-66179-9.00009-9

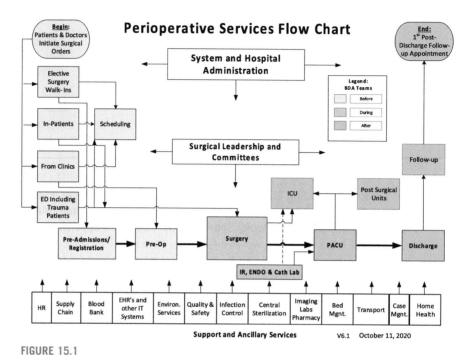

FIGURE 15.1

Perioperative services flow chart.

workflow, maximizing throughput, and ensuring surgery is performed in the safest environment for the patient.

This case study is based on the work at a Level One trauma healthcare system during the years 2020–22. We have changed the name to Muda Health (MH), part of the MH system, with a suburban and rural market presence. The work was sponsored by MH hospital leadership along with the engagement of surgical and nursing clinicians, quality management and infection control staff, and guided by external quality improvement and system change consultants.[1] The project was initiated due to increased surgical adverse safety events, inefficient services, low national quality ratings, and surgical site infection rates above the national averages.

The case study describes the transformation efforts, provides an overview of the new governance structure put in place to facilitate the transformation, details the methods, tools, and analytical approaches to the safety management of perioperative services, and discusses the results of the transformation efforts. The purpose of the transformation was to engage leadership and staff by leading, facilitating, and lending real-time support to ensure nurses and surgeons are teaming up in a highly aligned collaborative environment. The external facilitation challenge was to

---

[1] https://jbarainnovation.com.

empower front line staff to work and deliver improved surgical outcomes, making the hospital more efficient, and leading to increasing levels of patient and staff satisfaction.

Case study
Muda Health

MH's flagship hospital is a 250-bed community-based urban safety net hospital with a stated mission "to make a difference, every day." MH traces its history over 100 years. The system offers care in over 30 medical specialties serving 12 communities. MH provides over 5000 physicians and caregivers in the five-hospital system. As surgical services are the primary revenue source for MH, it is a high priority for driving performance improvement. Surgery schedules at MH drive the operations of many other departments. Three significant challenges to creating an efficient MH surgery schedule include the following:

- Estimating the duration of surgery;
- Scheduling cases to maximize the utilization of all ORs; and
- Clearing patients for surgery well ahead of the scheduled surgery to avoid any delays in the start of the scheduled surgery.

Scheduling and follow-through utilization of ORs impacts high cost resources within both the postanesthesia care unit (PACU) and intensive care unit (ICU), while potentially leading to wasteful utilization of supplies. Scheduling of the OR suites affects nursing schedules along with inpatient bed capacity. The VP of surgical services fields numerous demands including surgeon requests, changing staffing requirements, and capacity issues, all of which challenge the surgical schedule. MH leadership expressed a clear need for a more effective surgical scheduling process that considers five key guiding principles: patient safety, access, OR efficiency, patient service, and physician satisfaction. In addition, timely patient clearance is necessary to avoid patients arriving at preop without complete documentation including patient history and physicals, test results, preop orders, or consents which could delay surgery if incomplete. Figure 15.1 represents a procoess map of pre-, intraop- and post-op surgical services.

What was done?

We used the Assessment—Discovery—Action—Manage—Sustain (ADAMS) framework in the case study (Fig. 15.2):

a) Assessment
    a. Evaluated key organizational, strategic, and structural elements of the surgical services, ensured alignment of the baseline governance structure/

ADAMS

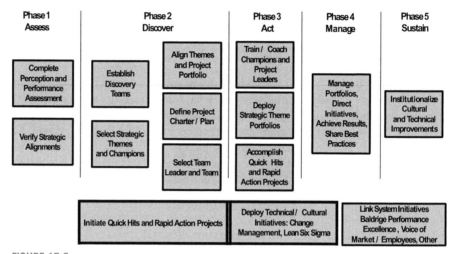

FIGURE 15.2

ADAMS change management model.
ADAMS—assess—discover—act—-manage—sustain.

leadership/operating performance with desired goals of developing highly reliable perioperative services delivery.

b. Identified and explored the factors that impede stable perioperative workflow.

b) Discover

a. Built consensus of the practices that help optimize OR team performance.

b. Brokered agreement on a new governance structure that will facilitate improvement in quality and patient/staff safety, cost/margins, and timeliness of delivery.

c) Action

a. Deployed a system of scorecards (high-level outcome measures) and dashboards (process performance measures) for quality/safety, cost (margin enhancement), time (surgical services throughput) that form the basis for improved decision-making.

b. Empowered physicians and staff to improve and innovate flow using a coaching model that used new teams that oversee the following:

  i. Presurgical process—we call the "before" phase,

  ii. During surgery process—we call the "during" phase,

  iii. Postsurgical process—we call the "after" phase.

    c. Provided a forum for receiving feedback and suggestions from other hospital stakeholders that support or benefit from the successful outcomes of surgical services (e.g., radiology, pathology, facilities, nursing units, ICUs, supply chain management, quality department, facility management, patient scheduling). A formal team called the "Voice of the Staff Team" (VST) was created to gather the feedback and suggestions that could be discussed and then relayed anonymously or without fear of retribution to the senior leadership team (SLT) and the **BDA (Before/During/After) teams.**

    d. Required the SLT to provide a structured forum to regularly (e.g., biweekly or monthly) receive updates from the BDA teams and VST regarding accomplishments since the previous forum meeting, anticipated next steps, along with challenges they face for which they seek leadership support and actions.

d) Manage

    a. Hospital and Physician Leadership agreed to take on the challenges to success that were identified by the BDA teams and VST so as to remove barriers to success.

    b. Deployed ongoing monitoring to ensure improvement and innovation efforts are borne out by the scorecards/dashboard system developed and put in place. Note: Scorecards provided outcome measures for all of perioperative services, while dashboards provided process and outcome measures for particular processes corresponding to the Before–During–After surgery processes.

    c. Held regular board and leadership review of perioperative services quality and safety efforts and results.

e) Sustain (Planned to be done in the future)

    a. Translated the governance structure for perioperative services to other service lines in the hospital including emergency medicine, women's and children services, outpatient diagnostic services including radiology and pathology, etc.

    b. Trained and engaged hospital staff and physicians in TeamSTEPPS training to enhance the transformation to a High Reliability Organization (HRO) for all MH Hospitals.

    c. Maintained a "parking lot" of project opportunities to improve/innovate that can be prioritized in order to sanction future projects to enhance MH ability to further drive its mission.

High reliability organization (HRO) framework for surgery quality improvement (Fig. 15.3)

HROs have characteristics that parallel many features of the surgical environment, including the use of complex technologies, a fast-paced tempo of operations, and a high level of risk, yet they have spectacularly low error rates. HROs are required

The Overlapping MH Surgical Process Metrics

The **J Bara Innovation** Group prepared, coached, mentored and supported MH project teams for each of the 4 metrics shown below, over an 18-month period to maximize and accelerate quantifiable improvements.

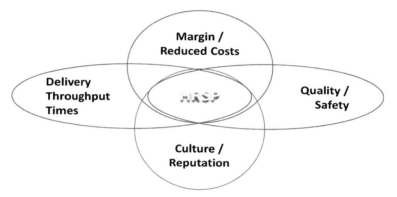

Great performances in the 4 main Metric areas can result in a
Sustainable and **High Reliability Surgical Processes (HRSP)**

FIGURE 15.3

Surgical quality compass model-high reliability surgical process metrics (HRSP-High reliability surgical processes).

to respond to a wide variety of situations under changing environmental conditions in a reliable and consistent way. The "pillars" of success for surgical process improvement are highly dependent on the interpersonal and group dynamics relative to communication, teamwork, shared goals, and an environment that fosters a "policy of no surprises" and zero defects. Mutual respect and shared responsibility are predicated on radical transparency of data and team performance, truth telling even when the news is not positive, and staff having psychological safety to speak up and out about safety concerns. They also use shared goals and knowledge of improvement to sustain a learning and trusting community.[2] Perioperative services depend on several communication handoffs including to and from inpatient floors and outpatient services, between physicians and nurses, in preop, surgery, PACU, tech staff and management, etc. Extensive research estimates that improving communication tools or methods can lead to an improvement of 80%—90% in patient handoffs and in surgical quality performance.[3]

---

[2] The more I know, the less I sleep, global perspectives on clinical governance. Lead author Berg M, Barach P, et al. KPMG Global Health Practice. 2013.
[3] Sanchez J, Barach P. High reliability organizations and surgical microsystems: Re-engineering surgical care. Surg Clin 2012;**92**(1):1—14. https://doi.org/10.1016/j.suc.2011.12.005.

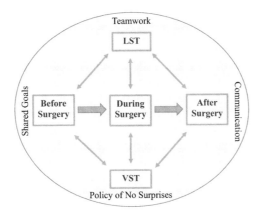

FIGURE 15.4

MH surgical improvement project new governance model.
LST—Leadership steering team; VST—Voice of the staff.

In this case study, the deployment of HRO methods facilitated the improvement of a surgical safe culture at MH that got more accustomed to "telling the truth" and addressing process variation in services or patient harm issues quickly and resolutely. Improvements in communication may lead to a significant level of quality performance improvement.[4] We used a just-in-time training approach with regular refresher drill downs as needed in concert with the Before—During—After (BDA) teamwork (Fig. 15.4) to enhance the HRO deployment, increasing awareness and engagement of leadership and BDA team members to address deployment deficiencies. We introduced the nationally acclaimed training program, TeamSTEPPS, a set of "Strategies and Tools to Enhance Performance and Patient Safety,"[5] to MH clinicians and staff through an online and in-person curriculum delivery supported by a dedicated project intranet website. This included role playing, case studies, and involvement of hospital personnel in enhancing both HRO and teamwork methods. The communication topics included active listening, empathic communication, interprofessional learning, conflict engagement, negotiation and relational coordination.[6]

[4] Amalberti R, Auroy Y, Berwick DM, Barach P. Five system barriers to achieving ultra-safe health care. Ann Intern Med 2005;**142**(9):756—764.

[5] Baker D, Battles J, King H, Salas E, Barach P. The role of teamwork in the professional education of physicians: current status and assessment recommendations. Joint Comm J Qual Saf 2005;**31**(4): 185—202.

[6] https://heller.brandeis.edu/relational-coordination/about-rc/index.html.

How was the quality improvement activity implemented?

MH recruited a multidisciplinary team of surgeons and other surgical team members, infectious disease specialists, and an antimicrobial stewardship pharmacist to create a core QI team and to conduct an initial analysis and identify opportunities for improvement. Problem characterization early is key (Box 15.1-Problem Statement) through fishbone analysis and process mapping, Supplier—Input—Process—Output Customer (SIPOC) analysis and Point-of-Pain analysis revealed that creating a clear, evidence-based guideline for surgical site infection mitigation and improved surgical flow required consistent definitions (Figs. 15.5 and 15.6).

Getting started. The team anticipated that acceptance and implementation of a new practice guideline with a large group of private practice surgeons and anesthesiologists working in surgical teams would be challenging. MH identified and engaged key stakeholders including nurses, physicians, pharmacists, and administrators through education sessions and regular team rounds led by MH surgical QI team leads and the consultant team. Teams agreed on clear and measurable goals (see Box 15.2-Goal Statement). All stakeholders were provided with an opportunity to raise their "points of pain," review, and provide early, often, and ongoing feedback throughout the project (Fig. 15.7). The MH core QI team met weekly to monitor progress through the cycles, sought feedback, to ensure success with implementation. The consulting team reviewed the literature as well as guidelines from other institutions and interviewed and surveyed MH clinicians. This information was used to create practice recommendations.

A focus was placed on reducing potential safety risks that contribute to adverse events, infections, delays, and returns to the OR. In doing so, we utilized a team of

---

Box 15.1 Problem statement

- The problem statement is a clear articulation of the problem that the organization is experiencing.
- It is intended to provide focus on the current problem or constraint that is hindering the attainment of an organizational objective.
- Describes the problem in sufficient detail for anybody to understand.
- Usually expressed in higher level terms rather than low-level details.
- Uses plain language with a minimum of jargon.
- Intended to help teams focus on a very specific issue to address.
- Usually takes more than a simple phrase or sentence to fully describe.
- States and quantifies the magnitude and impact of the problem.
- Helps to prioritize resources and funding.

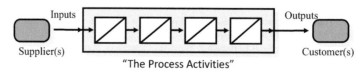

FIGURE 15.5

Identify the customers, suppliers, input, and outputs (SIPOC).

Mapping of the Work Flow Process (SIPOC Diagram)

Suppliers	Inputs	Process Requirements	Processes	Outputs	Customer Requirements	Customers
Who supplies the required process inputs?	What inputs are required?	What do the workers in the process require from each input?	What are the major steps in the process?	What are the process outputs/deliverables?	What does the customer expect from each output?	Who receives the outputs?
-Emergency Dept -Surgery Clinic -Inpatient Units -Admissions -Anesthesia -Biomed Engineering -HR -Supply Chain -Central Sterile	-Surgical order placed -Prep for case	-Appropriate and complete	Scheduling	-Scheduled surgery -Pre surgery education/instructions -Patient procedure type/class -PAT patient calling list -PAT patient review list -PreOp clearance	-Scheduled based on patient need/availability -Clarity on what they are supposed to do and when/where	-Patient -Surgery Scheduler -Surgeon -Central Sterile -PreAuth Team -PreAdmit Team -PCP -Specialists -PreOp
-IT -Bed Mngt -Transportation -Imaging, Labs & Pharmacy -Case Mngt -Primary Care Physician	-Scheduled surgery -Detailed surgery info (equip, supplies) -Patient medical history -Patient financial information -Trained staff -Appropriate # of staff	-Time to complete clearances prior to day of surgery, if non-emergent -Complete and accurate info	PreAdmissions/ Registration	-Medical clearance -Financial clearance -Registered patient -Patient ready for PreOp -Identified gaps in PreOp	-Completed accurately and timely -PreOp gaps addressed timely	-PreAuth Team -PreAdmit Team -PreOp -Lab -Imaging -Volunteer in Lien Waiting Room -Patient -Surgeon -Case Management
	-Patient ready for PreOp -H&P & consents -Equipment Prepped -Beds -PreOp orders -Meds/Equip/Supplies -Trained staff -Appropriate # of staff -Patient procedure type/class	-Arrives on time -Complete & timely -Sterile, timely & complete -Available -Bed assigned prior to surgery -Patient well informed and knows of expectations	Pre-Op	-Prepped patient -Patient wheeled into OR -Need for inpatient bed -Personal items collected -PACU orders entered by MDA	-Complete & timely -On time -Personal items secured -Orders for PACU entered prior to surgery	-Patient -OR -Hospital Coordinator -Patient family/point of contact -PACU

FIGURE 15.6

Mapping the work flow process of the before surgery team (SIPOC diagram).

Box 15.2 Goal statement

- Goal statements should broadly define improvement objectives—what will be accomplished by what dates, and by the end of project.
- The problem and goal statements provide the essential components that will define the scope of a project.
- Goal statements should reflect the same level of detail as the problem they address.
- Goals should be guided by the *SMART acronym:*
  - Specific
  - Measurable
  - Attainable
  - Relevant
  - Time bounded

Infection Prevention, Quality, Risk Management, and Operating Management personnel who implmented the initiative. An emphasis was placed on reinforcing risk management, sterilization techniques, proper hand scrubbing, and patient flow optimization as the patient moved through all phases of the surgical service line. Traffic in and out of the individual operating suites was minimized and monitored with door counters. Vendors were monitored to ensure scrubs were changed, movement in and out of the operating suite was reduced, and a reeducation program was reiterated to not violate the sterile field and to reduce unnecessary traffic in and around the perioperative suites (correlated with patient infection rates). Descriptive statistics were used to describe baseline data. Outcome and process measures were

BST-Points of Pain

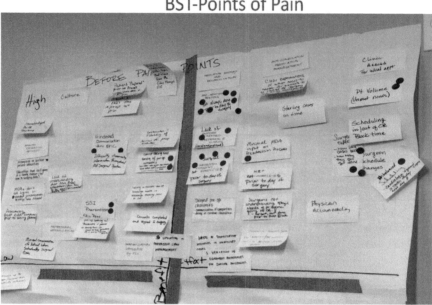

FIGURE 15.7

Before surgery team (BST)-Points of pain (POP).

evaluated using statistical process control charts with signals, indicating special cause, were identified by using standard control chart rules (Fig. 15.8).

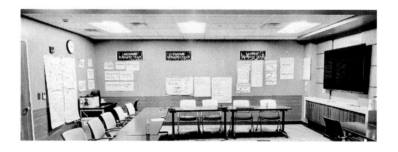

Description of the quality improvement activity

The consulting team used a multiphased approach called **ADAMS** (Fig. 15.2) and the projet was run out of a dedicated situation room ("war room") as seen above. The continuous improvement strategy included a series of Plan-Do-Study-Act (PDSA) cycles. ADAMS served as a model that hospital leadership was able to leverage to stage the deployment of a safe and "just culture" that consistently builds political capital by increasing staff and patient buy-in to support the deep drive

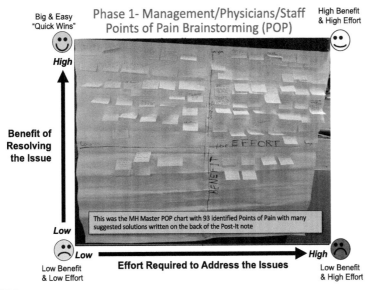

Phase 1- Management/Physicians/Staff Points of Pain Brainstorming (POP)

Big & Easy "Quick Wins"

High Benefit & High Effort

High

Benefit of Resolving the Issue

Low

This was the MH Master POP chart with 93 identified Points of Pain with many suggested solutions written on the back of the Post-It note

Low

Low Benefit & Low Effort

Effort Required to Address the Issues

High

Low Benefit & High Effort

FIGURE 15.8

Management and staff points of pain brainstorming.

toward achieving the quadruple time at MH. The ADAMS model approach was deployed through two phases (Fig. 15.2):

Phase 1 Assess – Discover

- Identify gaps between market perception and baseline performance.
- Identify "what keeps you up at night" (Fig. 15.9).
- Reality check–regularily assess the difference in perceptions between leadership and field.
- Conduct a Discovery workshop to identify a slate of projects aligned with key strategic themes.

Select Insights from the Medical Clearance Project

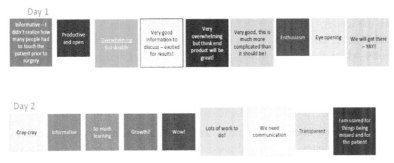

Day 1

Informative – I didn't realize how many people had to touch the patient prior to surgery | Productive and open | Overwhelming but doable | Very good information to discuss – excited for results! | Very overwhelming but think end product will be great! | Very good, this is much more complicated than it should be! | Enthusiasm | Eye opening | We will get there – YAY!

Day 2

Cray-cray | Informative | So much learning | Growth? | Wow! | Lots of work to do! | We need communication | Transparent | I am scared for things being missed and for the patient

FIGURE 15.9

Insights from before surgery team focus group brainstorming (BST)-"what keeps you up at night".

BST-Points of Pain

BEFORE SURGERY TEAM

High Benefit/Low Effort	Votes	High Benefit/High Effort	Votes
Process		*Process*	
Variation in preference card management		Unbalanced scheduling of surgeries	
Lack of understanding that anesthesia pre-op assessment/plan has to be done/documented before pt goes to OR		Scheduling in/out of OR block time	4
Where does pre-op bathing happen if patient is coming from the EDT ED or PreOp?		Surgeon schedule changes	
Hardwired communication to Epic; difficult to disseminate info across Surgical Services	2	Surgeon expectations for how long cases take and how many they can get done	
Communication & scheduling of services for pre-op evaluation		Starting cases on time	
Ability to communicate within Epic that flows from the clinic through to the OR		Clear expectations of what needs to happen for patients to be cleared medically and financially for surgery and timely management of those	
		Delayed pre-op clearances due to lack of communication of completion and delays in cardiac clearance	
Pt Care & Quality		PAT chart review workarounds & rework	
SSI Prevention - skin prep, pre op bathing	1	Waste of sterilization resources in unutilized items in instrument sets	
Nutritional Optimization		Lack of uniform, defined preference cards (currently unstandardized)	
Having a realistic idea of discharge needs i.e. discharge teaching prior to OR		Variation in equipment preferences for similar procedures	2
Consents completed and signed at day of surgery		*Pt Care & Quality*	
Lab work & EKGs done in PreOp, not prior to day of surgery		Medication history and reconciliation	
Standardized pre-op teaching		Inconsistent Anti-Coag Medication Management	
Immunizations up to date i.e. flu		Standardize expectation/process for anesthesia pre-procedure review of scheduled surgery patients	
Smoking Cessation program		Minimal MDA input on preadmission process	1
Incomplete or unclear patient education		H&P completed minutes before case start time	
Education that isn't given in a timely manner (too close to surgery date)		H&P not completed prior to day of surgery	
MDAs don't all agree on needed preanesthesia testing/labs		Surgical informed consent not completed prior to day of surgery	5
Anesthesia pre-op eval completed prior to seeing patient		Pre-Admission testing not always done prior to day of surgery	7
Patient "prepared" prior to PreOp (labs/tests done & in Epic, H&P in Epic, consents done & in Epic)		Surgeons not understanding specific needs of pt before going to OR (consents, H&P done prior to PreOp)	
Correct dosing and timing of antibiotics (too often given too close to cut time)	2		
Culture		*Culture*	
Minimal consideration of patient when scheduling surgical times		Physician Accountability	
		Culture	
Staff		*Staff*	
Leadership		Clinic access for initial appt	
		Patient Volumes (unmet needs)	1
		Leadership	
	Votes	Low Benefit/High Effort	Votes
Low Benefit/Low Effort			
Culture			
Manage up the surgeon/surgical team (ED specific reference)			

(Legend: Clearance; Scheduling of procedures; Central Sterile/Equipment; Day of Surgery; Patient Education; Internal Communication; Medication History)

FIGURE 15.10

Potential quick hits "points of pain" ratings before surgery team (BST).

- Identify candidate "Quick Hit" projects/rapid improvement events for short-term Return on investment (ROI) (Fig. 15.10).
- Categorize project types (e.g., process improvement, marketing, strategic, standardization, monitoring, new design of service delivery).

Benefits of phase 1: Assess and Discover

- Provides an assessment of the organization as it is perceived by others and how it performs in the marketplace.
- Involves senior leaders from all functions in understanding gaps or opportunities that can lead to better performance.
- Conduct reality check using interviews/observations/and data from staff and field observations to compare the workflow as seen by front-line clinicians versus how the leadership view the reality of surgical services.
- Establishes a baseline including of the actual workflow (time motion milestones) against which the effectiveness of various initiatives and corrective actions can be compared (Fig. 15.11).

Phase 2 Action—Manage—Sustain

- Assign strategic theme champions and new governance model for BDA and voice of staff teams for each aligned set of projects selected in the discover phase (Fig. 15.12).
- Enhance project portfolio management so that projects support each other.

Time Motion Milestones Map of the Perioperative Value Stream at Muda Health

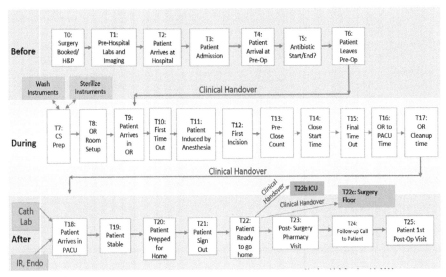

FIGURE 15.11

Time motion milestones on the value stream map.

Governance Structure – Graphic Description

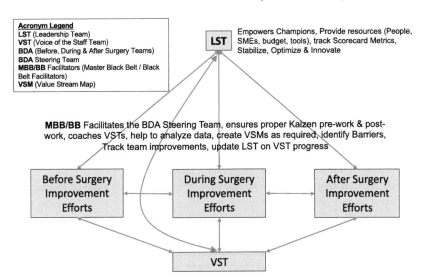

FIGURE 15.12

Graphic description of the new governance structure.

Sample Main and Sub-Metrics Targets for Improvement

Main Metric Category	Detailed Metrics
Margin / Costs	Revenue
	Operating Margin
	Block Usage %
	% Cases Starting on Time
	# of Suppliers
	Waste Reduction % (TIMWOOD: Transportation, Inventory, Motion, Waiting, Over-processing, Over-production, Defects)
	# of sterile kits not used
	# of SKUs
	Before Surgery:
	–Staffing levels (Volunteers and Employees)
	During Surgery:
	–Higher cost supplies / instruments substituted for less costly version
	–Pharmacy costs
	After Surgery:
	–Length of Stay in PACU
	–Staffing levels for monitored beds, transporters

Main Metric Category	Detailed Metrics
Delivery Throughput Times	**Before Surgery:**
	–Patient Arrival to Pre-Op cycle time
	–Pre-Op to arrival at OR cycle time
	–Equipment / instrument Order to Fill cycle time
	–Case book request to fill cycle time
	During Surgery:
	–OR arrival to Surgery Start cycle time
	–Surgery Start to Surgery Finished cycle time
	–OR room turnaround time
	–Unused block time after surgery / room turnaround time
	–First Case Start time (minutes early / late)
	After Surgery:
	–OR surgery complete to OR depart cycle time
	–OR depart to PACU arrival cycle time
	–PACU arrival to PACU depart cycle time
	–PACU depart to Patient depart cycle time

Main Metric Category	Detailed Metrics
Quality / Safety	Perioperative Adverse Events, Numerator:
	Perioperative adverse events, Denominator:
	1000 patient days using IHI. Trigger Tool for Measuring ADEs
	SSI, SIR
	SCIP Measures
	Transfusion Utilization data
	Safety Measures:
	Retained sponges/instruments
	Adverse drug events
	Fires in the OR
	Hemorrhage
	VTE and PE
	Near Misses
	Mortality (HSMR): Decreased mortality (hospital standardized mortality ratio, or HSMR)
	Before Surgery:
	–% Consents completed before patient arrival
	–% of sterilization carts filled accurately, completed on time
	–# Arrivals by route (e.g., Emergency, add-ins, scheduled)
	–% Arrivals that are ambulatory
	During Surgery:
	–Infection Control Measures
	–Near Misses, Adverse Events
	–Waivers of recommended sterilization times or methods
	–Physician, Anesthesiologist, Nurse not together at patient induction
	–3 time outs completed and documented
	After Surgery:
	–# Patients with post-surgery concerns
	–# Outpatients admitted rather than discharged
	–Infection Control audits with weekly
	–Risk management data on transitions out of post surgery, bounce back to OR, and to ICUs

Main Metric Category	Detailed Metrics
Culture / Reputation	**External Measures:**
	CMS Scores
	HCAP Scores
	Leapfrog Scores
	Healthgrades Scores
	Internal Measures:
	Patient Satisfaction Surveys internal
	HRO Maturity
	TeamSTEPPS Maturity
	Average Scores from Cultural Interview for a select group of individuals
	Leadership Climate Survey
	Staff Turnover
	Surgeon Satisfaction Survey
	Surgeon leadership effectiveness tool
	External Certifications:
	Magnet Hospital Cert Readiness
	SD Business Excellence Award

FIGURE 15.13

Surgery teams data dashboard—targets for surgical team improvement.

- Develop a data dashaboard with the QI teams with better metrics and review systems to ensure progress toward goals with obstacles identified and removed (Fig. 15.13).
- Institutionalized deployment as a "way of life" through BDA reports to the leadership steering team (LST) (Appendix VI).
- Improved communication internally and externally.
- Reward and recognize alignment with project themes.
- Conduct ongoing system audits to insure no slippage in Key Performance Indicators (KPI).
- Conduct ongoing training and education through seminars, one-on one coaching and dynamic intranet website. (Appendix IX)
- Focus on staff empowerment and ownership of all project phases and actions.

Benefits phase 2: Action-Manage-Sustain

- Provide a formal method to identify, prioritize, and select specific strategic themes for initiating project portfolios. (Figs. 15.14–15.16)
- Identify "quick hits" and rapid improvement projects (e.g., rapid cycle tests) that will drive short-term results (Fig. 15.17).
- Strategically align the QI project portfolio to bridge the ROI with long-term sustainability.

DST Process Mapping

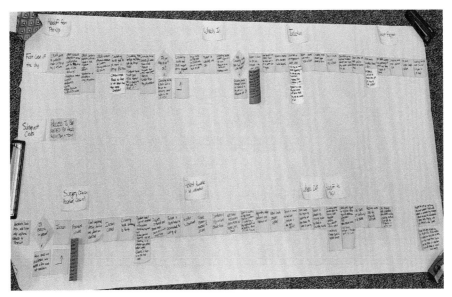

FIGURE 15.14

During surgery team (DST) process mapping.

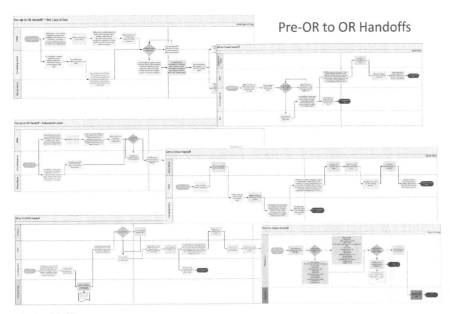

FIGURE 15.15

Preoperating room (before surgery team) to operating room (during surgery team) patient handoffs map.

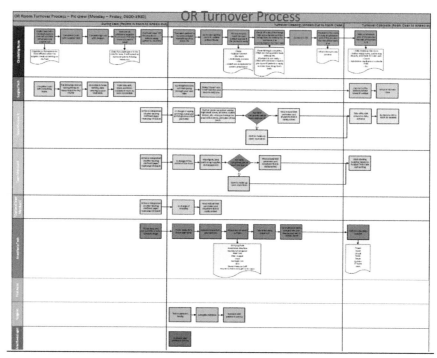

FIGURE 15.16

Operating room turnover process map.

PICK-DST Points of Pain

DURING SURGERY TEAM POINTS OF PAIN

High Benefit/Low Effort	Pts	High Benefit/High Effort	Pts
Leadership		Leadership	
Culture		Culture	
Not everyone participates in time-out/Not everyone is present for time-out	2	Low event reporting	
Process		Process	
Hearing that a surgeon arrives through word of mouth rather than a standard announcement	1	Phase of care orders can't be seen/limited Epic views in phases of care	1
Commonly dropped instruments are stored in Central Sterile instead of the core		Add-on cases (not scheduled)	1
Unknown ahead of time whether a foley will be needed or not		Consent and H&P are not available (ex. Anesthesia plan and testing complete)	1
No standard skin prep process/Use of wrong skin prep		Unexpected instrument needs are not on preference cards	
Pre-op antibiotics are not given within 60 minutes of time/Antibiotics not address and initiated	4	Non-standard handoff process to PACU	
Wrong pre-op antibiotic used for case		On-time starts	4
Consents are not completed	3	Preference cards are inaccurate/out of date	3
Inconsistent hand hygiene process	1	No dedicated general surgery room	3
No standard instrument cleaning process after case		PACU/ICU bed availability	
		No streamlined turnover process/no standard OR turnover cleaning process	6
		Lack of space in the OR	
Staff		Staff	
		Need more staff on weekends/in general	8
Patient Care & Quality		Patient Care & Quality	
		Organ space/deep surgical site infections	
Low Benefit/Low Effort	Pts	Low Benefit/High Effort	Pts
Leadership		Leadership	
Culture		Culture	
		Monitors outside each room displaying team metrics, FCOTs, turnover times, unused trays	
Process		Process	
Refine booking process with scheduling and office staff; web-based scheduling (i.e. Lean Taas)	1	Do not have individual instrument tracking/locating	
		Needing to turnover sets, same items used multiple times in a day	1
Staff		Staff	
Patient Care & Quality		Patient Care & Quality	

FIGURE 15.17

During surgery team (DST) points of pain (PICK chart).

- Establish a baseline against which the effectiveness of various initiatives and corrective actions can be compared.
- Balance program, process, and cultural improvement in order to institutionalize the changes and improvements.

Quality guiding principles adopted by Muda Health leadership and staff

Transforming complex surgical services first requires agreement by leadership, clinicians, and staff on the guiding principles of the QI project. MH held numerous town hall and department meetings facilitated by the consultants in which the following essential "pillars" were agreed upon to help MH facilitate a successful surgery quality improvement effort including the following:

1) Accountability and responsibility
   a. Establish cross-level and cross-functional accountabilities and responsibilities for taking positive steps toward improving perioperative performance.
   b. Plan clear and accountable timetable for the perioperative quality improvement project.
2) Data Transparency
   a. Process data would be shared with all project members in meetings, online, using data dashboards available in new perioperative wall monitors.
3) Decision-making
   a. Foster a transparent decision-making process and culture that is data driven and aligned with MH system values.
4) Teamwork
   a. Ensure all project levels are working together to implement changes that will drive performance improvement benefiting patients/families, MH, staff at all levels across perioperative services, and physicians.
5) Communication and discussion
   a. Encourage input from all levels within the organization so as to increase buy-in from all involved in perioperative service delivery.
   b. Build trust through clear and honest "truth telling" that is focused on facts not personalities, and that involves all staff levels within the hospital including nonemployed staff and physicians.
6) Change management
   a. Recognize that change is difficult although necessary, therefore, participation and buy-in by all individuals and teams involved is required and ongoing.
7) Keeping score (Fig. 15.18)
   a. Define current state performance as the baseline against which future performance is compared using agreed upon metrics.

BDA Metric Data Dashboard

Area	Metric	Calculation	Initiative Priority	Is it Defined?	Clinical Quality	Throughput/ Efficiency	Patient Experience	Cost of Care	Effort of Data Collection	Phase 1	Phase 2	Phase 3
Before	First Case On-Time Starts	Percent On-Time	Critical	Yes	*	***	*	**				
Before	Consents Completed before day of surgery	Percent Complete	Critical	Yes	**	***	**	*				
Before	H&P's Signed before day of surgery	Percent Complete	Critical	Yes	**	**	*	*				
Before	Pre-Op Orders completed before day of surgery	Percent Complete	Critical	Yes	**	***	*	*				
Before	Prophylactic antibiotic selection/ administered 30-60 min before incision	Percent Administered	Critical	Yes	***	*	**	**				
Before	Add-Ons after 1PM day before surgery	Percent Add-On's	Critical	Yes	**	***	*	*				
During	OR Turnover time	Average Minutes	Critical	Yes	*	***	*	**				
During	OR Case Length Bias	Percent 20+% deviated	Critical	Yes	*	***	*	*				
During	OpTime Supply and Pharmacy Costs	No KPI definied (Delta surg/proc)	Critical	No	*	*	*	***				
During	OR Cleaning Turnover vs Delta Turnover	Average Minutes	Medium	No	*	***	*	*				
During	Block Time Utilization	Percent Utilization, Minutes/Percent Overbook	Medium	No	*	***	*	*				
During	Preference Card Accuracy	Percent cases with added supply, in or out cans	Medium	No	*	***	*	**				
After	Press Gainey Metrics - Overall Experience	Percent 4+	Critical	Yes	*	*	***	*				
After	Press Gainey - Refer a Friend	Percent 4+	Medium	Yes	*	*	***	*				
After	Press Gainey - Effortless	Percent 4+	Medium	Yes	*	*	***	*				
After	Unplanned admissions - OP or Obs - Percent	Percent Admitted, changed to Obs	Critical	Yes	***	**	**	**				
After	PACU Holds	Percent held < 10 min.	Critical	Yes	**	***	**	**				
After	Post-Op visit planned before discharge	Percent scheduled before discharge	Critical	Yes	***	*	***	*				
After	Post-Op visit planned before admission	Percent scheduled before admission	Critical	Yes	***	**	**	**				

*** High impact metric to improve goal
** Some impact possible towards goal
* Low indicator / driver for goal

Data is easily linked to surgical episode in OpTime
Data is collected, but may require logic to link
Data is not collected and would require workflow modifications

FIGURE 15.18

Before/during/after (BDA) surgical outcomes metric data dashboard.

    b. Enhance a data-driven performance tracking system that focuses on quality, cost, and time scorecards (e.g., high level often lagging indicators) and dashboards (e.g., proxy real-time measures at the process detail level linked to the scorecard indicators).

8) Shared goals and goal setting (Fig. 15.19)

    a. Establish and commit to shared goals within the hospital in collaboration with nonemployed staff including physicians.

    b. 6-month and 12-month targets established in terms of quality, cost, time indicators.

    c. Set targets for weekly and monthly improvements in Before Surgery—During Surgery—After Surgery processes (i.e., simpler terminology for preoperative, intraoperative, postoperative processes).

9) Strategic project deployment

    a. Prioritize and cascade projects within Before/During/After surgical processes to ensure what needs to be done first while laying the foundation for ongoing future projects.

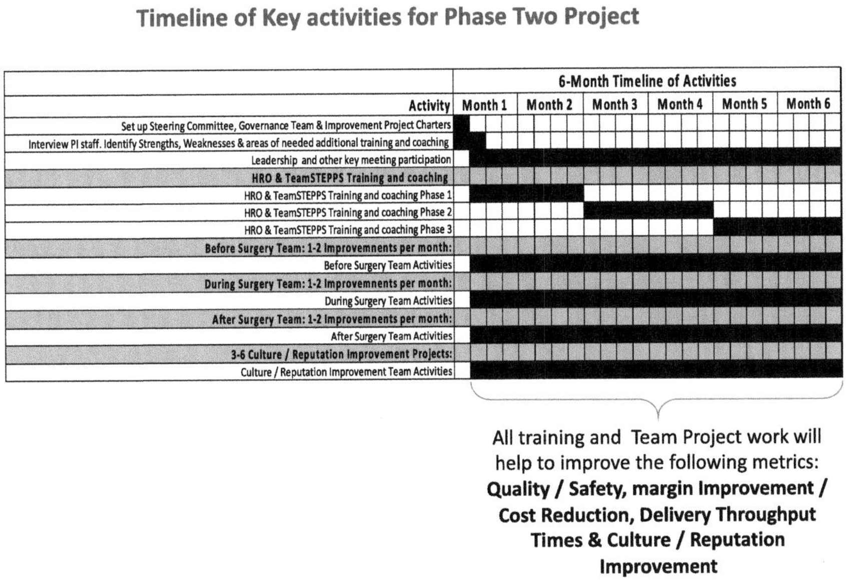

Timeline of Key activities for Phase Two Project

	6-Month Timeline of Activities					
Activity	Month 1	Month 2	Month 3	Month 4	Month 5	Month 6
Set up Steering Committee, Governance Team & Improvement Project Charters						
Interview PI staff. Identify Strengths, Weaknesses & areas of needed additional training and coaching						
Leadership and other key meeting participation						
HRO & TeamSTEPPS Training and coaching						
HRO & TeamSTEPPS Training and coaching Phase 1						
HRO & TeamSTEPPS Training and coaching Phase 2						
HRO & TeamSTEPPS Training and coaching Phase 3						
Before Surgery Team: 1-2 Improvemnets per month:						
Before Surgery Team Activities						
During Surgery Team: 1-2 Improvemnets per month:						
During Surgery Team Activities						
After Surgery Team: 1-2 Improvemnets per month:						
After Surgery Team Activities						
3-6 Culture / Reputation Improvement Projects:						
Culture / Reputation Improvement Team Activities						

All training and Team Project work will
help to improve the following metrics:
**Quality / Safety, margin Improvement /
Cost Reduction, Delivery Throughput
Times & Culture / Reputation
Improvement**

FIGURE 15.19

MH project timeline for the perioperative quality improvement project.

    b. Honest and accountable resourcing of projects in terms of staff time and
budget support.

    c. Identify and engage Champions and leaders for the Before/During/After
surgical projects.

10) Policy of No Surprises

    a. Ensure that all key data are transparently shared especially when they
portend to risky, and costly impacts.

    b. Ensure all surgical staff members are involved and participate in consensus
decision-making processes allowing for individuals to agree or disagree in
order to work together toward buildng support for implementing decisions.

New governance structure and timeline for perioperative services transformation (Appendix I, II, III, IV, V)

Significant surgical QI projects require alignment of governance and values to
ensure the project obstacles are addressed early and clearly. A Perioperative Services
Leadership Steering Team (LST), comprised of senior executives and physician
leaders, was established to drive safety and improvement across the perioperative
services. To increase the opportunity to involve more staff in the transformation,
the consulting team facilitated the initiation of a cross-function Voice of the Staff

(VST, which was built on MH foundational belief that "change is not what we do **to** people" rather "change is what we do **with** people."

The VST members were selected using the following guidelines:

- cross-functional, cross-level of representatives from various surgical service line functions with the only restriction being the level of those from perioperative services department being no higher than manager.
- viewed as respected peers and colleagues.
- known to be focused on what is in the best interest of MH staff and patients.
- not afraid to voice their opinions.
- those that peers seek out for help or support.

The VST team was expected to meet biweekly with subgroups of participants that meet daily in huddles. By having both the LST and a VST in place, meeting regularly, tracking relevant metrics, and transparently addressing issues helped to foster communication and trust across, down, and up within the organization. Needed improvements in culture were incorporated such as having a supportive environment to ensure positive engagement of all staff, volunteers, patients, and families in truth-telling, speaking up when poor behaviors were exhibited and seriously considering positive suggestions. The goal was for MH to increase ownership, employee engagement, and accountability at all levels.

The BDA teams were established to identify and implement improvements using various performance improvement (PI) methods, for example, via:

- "Do Its":
  - Obvious or easily understood changes to be quickly implemented.
  - Waste points identified in the process that can be reduced or eliminated.
- Rapid Improvement Events (RIEs)—called Kaizen Events:
  - A Kaizen event may totally change many process steps or the entire process
  - Bottlenecks or failure points are identified with solutions developed.
  - Remove bottlenecks that inhibit process flow efficiency/effectiveness.
- PDSA (Plan–Do–Study–Act) cycles:
  - Continuous process improvement cycles used for ongoing process learning and change.
  - Process owners and participants continually seeking ways to improve.
  - Deploy analysis tools to better understand the process data.
- Lean Six Sigma:
  - More advanced qualitative and quantitative tools to develop solutions.
  - Solutions are typically not obvious and require more process study.
  - May involve several steps in the process.

The governance structures in Figs. 15.4 and 15.12 depict the reporting relationships of the newly created project leadership teams.

Designing the new workflow

It is well known that for many hospitals the emergency department is often viewed as the "front door" to the hospital as many patients' first encounter with a hospital is through personal or family visits originating in the emergency department. For many others, their early encounters with the hospital are through outpatient or elective surgeries. Data show that 60%–80% of patients have their first encounter with the hospital through the emergency department or through outpatient/elective surgeries.

What might this mean for MH? The patient experience/satisfaction metrics are likely highly influenced by the hospital performance of the emergency department leading to the perioperative services. In this section, we will discuss the subprocesses that represent components of the period of time before the patient enters the OR. The following components are not meant to be a detailed and exhaustive list:

Admissions into surgical services

- Hospital admissions for inpatient stays.
- Emergency department transfers either directly to inpatient areas or to the surgical department (e.g., trauma cases).
- Outpatient arrivals and admissions.

Internal transitions

- Transportation from inpatient settings to surgical department.
- Patient arrival to outpatient registration.
- Signing patient/legal guardian consent forms.
- Outpatient registration to patient surgical preparation.

Patient family/friends care

- Family/friends waiting areas and comforting environment.
- Communication or information regarding patient status.
- Availability or proximity to access for food or beverages.

Scheduling of staff and surgical suites

- Physician/practice input as to preferred schedule or block times.

- Schedule constraints of surgeons, anesthesiologists or anesthetists, surgical nurses and techs, environmental engineering staff, sterilization staff/techs, others.
- Schedule constraints due to equipment availability, supplies, sterilized packs/trays.
- Add-on policies and enforcement.
- Trauma schedule impact mitigation policies.

Supplies

- Supply choice and purchase guidelines.
- Surgeon preference cards and consistency with supply policies among physicians, hospital supply chain management, and sterilization staff.
- "Just in Case" versus "Just in Time" supply management balance.
- Obsolescence policies for supplies.
- Supply disposal processes.
- Supply storage, infection control/management.
- Capital expense policies.
- Consumable expense policies.

Sterilization

- Preference card management policies.
- Add-on lead time policies and enforcement.
- Sterile process lead-time guidelines and enforcement.
- Sterile pack utilization policies and processes to minimize lack of pack/tray utilization.
- Processes to address sterile equipment demand conflicts.
- Collaboration with infection control to reduce surgical site infections (SSIs).
- Sterilization staff input (voice of sterilization) requested and considered by physicians and surgical staff in managing surgical demands and timelines.
- Weekday and weekend staffing process. The staffing HR dashboards showed between 30% and 40% of OR staff—nurses, technicians, and nursing aids were agency staff.

Surgical preparation

- Core measure policies enforced (e.g., administration of antibiotics before "first cut").
- Patient safety policies enforced.

- Patient communication/comfort checklist followed prior to anesthesia.
  - Patient consent forms signed.
  - Patient needs addressed.
  - Reason for surgery verified if possible
- Patients moved to OR suite (wheels up) 5 min before scheduled start.

Physician preparation

- Physicians prepped at least 5 min before scheduled start of case defined as entering in the OR.
- Surgeon present at anesthesia administration as required by the joint commission.
- Presurgical checklists completed.

In summary, the before surgery components are key in setting the stage for reliable surgical outcomes along with detailed consideration of the patient/family/friends' experiences. Poor scheduling and adherence to policies for scheduling including add-ons, rushing/skipping over checklist elements, poor teamwork among the employed and unemployed staff, poor supply, and sterilization management, and otherwise any lack of preparation can lead to shoddy teamwork, bruised egos, poor surgical outcomes, and ultimately-litigation.

Quality may not be of prime importance

The consulting team heard comments from those involved in the before surgery processes that they are often either directed to "make it happen" whether there was enough lead-time or staff on board to ensure that "safe" practices would be followed. There have been other times that front-line staff have been pressured to not report safety concerns and policy violations and that they were not provided sufficient time to carry out their job and patient preparation according to safe and accepted guidelines. It was suggested that "physician time" is more valuable than their time so they must do their best to accommodate the demands of surgeons.

Costs can be better managed

From detailed observations of management meetings in which decisions were made about which new supplies to order, the consulting team observed decisions that were weighted more on qualitative perceptions rather than being guided by robust cost/quality and effectiveness industry-wide measures with little input from teams (not individuals) of physicians and hospital experts in logistics. We observed a laissez-faire style of decision-making.

The consulting team observed that there was an inordinate number of SKUs (stock keeping units) for many supplies (total of 24,000 SKUs for MH). For example, for surgical sutures there were over 580 SKUs, yet by national standards surgical services of this size would expected to have not more than 100–150 SKUs relative to the surgical volume in all of MH locations. The greater the number of SKUs for the same type items, the greater the complexity of managing and costs in maintaining the inventory levels, usage, and reordering points for each individual SKU.

The costs of sterilization were higher than they should be. The consulting team understood that 30%–40% of sterile packs/trays go unused during surgeries rather than the inustry aeverage of only 5%–10% of unutilized sterile packs/trays. Important questions include the following:

- How much staff time is consumed in preparing sterile packs/trays? How much staff time is not available to prepare pack/trays for other surgeries?
- How often do sterilization staff rush to prepare for other surgeries as their time was consumed with needless preparation for previous surgeries?
- Is there an impact on the quality and safety as a result of not having sterile packs/trays prepared well or being sent to a OR suite that ultimately does not use them?
- What are the opportunity costs of cutting the percentage of unutilized sterile packs/trays by 50% which in fact will still be twice as much as what is considered best practice across the United States?

Time or timeliness

The scheduling of cases seeks to optimize surgical suite time and surgeon utilization. However, block time utilization at MH was as low as 50% or sometimes lower, indicative of poor utilization. There were examples of utilization of about 80% with some physicians but it was not consistent. Patient case add-ons sought to increase OR utilization, yet the operational definition of what constitutes a practical lead time for an add-on was not clear and seemed to vary by surgical services causing schedulig confusion. The baseline measure of add-on surgical cases was as much as 40% of all surgeries.

- Questions arose such as:
  - Do add-on cases take into account the availability of staff, or the time needed to schedule staff?
  - Are there deficiencies in established complete sterilization protocols?
  - Are there shortfalls in completion of preparation time including OR suite turnaround?
  - Are there deficiencies in documenting signed patient consent forms and insuring patients are educated as to what is entailed by the surgeries along with necessary postoperative care and follow-up?
  - Do the add-ons increase the likelihood of rushing to "make it happen" thus not ensuring that the preparation checklists or timeouts are managed well? (see Appendix VIII for more details).

- Do the schedulers know how long it takes to sterilize and turn over vital equipment and that downtime needs to be part of all scheduling decisions (especially for back-to-back cases)?

Keeping score—construction of the data scorecards and leadership dashboards

During the summer of 2020, The Leapfrog Group, a nonprofit organization that provides consumers with an assessment of the quality performance of hospitals nationwide, reported (https://www.leapfroggroup.org) that the surgical site infection (SSI) rate at MH had declined from a grade of "B" to a grade of "D." The Leapfrog national grade was matched by the Centers for Medicare and Medicaid Services report of two stars (out of five stars) for MH.[7] The public perception and reputation of a hospital can be impacted by outside reports and patient stories. Creating an internal scorecard system that represents performance outcomes along with a dashboard system of internal process performance can help support the change management efforts. It was decided that these two systems could be utilized to help MH prioritize and direct process improvement efforts that could positively improve outcome performance.

Key components of a balanced scorecard approach

The MH operations plan outlined the key strategy, priorities, areas of responsibility, and critical performance measurements through responsible leadership and team performance focused on measurable areas. Critical plan components included strategy, deliverables, performance indicators, and organization change. The key components for the MH surgical services plan included the following:

- **Operating plan strategy:** Understand why and how the targets will be met.
- **Deliverables:** Know the performance measurement targets.
- **Performance indicators/measurements:** Show how to meet targets.
- **Organization:** Understand who is accountable for targets.

The **scorecards** represent outcome measures that the LST must manage and oversee. The **dashboards** represent process measures associated with the BDA aspects of perioperative services. For example, an SSI rate is an outcome measure that is impacted by the quality of the handoffs within perioperative services, performance to core measures such as antibiotic administration less than 60 min before first surgical incision, infection control processes, sterilization of equipment, management

---

[7] CMS uses a five-star quality rating system, with 5 being the highest, to measure the experiences Medicare beneficiaries have with their health plan and health care system.

of sterile fields, effectiveness of surgical timeouts, and many other factors. All these factors can be measured and represented as possible dashboard metrics. If the dashboard metrics continue to show poor results over time, then the SSI rate at the scorecard level will be impacted.

The metrics should be impartial to **ensure trustworthiness of quantifiable results,** and should match the leadership concentration areas of MH. However, a critical focus on key concentration areas and requirements can enhance patient safety, surgical services and financial objectives. Metrics have to be viewed as **reliable sources of data**. The MH surgical performance metrics should ensure alignment with the MH corporate financial performance targets and link to the MH clinicians and staff performance.

In general, the LST needs to be accountable for the scorecard metrics, while the BDA teams provide ongoing (e.g., weekly) reports regarding the dashboard metrics (Appendix VI) using agreed upon project charter worksheets (Fig. 15.20). The BDA teams can more quickly highlight positive performance improvement and similarly address downturns in performance by understanding variance in the dashboard performance metrics (Fig. 15.21).

The major categories for scorecards and dashboards along with some examples are as follows:

- Quality
  - Scorecard example—SSI rate, infection control metrics.
  - Dashboard example—Core measure for antibiotic administration.

Why Construct a Project Charter.

LEAN SIX SIGMA PROJECT CHARTER WORKSHEET

Project Title:		Date:	
Business Case/Problem Statement:		**Initial Goal Statement(s):**	
What is the problem? Be specific and include data, etc.		Create 1-3 goals addressing time, defects, and/or money, etc. Make them SMART and include baselines and targets if possible.	
What specifically will happen if you do not do the project?			
Project Scope & Constraints:		**Customers/Stakeholders:**	
What are you going to do? What specifically should be included in the project?			
What specifically should be excluded or limited?			
Resources Needed for Project		**Project Start Date**	**Completion Date**
Team Members	**Role**	**Team Members**	**Role**
	Champion		Member
	Leader		Member
	Facilitator		Member
	Member		Member
	Member		Member
Leadership Approval			
Signature of Sponsor			
Name of Sponsor		Date Approved:	

FIGURE 15.20

Lean six sigma project charter worksheet.

Charter for: Muda Health
Surgery Improvement
Date: 10/15/20   Version: 2

Process/Area: "During Surgery Team"   Champion: Dr. PK

Strategic Alignment: Deliver High Quality Care - Monument Health Surgical services is committed to achieving the Quadruple Aim to provide for systems improvement in patient safety, cost reduction, and preservation of the workforce.

Problem Statement: Measured over the last 24 months, year on year, the quality, infection (high nationally benchmarked rates of SSI, CLABSI, MRSA measures), productivity (i.e, @40% late starts, 40% add-on cases, 30% wasted sterile packs, etc.) and reputational challenges (i.e, CMS 2/5 star rating; Leapfrog D grate; MH ranked 12/12 in South Dakota) related to the intraoperative phase of the Surgical Services processes at MH RCH continues to be subpar. If this continues, we may lose patients/revenue to our competitors.

Objective Statement: Improve quality, time, and culture aspects of intraoperative areas through focused efforts on decreasing SSI rates, OR turnover time, and the number of instrument SKUs; increasing completion rates of time-outs (before & after surgery), the rate of appropriate antibiotic administrations, and on time starts. In addition, the intraoperative team members will complete Lean White Belt training and the TeamSTEPPS program, as well as evaluate patient experience and employee engagement scores.

Define Project: Intraoperative Process for Muda Health Hospital

In Scope: All patients from the time they are brought into the operating room until they are ready to leave the operating room. This includes the physical, organizational, cultural, and financial aspects related to the surgical process.

Out of Scope: All aspects prior to entering the operating room, from patient diagnosis//decision to undergo surgery to the time they are brough into the operating room, and, after leaving the operating room, including recovering room to home discharge

Improvement Metrics

Metrics / Objectives / KPIs	Current	Target	% Change
1 OR turnover time (max)	**31 min** **36.13% (0-24 min)**	<25 min	
2 Sign-in Completion rate	**99.83%**	100%	
3 Time-out Completion rate	**99.79%**	100%	
4 Sign-out Completion rate	**96.43%**	100%	
5 Number of Suture SKUs	**290**	100	**-65.52%**
6 Number of Mesh SKUs	TBD	TBD	
7 SSI rate for Colorectal Surgeries	**10.43**	TBD	
8 SSI rate for All Surgeries	**1.93**	TBD	
9 % of Appropriate Antibiotic Administrations	**72.78%**	TBD	
10 % of First Case On Time Starts	**58.71%**	TBD	
11 % of Subsequent Case On Time Starts	**51.99%**	TBD	
12 PSI 05 – Retained Surgical Item or Unretrieved Device Fragment count	TBD	TBD	
13 PSI 09 – Perioperative Hemorrhage or Hematoma rate	TBD	TBD	
14 PSI 16 – Transfusion Reaction count	TBD	TBD	
15 Epic Predicted vs. Surgeon Predicted vs. Actual Time for surgery* (Case Length Accuracy)	**40.97%**	TBD	
16 % White Belt Completions – Core Team	**69.23%**	100%	**+30.77%**
17 % of team members through the TeamSTEPPS Program	**0%**	100%	**+100%**
18 Patient Satisfaction – Area to be identified	TBD	TBD	
19 Surgical Services Employee Engagement Score	TBD	TBD	

Sponsoring Team: RCH Surgery Improvement Leadership Steering Team (LST)

Team Members:

FIGURE 15.21

Example of a During Surgery Team (DST) project charter completed worksheet.

- Cost/Margin
  - Scorecard example—Ratio of surgical inventory relative to surgical revenue.
  - Dashboard example—Ratio of obsolete surgical inventory to all surgical inventory.
- Time/Timeliness of Delivery/Throughput
  - Scorecard example—Number of outpatient/inpatient surgeries performed per week or month.
  - Dashboard example—Lead time from patient arrival to patient preop complete.

The LST oversees the scorecards for quality (e.g., SSI), cost, and time metrics. As the scorecard metrics are typically high-level outcome metrics, each of the BDA teams will use a dashboard of quality, cost, and time process metrics that are related to the scorecard metrics. The BDA teams are responsible for focusing their efforts on improving the dashboard metrics which in time are expected to positively impact the scorecards that the LST is overseeing (Appendix VI) (Figs. 15.22–15.24). The three figures represent three types of work assessments.

Keep in mind that data scorecards are high-level outcome metrics and as such are typically lagging indicators. A lagging indicator is a quality, safety, or financial sign that becomes apparent only after a large shift has taken place over time. Therefore, lagging indicators confirm long-term trends, but they do not predict them. In other words, improvements in the underlying BDA processes may be noticed more readily with the dashboard metrics, yet there may be a delay of weeks to months before they show up in the scorecard's "leading" metrics.

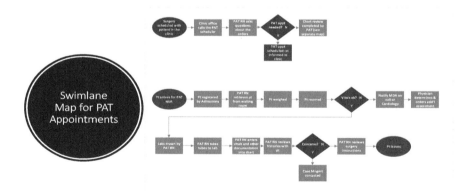

FIGURE 15.22

Swimlane assessment of before surgery pre-operation clinic (PAT) appointments.

Map and Waste Analysis

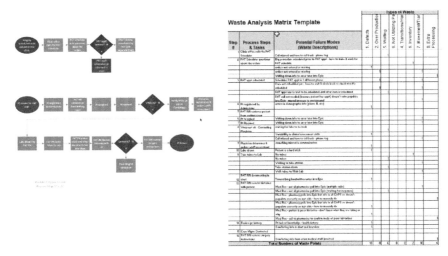

FIGURE 15.23

Before surgery preoperation clinic (PAT) map and waste analysis.

Failure Mode and Effects Risk Analysis for PAT Waste Points and Quick Hits

#	Process Step or Function	Failure Mode	Effect of Failure	Severity	Cause (s) of Failure	Occur.	Controls / Detectability	Detect.	Risk Priority #	Recommended Corrective Action/Status
1	Clinic office calls the PAT Scheduler	Call missed and have to call back - phone tag		3		7		1	21	
2	PAT Scheduler questions about the orders	Big procedure scheduled prior to PAT appt - have to make it work for PAT schedule		1		10		1	10	
		orders not entered or missing		10		3		3	90	
		orders not entered or missing		7		3		3	63	
		Writing down info to enter later into Epic		3		10		1	30	
3	PAT appt scheduled	Schedules PAT appt in 3 different places	Delays	10	No solution w/Epic	10		3	300	
		Case not scheduled yet - have to wait & circle back to check that it's scheduled	Delay, Cost,	10	Office scheduler calling too early	3		7	210	
		PAT appt has to wait to be scheduled until after case is scheduled								
		PAT call not needed (because patient has appt) doesn't auto populate into Epic - manual process to workaround								

FIGURE 15.24

Before surgery preoperation clinic (PAT) failure modes and effects analysis.

Training of the MH staff, clinicians and leadership (Appendix IX)

Ongoing learning about patients, customers, processes, ideas, and each other propels the lead improvement engine. The MH Surgical Improvement Training Program relied on lean tools and concepts and covered the major approaches to surgical safety and quality improvement. Program participants were taught to understand the advantages and disadvantages of various ways of organizing surgical services according to a range of tools, criteria, and approaches for improving cost, quality and service.

The consulting team designed a training program to help MH clinicians, healthcare risk management, and patient safety professionals understand and apply their key contributions to improve surgical patient care and outcomes. The consulting team collaborated closely with the Operations Performance Management Department (OPM) to deliver a consistent approach toward improving MH surgical services. The HR department learning management system (LMS) system facilitated access and oversight to the training materials. The consulting team designed the training with a "bias toward action" approach that was conducted "just in time" for MH and BDA teams to immediately apply the new system's knowledge and skills as they lead the BDA surgical improvement work.

Communications and messaging—internal and external

Vigorous daily and regular communications are essential for any surgical improvement program to succeed. The consulting team heard from front-line clinicians and senior executives about their deep and emotional commitment to care for their communities. The consulting team crafted the surgical improvement project to closely align with these bedrock values. The larger story of the project was aligned with the key messages of commitment to patient and community centered care, deep investment in the staff wellness and loyalty, lean/six sigma operations, and above all-being a good steward of community financial resources. These core messages need to be explained and articulated in the messaging. This transformation effort was complex and fast moving with multiple stakeholders and audiences. The consulting team identified several practices believed as success factors. The following steps were done.

- Hospital President public messaging to community-August 2020
  - "Over the years our surgical performance has not met the highest expectations of our patients, our medical staff, and industry best practices. That must end now!"
  - "We are launching a large, focused effort to redesign and change the culture of this organization."
  - "We will focus on delivering:
    - Safest and high-quality outcomes

- Improved efficiencies
- Improved patient experience
- Better caregiver and surgeon work environment"
- "Muda Health and the current leadership is committed to making a difference to everyone we serve."
- A dedicated intranet website was launched at the beginning of the transformation project:
  - serving as a repository for all facets of the SSI improvement project,
  - supporting the work effort by the LST/BDA/VST teams,
  - featuring the latest news, work products, photos, videos, and frequently asked questions.
- Learning Management System (LMS)—The consulting team developed training materials for the MH LMS for ease of access and learner follow-up and to support the training of all MH members in lean and HRO methods of improvement and reliable outcomes.
- Monthly workshops and seminars (see Appendix IX) were conducted throughout the project.

What were the results
Early baseline observations and improvement recommended opportunities (Appendix VII)

1. Large variation in clinical practices is critical (Appendix VIII)
   a. Daily Variations in input/output processes for patients was too high
      i. Infrequent on-time starts (@60%−80% on time starts)
      ii. Excessive add-on cases (@40%) (see below)
      iii. Missing Patient health information (PHI) prior to surgery
      iv. Variable surgical block time utilization (50−80%)
      v. # of surgical procedures per day/week/month, # of endo procedures per day/week/month using PACU and D/C units, # of IR procedures per day/week/month using PACU and D/C unit, and # of caths/cardiac procedures using PACU and D/C units.
      vi. Info needed to predict staffing, patient flow, and bed assignments.
   b. OR scheduling/patient throughput is unstable, high add-on roster
   c. Discrepancies in definitions and lack of knowledge of volumes
   d. Addressing black holes
2. Relentless focus on following best surgical care practices
   a. Violations of surgical infection control policies must be addressed
   b. Too many patient handoffs which are mostly done in ad hoc, nonstandardized manner
   c. Preventable surgical errors and patient harm are too common
3. Waste identification and redesign
   a. Scheduling inaccuracies (see below)

    b. Variability in OR product utilization (e.g., underutilized sterile packs/trays during surgeries, unnecessarily high inventory)

    c. Overused nonbillable supplies

    d. Suboptimal use of expensive technology

    e. Labor costs during idle OR time

    f. High staff turnover, high traveler/agency staffing

Massive variation with pre-operation clinics operations

Deep dive into surgical site infections (SSI)

We focused on SSI because they are preventable and result in devastating complications with significant morbidity after surgery (Figs. 15.6—15.10). MH reported greater than 200 SSIs in 2020 with an estimated cost to the hospital of approximately $4.2 million.[8] First, a champion was designated to represent their project to the SLT (Fig. 15.25). The champion is the "rock removal" leader who sought to eliminate the barriers to success. With the support of the consultants, a deep dive into SSI identified SSI risk factors using evidence-based practices while applying a lean six sigma approach to problem solving.

    We mapped the patient processes to help understand where the SSI might be originating from (before—during—after surgical processes) (Fig. 15.26). The data

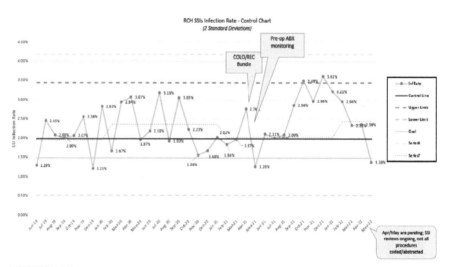

FIGURE 15.25

Surgical site infections (SSI) prevention, 2019—22.

---

[8] National estimated SSI average cost: $20,785.

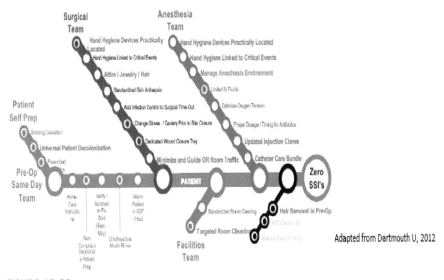

FIGURE 15.26

Fishbone template to address SSI prevention efforts.

collected included the patient-related factors, sterilization and the hygiene practices in the OR and OR flow and traffic, and compliance to the bundle of care. The gap analysis helped identify the potential risk factors.

Gap Analysis (Fig. 15.27): A comprehensive gap analysis was completed that compared national best practices with the perioperative processes currently in place at MH in order to determine the "gaps" and help MH best focus on improvement efforts most at need at MH.

- Antibiotic Administration and Redosing Guidelines (Table 15.1): Wide antibiotic fallout was noted by time of day and day of week with over 50% of patients not receiving full antibiotic coverage from midnight to 7 a.m. and over 40% did not get their required antibiotic on Saturday surgeries. Variation was found. A dosing and redosing guideline for prophylactic antimicrobials during surgery was agreed upon and a review of all antibiotic fallouts from clinical practice guidelines was done weekly.
- SSI Case Review/Investigation tool (Fig. 15.27): A robust peer review template was developed with standardized definitions for SSI that provides reviewers (physicians and nurses) with a series of agreed on data points and pictures to help identify SSI risk factors and discussion questions to determine trends and opportunities for improvement related to SSI.
- SSI Team and Focused Subgroups (Figs. 15.28—15.30): The data showed that colonic and small bowel surgery had the most variation and higher than standard infection (SIR) national rates. Multidisciplinary teams were dedicated to

Best Practice	Best Practice Strategies	How to Achieve Recommendation	How Our Practices Differ From Best Practice	Barriers to Best Practice Implementation	Will Implement Best Practice (Yes/No; why not?)	Tracking Method
Give Prophylactic Antibiotics Based on Clinical Practice Guidelines	Antibiotics given prior to surgery on clinically indicated cases, administer antibiotics only when indicated by guidelines	Give ABX appropriately and timely	~95% of cases receive appropriate and timely prophylactic antibiotics	Phase of care, Patient already on scheduled abx	Yes	Antibiotic fallout report and review. Moved to quarterly monitoring as we have several Months >95%
Preoperative Bathing	Bathe each patient before surgery	Use Theraworx for every patient before surgery	89% of Surgeries had Preop bathing (Theraworx)	Consistency, documentation	Yes	Theraworx report with denominator
Surgical Site Skin Preparation with Alcohol-Based antiseptic agent unless Contraindicated	Alcohol-based antiseptic solutions based on CHG for Surgical site skin preparation. Skin Prep must be dry before incision	Use Chloraprep or alcohol based skin prep (Dual agent Skin Prep)	Lack of Standardization	Obtaining accurate data	Yes.	Skin Prep report with denominator, Will check data in 90 days.

Best Practice	Best Practice Strategies	How to Achieve Recommendation	How Our Practices Differ From Best Practice	Barriers to Best Practice Implementation	Will Implement Best Practice (Yes/No; why not?)	Tracking Method
Implement perioperative glycemic control and use blood glucose target levels less than 200 mg/dL in patients with and without diabetes.	Monitor blood glucose levels perioperatively Audit tool to determine fallout	Maintain levels below 200 mg/dL in all patients	Completed on Colons and Small Bowels	Optimum Patient before surgery from floor, time and equipment	Yes on COLO and SB	Audit Tool
Maintain perioperative normothermia	Confirm temp probes are accurate Use of forced warm air.	through all phases of surgery Maintain temp >35.5° C postoperatively	Monitored on any surgeries over 2 hours	Baier hugger limitations.	Yes	Audit Tool
Consider the use of triclosan-coated sutures for the prevention of SSI.	Use triclosan-coated sutures	Standardize inventory	Do not currently use	Antimicrobial resistance and only effective for superficial SSI	No, ABX resistance thru Efflux pump activation	NA

FIGURE 15.27

Surgical site infection prevention gap analysis.

Table 15.1 Effect of night surgery on antibiotic fallout- time of day.

Time range of surgery case	Fallouts	Total	%Rate
00:00–>07:00	2	4	50.00%
07:00–>12:00	8	55	14.55%
12:00–>17:00	5	40	12.50%
17:00–>24:00	6	21	28.57%
Total	21	120	17.50%
Antibiotic fallout by day of the week			
Day of the week	Fallouts	Total	%Rate
Sunday	1	10	10.00%
Monday	4	32	12.50%
Tuesday	8	23	34.78%
Wednesday	2	23	8.70%
Thursday	3	18	16.67%
Friday	0	7	0.00%
Saturday	3	7	42.86%
Total	21	120	17.50%

New and Redesigned SSI Case Review Investigation tool

COLON Surgical Site Infection (SSI) Drilldown Tool

Instructions:
1. Review case information and surgeon to complete the last section of the form
2. Return completed form to Dr. Patrick Kenney (pkenney@monument.health) and Candice Holzer-Infection Preventionist (cholzer@monument.health) by the due date

DRILLDOWN COMPLETION TRACKING	
DUE DATE	
DRILLDOWN COMPLETED BY SURGEON (DATE)	
DEMOGRAPHICS	
MRN	
NAME (LAST, FIRST)	
SEX	
AGE	
DATE OF ADMISSION	
DATE OF SURGERY	
SURGEON	
FIRST ASSIST	
PROCEDURE	
PRE-OP DIAGNOSIS	
POST-OP DIAGNOSIS	
SURGERY SCHEDULED AS	
ACTUAL SURGERY PERFORMED	
OR SUITE (room #)	
Lap/Open/Robotic	
CASE CLASSIFICATION	
CPT or ICD-10 Code	
WOUND CLASSIFICATION	

RISK FACTORS		
BMI	Weight Status	
Below 18.5	Underweight	
18.5 – 24.9	Normal or Healthy Weight	BMI
25.0 – 29.9	Overweight	
30.0 and Above	Obese	
SMOKER		
DIABETES		
IMMUNOSUPPRESSED		
OTHER		
INFECTION REVIEW		

READMISSION DATE (OR N/A)	
INFECTION TYPE	
DATE OF INFECTION	
SIGNS AND SYMPTOMS	
PATHOGEN	
PATOS?	
SSI FOUND	
CASE DETAILS	
HAIR REMOVAL IF NECESSARY [WAS HAIR CLIPPED VS SHAVED? WAS HAIR REMOVED IN PRE-OP OR IN OR?]	
Theraworx Bath done in Pre-Op?	
SKIN PREP (WHAT WAS AGENT WAS USED)	
CUT TIME (DATE/TIME)	
END TIME (DATE/TIME)	
DURATION OF SURGERY	
ANESTHESIOLOGIST	
CRNA	
ASA SCORE	
GLYCEMIC CONTROL (110-150MG/dL):	
WAS OXYGENATION IN PACU AT 80% FIO2?	
NORMOTHERMIA MAINTAINED DURING THE PERIOP PERIOD (T=>36 C)?	
COMMENTS	
ANTIBIOTICS	
ANTIBIOTIC ALLERGIES (PLEASE LIST)	
PRE OP ANTIBIOTIC GIVEN (LIST ANTIBIOTIC)	
WAS PRE-OP ANTIBIOTIC ADMINISTERED WITHIN 1HR OF CUT TIME (2 HR FOR VANCO)	
WAS CHOICE OF ANTIBIOTIC CONSISTENT WITH PUBLISHED GUIDELINES?	
WERE ANTIBIOTICS RE-DOSED AT APPROPRIATE TIME IF INDICATED?	
SURGEON TO COMPLETE:	
WERE WOUND PROTECTORS USED?	
IRRIGATION USED?	
WAS A NEW TRAY USED FOR CLOSING?	
WERE GLOVES CHANGED PRIOR TO CLOSING?	
WAS ASEPTIC TECHNIQUE EVER COMPROMISED?	
WERE THERE ANY ISSUES DOCUMENTED OR RECALLED DURING THE PROCEDURE?	
COMMENTS	

FIGURE 15.28

Redesigned surgical site infections (SSI) case review investigation tool.

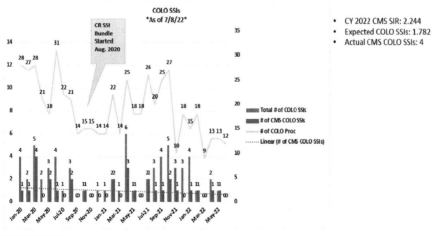

FIGURE 15.29

Surgical site infections (SSI) for colon surgery by SSI, 2019—22.
SIR—Standardized infection rates.

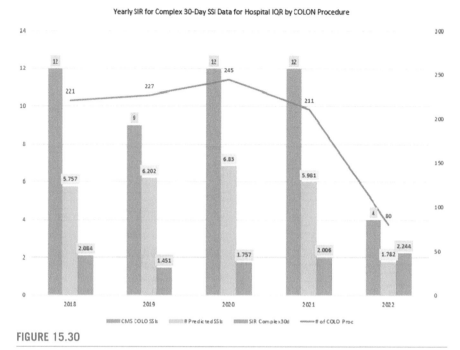

FIGURE 15.30

Surgical site infections (SSI) yearly SIR for complex 30 day for colon surgery.
SIR—Standardized infection rate.

eliminating preventable SSIs, GI subgroup reviews data, and case reviews of
SSIs were done weekly.
- Environmental Cleaning Process: Standardized process and checklists for OR
cleaning prior to first case of the day, end of case, and terminal cleaning (end of
day) were implemented. The consulting team facilitated a focus on quality with
ATP testing as the quality metric.
- Surgeon Report Cards: The chair of surgery introduced surgeon report cards to
include individual SSI rates and comparisons with MH peers, and this was
agreed to by a majority vote of the surgeons.
- Patient Education: Patient education materials were created with the purpose of
addressing what patients can do to prevent SSI and how to perform preoperative
cleansing either through showers and skin wipes.
- Routine Audits: Scheduling and conducting of unannounced audits was implemented to document infection control in the perioperative service line with
agreed to reporting back to surgeons, nurses, anesthesia, Cliically registered
nurses anesthesists (CRNAs), and to the senior leadership team (SLT).
- Leadership SSI goals were crafted and reviewed regularily (Fig. 15.31,
Fig. 15.32).

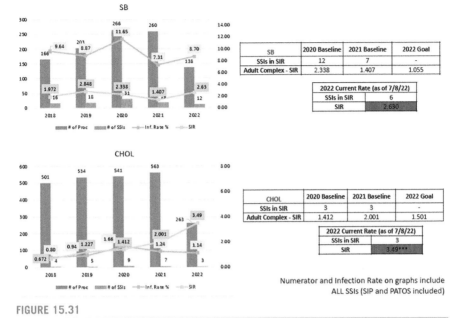

FIGURE 15.31

Summary of SSI for small bowel (SB) and colon surgery (CO) 2018—22 by SIR. SIR—Standardized infection rate.

Postoperating room results and analysis

Scheduling deep dive improvement analysis (Appendix VIII)

Scheduling surgeries is a complicated process. Variability among surgery, anesthesia, and cleanup durations affects the OR schedule. Surgery schedulers must also take into account varying priorities in the schedule. The OR managers want to keep the surgeons satisfied and have high utilization of the rooms. The surgeons do not want downtime between surgeries and prefer to have their surgeries scheduled at times that work around their clinic schedules. On the other hand, surgeons need to be on time for the scheduled surgeries or their tardiness can cause rippling delays throughout the day. In addition, case add-ons can also impact the schedule and available resources. Nurses want evenly dispersed patient flow so there are not peaks where are they are busier. Patients want minimal indirect and direct delays. These varying priorities are difficult to balance when scheduling surgeries, as they often conflict. The project goal was to propose a more effective surgical scheduling process in which schedulers consider five key guiding principles: patient safety, access, OR efficiency, patient service, and physician satisfaction. Finally, timely patient clearance was important because patients that arrive at preop without H&Ps, testing, preop orders, and/or consents add time to the preop schedule (Figs. 15.33—15.34 show Failure Mode and Effect Analysis and Scheduling Analysis).

SSI Goals 2022

1. Reduce SSI rates in colon surgeries by 25% (SIR) by December 31, 2022

COLO	2020 Baseline	2021 Baseline	2022 Goal
SSIs in SIR	12	12	-
Complex 30 Day - SIR	1.757	2.006	1.505

2022 Current Rate (as of 7/8/22)	
SSIs in SIR	4
SIR	2.244

2. Reduce SSI rates in small bowel surgeries by 25% (SIR) by December 31, 2022

SB	2020 Baseline	2021 Baseline	2022 Goal
SSIs in SIR	12	7	-
Adult Complex - SIR	2.338	1.407	1.055

2022 Current Rate (as of 7/8/22)	
SSIs in SIR	6
SIR	2.630

3. Reduce SSI rates in cholecystectomy surgeries by 25% (SIR) by December 31, 2022

CHOL	2020 Baseline	2021 Baseline	2022 Goal
SSIs in SIR	3	3	-
Adult Complex - SIR	1.412	2.001	1.501

2022 Current Rate (as of 7/8/22)	
SSIs in SIR	3
SIR	3.49***

4. Decrease monthly average of SSIs (Ø PATOS) by 25% by December 31, 2022

AVG	2020 Baseline	2021 Baseline	2022 Goal
SSIs	13.66	13.33	10.00

2022 Current Average (as of 7/8/22)
73
11.66

5. Obtain an SSI SIR of <1.3 for all NHSN procedures by December 31, 2022 (25% reduction)

Adult Complex SIR	2020 Baseline	2021 Baseline	2022 Goal
	1.448	1.733	1.3

2022 YH SIR (as of 7/8/22)	
SIR	1.695

FIGURE 15.32

Muda Health SSI goals for small bowel and colon surgery 2020—22.
SIR-Standardized infection rate.

Project Setbacks

The COVID-19 outbreak showed the vulnerabilities in the US healthcare system, and MH was not spared, with procedures canceled, tests postponed, and many patients' elective cases postponed. It is important to be honest and realistic with hospital staff about missed targets and internral or external factors that are delaying the project goals. Phase I of the project was curtailed due to the growing infections caused by COVID-19 which forced canceling of a second on-site visit, patient interviews, and postsurgical/ambulatory site observations.

The major barriers encountered during the QI activity implementation centered around the complexity of coordinating all personnel in every phase of care. Busy surgeons and surgical groups with many rotating on-call providers and demanding private practices evoked a natural variation in familiarity with the SSI, Enhanced Recovery After Surgery (ERAS), and other protocols for reliable and safer outcomes.

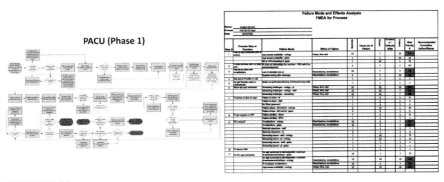

FIGURE 15.33

Postanesthesia care unit (PACU)—failure modes and effects analysis (FMEA).

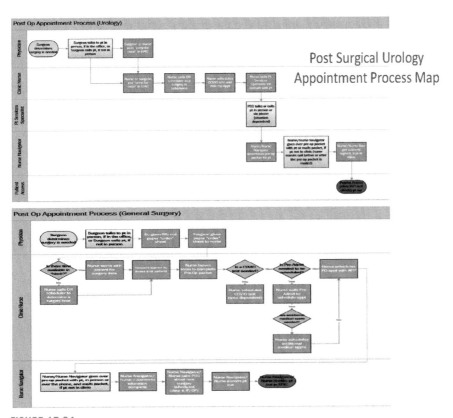

FIGURE 15.34

Postsurgery urology appointment process map.

We experienced setbacks mostly related to lack of communication or unwillingness of some surgeons and anesthesiologists to participate in improvement opportunities with potential changes to their practices. These experiences reiterated the need for providing data in support of the initiative. For example, when resistance was met regarding revising the guidelines for elective cases regarding appropriate and timely antibiotic preoperative administration, instead of demanding adoption of the recommendations, we relied on surgical service line meetings to discuss among themselves, provide the most current guidelines/recommendations, and vote them into acceptance. Utilizing experts including the consultant clinicians and experts in systems improvement facilitated buy-in and lent overall credibility to the initiative.

Regular meetings (every 1 to 2 weeks) of the multidisciplinary team allowed for discussion of the data and for addressing setbacks as they were encountered. For example, a decrease in compliance was noted on particular surgical wards where there was high staff turnover, and this was remedied with intense staff education by nurse educators. Additionally, certain aspects were not being documented adequately such as the complexity of the surgical wounds. This was ameliorated with regular audits by infection control staff. This improved documentation did not increase nursing workload.

Frequent communication between the surgeon champions and individual hospital providers was essential in establishing hospital-wide compliance of protocols and to mitigate and reducate variation that was secondary to physician preferences and was not aligned with best practice guidelines. Sharing of data and up to date literature at meetings with hospital providers helped assuage concerns and increase clinician trust, support for the project, and compliance.

Cost savings

- We demonstrated using a robust ROI framework that MH saved **well over $1 million in phase 1 and over $2.6 million by the project end. Several recommendations were made regarding sustaining these improvement gains:**
- Costs can be better managed and should be guided by common robust cost/quality and effectiveness industry-wide measures for example to include:
  - Formulary—We found no research that Sugammadex leads to less occurrence of reintubation than other reversal drugs (real cost savings of $341,000).
  - Equipment
  - Supplies
  - Instruments
  - Implants
  - Scrubs
- The analysis recommended curbing unnecessary use of the drug vasopressin leading to an annualized cost avoidance of nearly $100,000 over the past 5 months.

- Getting the CFO and VP for supply chain and contract management working together to examine all surgical capital assets' strategic use, including supplies and human capital (e.g., detailed return in investment assessments and costs management, and investments made strategically including investment in staff).
- The following should be regularly calculated:
  - Cost per case by specialty and surgeon.
  - Scrubs—usage per case, cost, "lost inventory."
  - Staffing—staffing model (circulator, tech).
  - Staffing—on-call—utilization.
  - Staffing—OT—# of hours per pay period, $ per pay period, right people right place, right time.
  - $ value of lost instruments annualized.
  - Staffing—agency, costs, culture leakage.
  - Quality outcomes—costs associated with SSIs, adverse events, readmissions, additional testing, follow-ups.

Tips for others planning surgical quality improvement initiatives

Getting started

A crucial factor for success was the early engagement of key stakeholders at the conceptualization stage, including healthcare providers from surgery, anesthesiology, nursing, infectious diseases, and pharmacy. When introducing the project, stress the WHY. No one wants to perform additional work, but by stressing how this project was impacting patient care and surgeon workflow helped to increase engagement. We included hospital leaders from the surgical program, emergency department, intensive care and hospital professional staff leadership together with the hospital Quality team. This proved essential to ensuring staff buy-in, not only by the surgical group but also the nonphysician staff through the VST working group. We did a comprehensive needs analysis and assessed the readiness assessment to better understand MH's organizational maturity and competencies for organizational transformation. The presentation of real-time local data, supported by external standards, and the most up-to-date literature, were key steps that increased the acceptability of the practice changes. Creating a common language and commitment in support of lean methods and adopting a HRO approach and terminology were essential for the project's initial success and sustainable gains.

Increasing buy-in

Get buy-in from staff by emphasizing the patient safety and quality improvement potential for organizational cost savings, decreased resource utilization, and improved patient outcomes. Establish surgeon champions who are invested in the project and can provide support from senior management. We regularly reviewed and presented preliminary audit results after each PDSA cycle to provide direct feedback and education to key stakeholders during surgical and BDA multidisciplinary rounds. We discussed solutions to unanticipated implementation hurdles. Embedding reminders and reinforcements via the dedicated intranet website and document repository helped to consolidate the change and facilitated sustainability of the planned interventions. We highlighted early wins and made sure local champions made the case to their clinical peers using leadership and data metric dashboards (Figs. 15.35 and 15.36). Bringing outside consultants helped to make an enormous difference the level of coaching and mentoring of surgeons, surgical staff, anethesiologists and the quality improvement staff. The most helpful interventions included reminders to stimulate discussion among staff about the duration and indication of perioperative antibiotics during rounds, and the prompts regarding perioperative checklists and computer monitors. These two interventions were seen as the most important to trust and support throughout the project. Spot audits to track surgical site infections, OR turnover, OR equipment sterility and cleanliness, and postoperative antibiotic use with feedback to front-line providers supported sustainability. It was essential to develop and sustain the QI skill set through training QI tools, seminars, and by creating a common project handbook that provided a common language and mindset. Creating a patient information booklet helped to set clear expectations and

Leadership Dashboard—Feb 19, 2021

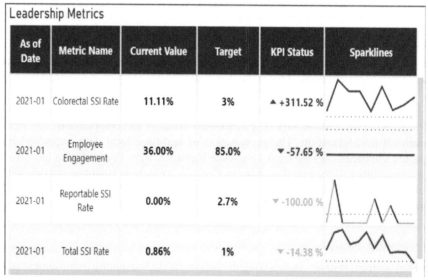

Leadership Metrics					
As of Date	Metric Name	Current Value	Target	KPI Status	Sparklines
2021-01	Colorectal SSI Rate	11.11%	3%	▲ +311.52 %	
2021-01	Employee Engagement	36.00%	85.0%	▼ -57.65 %	
2021-01	Reportable SSI Rate	0.00%	2.7%	▼ -100.00 %	
2021-01	Total SSI Rate	0.86%	1%	▼ -14.38 %	

FIGURE 15.35

Leadership data dashboard snapshot.

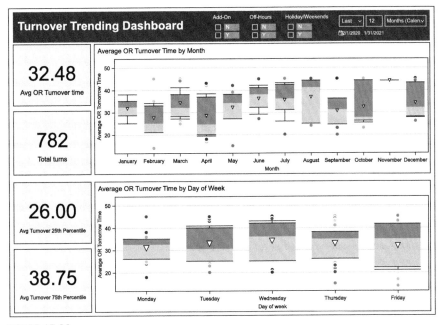

FIGURE 15.36

Front-line clinical data dashboard.

answered most common questions regarding SSI prevention. Reviewing this booklet with each patient in the preoperative evaluation was seen as key to success.

Sustaining the project

One of the keys to sustaining the patient safety gains and improvements was frequent feedback, particularly sharing the successful results in the reduction of SSI, OR turnover times, and other productivity metrics on a daily/weekly basis during the implementation period. It is important to always remain supportive and not judgemental in all interactions. Individuals take data very personally and often will self-motivate once the data are available. The standardized paths and surgical equipment card sets made it easier to follow the protocol than to deviate. The frequent vocal reports of caregivers at weekly meetings about "how (the process) was better and so much easier than they thought it would be" reinforced the care teams' committment.

The success of this intervention—like any novel model of care—can also be attributed to buy-in from key stakeholders and leadership from the outset. While there was some leadership pushback which slowed down the project and coupled with the COVID-19 pandemic-imposed travel restrictions, imposing huge increased demands on staff, delayed the project significantly. Continued commitment at senior levels and ongoing support from clinical champions were essential to ensure that a collegiate and collaborative environment was maintained, along with regular communication with key stakeholders such as surgeons, OR nursing and technical staff, assisted with the successful implementation.

Conclusions—path toward high reliability and safe surgical care

Quality improvement is not an exact science; however, this case study serves as a starting point to assist surgical teams and departments in developing their own surgical safety and quality improvement initiatives. The case study provides details of the quality improvement efforts that hospitals can implement at their own facility. The project led to remarkable results over an 18-month period and continues to demonstrate continuous improvement 28 months after initiation. The project was able to:

- Improve safety and reduce surgical infection rates
- Improve quality metrics
- Maximize operating room uptime
- Reduce supplies expenses
- Eliminate staffing hassles
- Increase surgeon and nurse satisfaction
- Grow a large number of staff (>1/3 of workforce) trained in lean six sigma and HRO principles.

The key recommendations from this case study to achieve and sustain surgical excellence include the need to:

1. Develop and deploy a new governance structure to facilitate improvements in safety, quality and effeciency by using a
   a. Leadership steering team (LST).
   b. Before/during/after process improvement teams (BDA).
   c. New VST.
2. Engage MH wide expertise and experience
   a. Engagement was key by assinging, individuals responsibility for clinical and financial outcomes of defined surgical care processes, including from operations PI, infection control, supply management, risk management, environmental services, and the physician utilization committee.
3. Focus on measurement and transparency
   a. Measure the outcomes that matter most to patients and clinicians, and the contributing processes and intermediate outcomes.
   b. Establish scorecard metrics and associated rate of improvements for each dashboards with rates of improvement to reach goals (quality/cost/time).
   c. Adopt the appropriate information technology (IT) to optimize measurement and processes improvement and be careful not to let the lack of a proper IT infrastructure act as an excuse for inactivity.

    d. Hardwire process optimization and standardization align measurement processes with your surgical care pathways and lines of reporting.

    e. Continually seek ways to risk-adjust measurements, to enable better benchmarking.

4. Culture of safety

    a. Train all surgical team members and support teams in TeamSTEPPS and HRO training approaches while embracing their building blocks of measurement, responsible and accountable governance, culture, process optimization, and standardization.

    b. Support and model safety reporting and methods to address behaviors/actions counter to a culture of safety.

    c. Create a culture that is zero tolerant to complacency, but also open and just, committed to excellence and joint learning.

    d. Remember culture is at the heart of all safety and quality transformation ("Culture eats strategy," Peter Drucker)

5. Seek independent assurance over the reliability of quality measures, via internal and external audits, while applying established assurance, lean six sigma and Baldrige excellence principles.

List of appendices

Appendix I. Team roles

Each of the three Before/During/After (BDA) teams should consist of a champion, a leader, perhaps an associate leader, a performance improvement (PI) facilitator, along with other staff members selected by the Champion and leaders to be involved on their team. The LST will ensure their ability to commit time and energy to the effort.

    The roles of the Leadership Steering Team (LST) members, champions, leaders, and performance improvement facilitators are explained and expanded on below.

Keep in mind that individuals may play more than one role. For example, a PI leader may serve a dual role as team leader and performance improvement facilitator.

What is an LST member? Here are some characteristics of an LST member

- A senior executive with direct or indirect responsibilities for championing the perioperative services of the future effort.
- A senior executive with ability to assign resources, mentor/coach staff involved in perioperative services, and budget authority.
- A senior executive with discretionary time that allows them to regularly visit perioperative services.
- A senior executive with ability to determine how resources are allocated in keeping with changes in project focus or priorities.

What is a champion? Here are some characteristics of a champion

- An individual with a history of successfully leading or deploying positive change at MH.
- A collaborator who is trusted within MH.
- A person with the wherewithal (e.g., budget, authority, resources, trusted network) to overcome obstacles in the way of those seeking to implement improvements—"rock/barrier removal experts."
- Champions often are executives and may be members of the LST. For the perioperative services project, the initial BDA champions will be members of the LST.
- A person who takes the time to mentor and coach other employees.

Who are the leaders of each team? The leaders should have the following characteristics:

- Someone with a vested interest in the success of their project.
- Someone respected and trusted by others in the team.
- Someone who is willing to listen to all involved and make "tough" decisions when it is difficult to get to consensus.
- Someone who cares for both the process and participants on the team as they prefer to implement win–win solutions.

Who are the performance improvement facilitators?

Consider the following characteristics:

- Staff with performance improvement training and experience (e.g., lean six sigma yellow belts, green belts, black belts).

- Staff with skills in data gathering, organizing data, and analyzing data that facilitate turning data into information to improve decision-making.
- Staff either familiar with or open and engaged in learning more about the processes in which the improvements are to be applied.
  - Muda Health Leadership Steering Team (LST)
    - Membership
      - CMO
      - CNO
      - CFO
      - VP Supply Chain
      - Ex-officio members—CEO, president
      - Physician Leaders (hospital employee, nonhospital staff)
      - Ancillary services representatives as needed (imaging, lab, pharmacy, housekeeping, transportation, bed management)
      - HR support as needed
      - IT leader and data analyst
      - VP Operations—perioperative service and project owner
      - Director of surgical services
      - Vice president quality, safety, risk management
    - Select champions for Before, During, After (BDA) teams
      - Before team (nursing leader and physician support)
      - During team (MD/DO leader with nursing support)
      - After team (nurse and bed management support)
    - Performance improvement facilitation
      - Establish scorecard/dashboard metrics
      - Establish baseline measures
      - Set SMART goals for each team
      - Each team to have performance improvement facilitator from hospital
      - Willingness to have support of volunteers, children of employees, high school/college interns—data gathering and observation assistance
    - Meetings with LST and or champions
      - Initially set up 1–2-hour meetings once every 2 weeks on a set schedule.
        - As BDA teams launch and move forward, once a week review meeting frequency is appropriate.
      - Team reviews
        - Review of dashboard metrics to date.
        - What was accomplished since last meeting?
        - What is planned to be accomplished before next meeting?
        - What is going well and new learnings?
        - What are "barriers" that need SLT or champions to address?
  - **Before Surgery Team (BST)**
    - Establish team membership
      - Champion assigned by SLT (can be a member of SLT)

- Performance improvement leader assigned to team
- Nursing leader, preop representative
- Pharmacy
- Laboratory
- Finance representative
- Central sterilization representative
- Clerical staff, scheduling representative
- Virtual team representatives (transportation, ED, physician)
- Materials management
- Patients and families
- Dashboard metrics
  - Quality
    - Sterilization carts filled accurately, completely, on time
    - Variances from best practices (e.g., sterilization time, lead times, preference card first time accuracy)
    - History and physical (H&P) and consents completed before patient arrival
  - Cost
    - Staffing levels
    - Supply costs that are high-end outliers when suitable alternative is available
    - Opportunity cost of unused surgical suite space
  - Time/delivery
    - Patient arrival to preop cycle time
    - Preop to arrival at OR cycle time
    - Equipment/instrument order to fill cycle time
    - Case book request to fill cycle time
    - OR block release time ahead of schedule time
- Process improvements
  - Kaizen events—1 or 2 incremental changes per month
  - Lean six sigma type efforts of 3–6 months in duration
    - Significant impact expected in quality, cost, and time
- During surgery team (DST)
  - Membership
    - Champion assigned by SLT (can be a member of SLT)
    - Performance improvement leader assigned to team
    - Surgeon leader (internal or external)
    - Anesthesiologist leader
    - Nursing representative
    - Infection control/quality representative
    - Environmental services
    - Materials management
    - Others as needed
  - Dashboard metrics

- Quality
  - Near misses
  - Adverse events
  - Waivers from recommended sterilization times or methods
  - Each time out completed and documented
  - % Surgeries with doctor, anesthesiologist, and nurse at patient induction
- Cost
  - Higher cost supplies/instruments substituted for less costly alternative.
  - Pharmacy costs
  - Unused surgical OR suite cost
- Time
  - OR arrival of patient to surgery start cycle time
  - Surgery start to surgery finished cycle time
  - Surgery finish to OR room turnaround started cycle time
  - OR room turnaround cycle time
  - First case start time (minutes early/late)
- Process improvements
  - Kaizen events—1 or 2 incremental changes per month
  - Lean six sigma type efforts of 3—6 months in duration
    - Significant impact expected in quality, cost, and time
- After surgery team (AST)
  - Membership
    - Champion assigned by LST (can be a member of LST)
    - Performance improvement leader assigned to team
    - Nurse leader (PACU)
    - Bed management representative
    - Admissions/finance representative
    - Transportation
    - Hospitalist representative
    - Data analyst
    - Clerical staff
    - Patients and families
  - Dashboard metrics
    - Quality
      - # and % patients with postsurgery concerns
      - # and % outpatients admitted rather than discharged (outpatient)
      - # and type of PACU patient concerns identified
    - Cost
      - Length of stay in PACU
      - Staffing levels for monitored beds, transporters
    - Time
      - OR surgery complete to OR patient depart cycle time

- OR patient depart to PACU arrival cycle time
- PACU arrival time to PACU depart cycle time
- PACU depart to patient depart cycle time
- VST
  - Membership
    - Champion—a senior leader (e.g., physician) who is well respected by front-line staff and supervisors in perioperative services.
    - Leader—an experienced staff member who is passionate about wanting to improve perioperative services and is well respected by front-line staff.
    - Nurse(s)
    - Technical staff
    - Sterilization staff member
    - Scheduling staff member
    - Supply chain staff member
    - Clerical staff
  - Meets as a group once per week for 30–60 min and has subgroup huddles every day of the week.
    - Daily huddles may include expected ED/ICU admissions and unusual situations in and around the OR. Does not last more than 10–15 min and is conducted while standing.
    - The huddles provide a structure for work in between weekly meetings.
    - Ideally, these huddles should happen in front of posted metrics on some type of huddle board.
  - Provides a vehicle to gather suggestions, issues, concerns, and opportunities from peers.
  - Suggestions made and implemented should be tracked.
  - Must be able to promise peers and others complete anonymity if they request it as their ideas, suggestions, issues, concerns, and opportunities are the focus not the individual providing the information.
  - Meets with LST minimally once every 2 weeks and more frequently when LST wants to communicate their issues, plans, and decisions throughout the organization.
    - VST provides input to the LST and vice versa.
    - The VST provides an additional conduit to communicate to those engaged in perioperative services.
    - A VST champion and leader may participate as an ex-officio member of the LST and should be invited to participate.
  - E3-Engagement everywhere, everyone. The more MH staff members who participate in the process change, the better the understanding and the higher the level of investment in the changes. High levels of ownership will result in higher achievement. The staff will want the changes to work, as they belong to THEM. This approach will also help mitigate some resistance to the changes. The more people know about the change, the less they will fear the change.

Appendix II. Before—during—after (BDA) surgery project charters

All of the initial preparations are collected together in a single document.

- This is commonly known as a "Project Charter." (see Figs.15.20 and 15.21).
- It contains the results of all key preparation and planning activities.
- The problem statement aspect of the project charter derives its clarity from aspects that were not aligned with the values statements of MH.
- Charters can be modified during the project. They are living documents.

Project charters are used in four key capacities:

- A guideline ensures that key planning activities are done.
- A tool to communicate and set project expectations.
- An authorization, *or contract*, between the project team and management
- A tool to hold executives and employees accountable to each other and the organization.

The author(s) of a draft project charter are the champions of the project and the leaders. The following are key elements of a project charter:

- Develop the problem statement
- Develop the goal statement
- Identify the process(es) and scope
- Identify the customer(s) and supplier(s)
- Identify the key players
- Develop a business case for the project
- Prepare the project plan
- Prepare the project charter

Appendix III. Meeting location and team etiquette

f. Expectations

    i. Clarity of aim

        1. Establish team rules and team guiding principles early to help scope discussions and decisions.

        2. Come prepared to meeting (review results, prereading)

        3. Agenda (time, method, item, aim/action):

           a. The agenda is an important part of your meeting. It should be sent out to the team members before the meeting. By setting the agenda, people are prepared for what work is expected to be accomplished.

           b. Specific tasks are listed and responsible persons noted. This way there is no question who is to follow-up with for action items.

      c. With the agenda, the first part of the meeting is to assign the roles listed for meetings. This helps you to stay on task before you get started. Jobs or participation are never assigned to absent team members because it does not allow for discussion or true ownership of the task.

      d. If someone is unable to attend the meetings, but is willing to take on a task, that should be announced to the team only if a firm commitment is made by the absent team member.

      e. Every meeting should be evaluated for its effectiveness during the last few minutes of the meeting. Those scoring should be prepared to express why they scored in the way they did. Using a scale of 0–10 with 10 being the best meeting ever and describing what went well and what could be improved helps develop open communication among the team and to also provide feedback on your meeting process.

  ii. Practice effective meeting skills

      1. Frequent, timely, and accurate communication

      2. Problem solving communication

      3. Encouragement

  iii. Clarifying

      1. Process improvement knowledge

      2. Expectations—different perspective

      3. Action plan:

         a. What tasks will be done?

         b. By whom?

         c. By when?

         d. How?

         e. Comments

         f. Completed action times

  iv. Meeting report-out templates

      1. Complete report out meeting sheet (meeting types; aim; day/time/location; notes; baseline, goals, etc.)

  v. Feedback:

      1. How to give it well

      2. Learn to use plus/delta assessment. Participants identify positive things as pluses and things that should be changed as deltas. Using deltas instead of "cons" reinforces that learning is part of all continuous improvement work.

      3. Group dynamics—promote and transition facilitator leadership to the clinical staff as they emerge.

g. The situation room—The BDA teams need to find an effective way to communicate and collaborate with other team members. We created a physical environment for innovation teams to colocate their work. Having the teams work together in this environment helps to keep a constant focus in the big room, large enough to gather the work of the three teams, and with lots of wall space for visual communication and collaborative facilitation of tools.

h. The big room enables two principles of lean thinking that speed up the design and improvement process: comprehensive and focused decision-making early in the process, instead of teams working in isolation and later addressing conflicting decisions, and concurrent processes, i.e., teams working simultaneously instead of with hand-offs back and forth and between steps. See below pictures of the situation room.

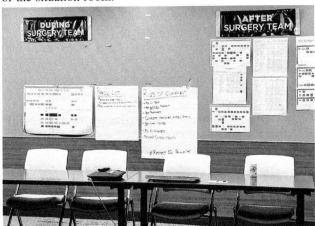

i.

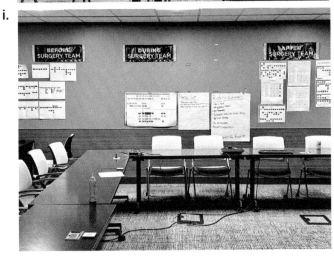

Appendix IV. Identify the process(es) and scope

- The project scope focuses attention on the boundaries (e.g., start and end points) and resources of the team's process improvement efforts.
  - A scope that is too broadly defined can lead a team to work outside of its sphere of influence and resource capacities.
  - A too narrow a scope can produce solutions with limited (disappointing) results.
- The SIPOC—high-level view of process, scope, and requirements (Figure 15.37 and 15.38)
  - Supplier: Internal or external provider of information, equipment, supplies
  - Input: What is needed to carry out the process
  - Process: Typically, four to six primary high-level steps to complete requirements
  - Output: What is expected to be achieved at each process step and overall
  - Customer: Internal or external beneficiary of the process

Identify the customers and suppliers—should be incorporated into SIPOC development.

Identify the key "players"

- Champions
- Leaders
- Performance improvement facilitator(s)
- Team members
- Process owners—those who are expected to sustain the improvements generated

Develop a business case

- The business case should answer the following key questions:
  - Why is this project worth doing now?
  - What are the consequences of not doing this project?
- Usually, the business case language will come directly from the champion.
- How does it fit with key business goals and initiatives?
  - Link to strategic business plan
  - Identify all of the financial implications
  - Quality, cost, and time
- Compare with other investment (financial or people) alternatives

Develop a project plan

- Draft an expected rollout plan for the project
- Include timing of resource demands (financial or people)

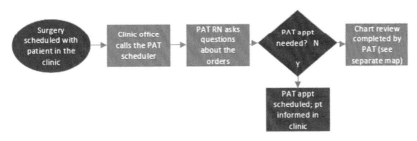

FIGURE 15.37

Pre-hospital (PAT) surgery scheduling process.

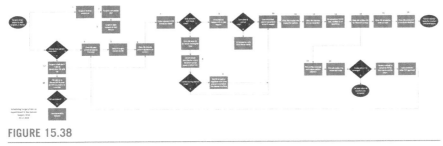

FIGURE 15.38

Surgery scheduling process.

Appendix V. Proposed timeline for a perioperative improvement project

Month 0—quick start for launch of perioperative services of the future

a. First month of LST meetings.
b. LST confirm membership
c. LST select members from LST to serve as BDA, VST champions
d. Executive leader/champion initial training workshop (2 h)
e. Champions meet with consultants and BDA PI (OPM) leaders
   i. Confirm core members of the BDA teams
   ii. Confirm candidates for ad hoc/virtual team members
   iii. Develop BDA draft charters (see charter section)
      1. Key metrics with targets
      2. Initial business case highlighting potential value to MH
      3. Determine initial project scope and needed resources
      4. Initiate project plan
f. BDA PI team leaders and consultants begin the mapping of MH surgical processes
   i. Value stream map
   ii. SIPOC

      iii. Process mapping
        1. High-level map
        2. "Swimlane map"
        3. Metric inventory associated with process
      iv. Process analysis
        1. "Downtime"
          a. Defects
          b. Overproduction (doing more than needed)
          c. Waiting
          d. Not put to use appropriately (underutilizing)
          e. Transitions/handoffs
          f. Inventory (supplies, sterilization kits)
          g. Motion
          h. Extraprocessing (e.g., too many steps)
        2. Process "black holes"—not knowing how it actually works
        3. Bottleneck identification or poor process flow
      v. Begin draft list of "Do Its"
        1. Opportunities identified from mapping process
        2. Opportunities identified by process subject matter experts
  g. VST meeting with J Bara and champions
    i. Discuss roles and high-level charter of the VST.
    ii. Begin identifying biweekly meeting times.
    iii. Identify those interested in leading frequent (e.g., daily) huddles

Month 1

a. 2 days of assessment for facilitators to conduct quick assessment of all BDA areas along with ancillary services, physicians, nursing, and possible patients/families.

b. Weekly BDA steering team meeting (consultants can participate by phone) including weekly report to LST
    i. Metric report—baseline, target, current
    ii. What was accomplished that week?
    iii. What went well and what was learned?
    iv. What did not go so well and where help may be needed?
    v. Actions for the next week?

c. Barrier busting by LST
    i. Address policy modification
    ii. Intradepartmental relationship (e.g., radiology and OR)
    iii. Resource limitations (capital and people)

d. Each BDA team is to accomplish a minimum of one change and test of the change per month with a goal of two changes per month per team. These changes may be small in nature (e.g., reducing first case late starts, location of wheelchairs, new monitoring methods).

Month 2

a. MBB/BB continues ongoing facilitation and coaching of each BDA team:

   i. Kaizen event opportunities (e.g., three-day focused change event)
   ii. Value stream mapping of each team area and overall process
   iii. Ongoing process improvement training to cover basic tools and data collection

b. MBB facilitates BDA steering team

   i. Barrier identification along with barrier busting execution
   ii. Observation and data collection
      1. Clinical personnel time barriers (e.g., printer jams)
      2. Administrative issues (e.g., IT, lack of cooperation)
   iii. Basic process improvement facilitation training.

c. A one-day meeting with the BDA steering team to recap previous month, plan for next month, and provide additional tools training appropriate to the work for each team. Review BDA scorecard.

d. As in month 1, continue weekly BDA steering team meetings and daily huddles.

e. Each BDA team is to accomplish a minimum of one change and test of the change per month with a goal of two changes per month.

Months 3–6

a. MBB/BB continues ongoing facilitation of each BDA team:

   i. Kaizen event opportunities (e.g., three-day focused change event)
   ii. Workflow changes
   iii. Ongoing process improvement training

b. MBB facilitates BDA steering team

   i. Major barriers being attacked

c. A one-day meeting with the BDA steering team to recap previous month, plan for next month, and provide additional tools training appropriate to the work for each team. Review BDA scorecard.

d. Move to biweekly BDA steering team meetings.

e. BDA steering team identifies larger more complex issues that may be appropriate for handling with a rigorous lean six sigma approach

f. More advanced tools may be brought to bear such as modeling such as "hospital physics" (e.g., axioms/laws that govern process flow).

g. Each BDA team is to accomplish a minimum of one change and test of the change per month with a goal of two changes per month.

Appendix VI. BDA reports to the leadership steering team

Each week of the project, each of the BDA team leaders reported the current status of their working group to the LST. Prior to reporting to the LST (e.g., one business day before the LST meeting), each BDA team leader is expected to review the report with the champions of the BDA teams. This is in keeping with the "Policy of No Surprises" as the champions are members of the LST. The presentation of the report should take no more than 5—10 min although the LST may wish to grant more time in order to ask questions, provide thoughts or suggestions, and discuss how they can further support the teams. See example report form on the next page.

The elements of the report consist of the following:

- Dashboard metrics chosen for focus
    - Baseline—this is the performance of the metric at the outset of the BDA project.
    - Target—this is the performance target (goal) for the metric with target date (e.g., 1 year, 6 months).
    - Current—this is the current performance of the metric which is equal to the baseline at the outset of the project and should move toward the target each week.
    - Percentage attainment (optional)—this is the percentage of the distance the current metric has moved from the baseline performance to the target performance.
- Accomplishments in the past week
    - The team highlights the actions completed since the previous weekly LST report.
    - Should be provided in a simple bullet list of actions.
- Actions planned for the next week before the next LST meeting
    - The team highlights their actions to be taken in the next week.
    - These actions may be ongoing actions started in previous week.
- What is going well?
    - Team provides stories or examples of what is going well for the project team.
- What are the barriers/obstacles/issues for which the team needs help?
    - Team highlights difficulties for which the team needs help (e.g., lack of resources, departments or personnel not responding to requests for support).
    - Any suggestions on the nature of help needed?
- What are opportunities outside scope of team that may be suitable for others to address?
- What do want to make sure does not happen again?

An example of a project charter form for a lean six sigma project follows. This includes all the major elements of a project charter except a project plan. The level of detail of a project plan is related to the project scope.

Appendix VII. Recommendations for the before surgery, during surgery, after surgery teams

The before surgery team needs to improve preoperative component processes as indicated in the governance section. The following is a suggested initial list of recommendations for MH leadership to consider relative to the BST although not necessarily in order of priority:

1. Supply chain management including reconciliation of SKUs—We were able to reduce capital expenditures and costs by seven figures.
    a. Reduce the number of SKUs to manage.
    b. Identify obsolete supplies/SKUs where obsolete is a supply item that has not been utilized in the previous 6 months and eliminate those that are consider nonessential or simply "nice to have" while keeping those that are a medical necessity although of infrequent use.
    c. Reconsider and apply previous supply chain management studies (e.g., Vanderbilt consultant report) and determine which make sense and are feasible to implement.
    d. Clearly define supplies as "vital," "essential," and "desired."
        i. *Vital supplies* are those that are critical to surgical services at MH as without them surgery cannot be effectively performed.
        ii. *Essential supplies* are those that impact the quality of performance of surgical services at MH.
        iii. *Desired supplies* are those that some may have a preference to have those supplies although they do not inhibit the performance of surgical services at MH if they are not available.
    e. Seek collaborative approach with physicians (e.g., surgeons and anesthesiologists) to determine which supplies are vital, essential, and desired but not necessary.
    f. Improve the preference card consistency with consideration of what is vital, essential, and desired as this can impact both the supplies and sterilization.
    g. Track closely unnecessary expensive shipping/overnight costs for urgent surgical supplies and ensure which surgical cases truly need this equipment and that it was not possible to order these supplies with standard shipping times and costs. This cost and details should be reported on a weekly basis to the LST.
2. Scheduling including add-ons
    a. Operationally define add-ons to consider the following:
        i. Sterilization weekday versus weekend staffing levels.
        ii. Lead times required to meet sterilization preparation protocols.
        iii. Lead time to schedule staff and ORs during weekdays and weekends.
        iv. Minimal preparation times for each type of surgical procedure.
    b. Improve block-time scheduling and utilization considering the following:
        i. Physicians/practices who are poor "consumers" of block time including those not available for first starts of the day or those who consistently are late to their first case or cancel their surgeries.
        ii. Day of week surgical suite hours of availability where an available hour is a suite hour that has simultaneously all three of the following "cleaned, ready, and staffed" characteristics.

      iii. Address and minimize disconnects between surgeon, anesthesiology services, nursing and tech staff, and sterilization staff availability so that OR utilization is less constrained by time of day.

      iv. Consider extending routine OR scheduling daily until 5 p.m.

3. Improve internal transitions of patients and equipment

   a. Gather data to establish baselines for transportation and hand-offs from inpatient settings to preoperative services and return from postoperative services.

   b. Determine hindrances leading to patients either spending too much time waiting for transport or arriving too early/late for preoperative procedures. Seek improvements.

   c. Gather data to establish a baseline for moving patients from outpatient arrival through to surgical preparation.

   d. Gather data on the outpatient experience in order to establish baselines and identify opportunities for improvement.

   e. Seek improvements in opportunities identified related to outpatient experience including family/friend's feedback (the patient and family interviews we planned were missed due to COVID-19 shutdowns).

4. Sterilization of instruments and surgical kits

   a. Create a forum to collaborate with physicians to minimize items on preference cards and increase consistency across each type of surgical procedure. Industry suggests savings of hundreds of thousands of dollars for the MH surgical volume.

   b. Establish a regular forum for physicians to meet with equipment sterilization staff to discuss issues identified and agreement on how to address. This is to be a two-way communication and improvement sessions to improve the appreciation and respect between the OR and CS staffs and mitigate the attitude that sterilization staff are "glorified dishwashers." They are vital contributors to surgical performance. Invite and encourage CS staff to visit the operating room on a regular basis to help build familiarity and trust.

   c. Reduce percentage of underutilized packs/trays in cooperation with physicians.

   d. Collaborate with infection control staff to highlight opportunities to report and invite them to do weekly infection audits.

   e. Optimize sterilization staff scheduling to consider weekday and weekend staffing models that support both scheduled and add-on surgical demands.

5. Physician surgical readiness

   a. Operationally define physician surgical readiness to include "garbed, washed, ready, present before administration of anesthesia, patient consent forms signed, and antibiotics administered before surgery."

   b. Gather data to determine the level of physician surgical readiness in order to identify opportunities to improve.

   c. MH/OR leadership to collaborate with physician leaders to identify and implement actions to improve physician surgical readiness.

    d. Metrics/graphs continually provided in near real time to physicians/practices to highlight physician surgical readiness performance with monthly meetings to review past month performance and effectiveness of actions taken to improve.

6. Infection control

    a. Infection control to conduct weekly audits of all relevant before (preoperative) processes and to present findings and recommendations to MH/OR/physician or practice leadership.

    b. Action items identified and followed up at weekly reports for status.

7. Performance improvement—lean six sigma

    a. LSS trained staff identified to support before (preoperative) recommendations and to facilitate Kaizens/rapid improvement events to drive improvements. Consider assigning several newly minted yellow belts to be officed in the operating room area.

    b. LSS staff to represent "listening posts" for which before surgical process staff can bring suggestions and issues to be addressed.

        i. Those who contribute suggestions or highlight issues are to be "anonymous" unless they specifically indicate that their name can be used.

        ii. When an issue is identified by one staff person, the LSS facilitator should seek to determine if the issue is backed up by data or with agreement by others in the organization.

        iii. Once the issue is validated or the suggestion is determined to be reasonable, the information can then be presented at a formal MH/OR leadership meeting.

The recommendations can be added to, reduced, or better formulated by the BST process improvement team as described in the governance section of this report. There are many potential opportunities for quality improvement that should be prioritized and sequenced over the next year.

Recommendations for the during surgery (DST) processes

  I. Revitalize the surgical services executive committee

    a. Review membership and remit—collaborative governing body held peers accountable by enforcing policies informed by analytics

    b. Cochaired by a surgeon and anesthesiologist

    c. Establish governing rules and definitions that are critical to success

  II. Establish surgical advanced analytics unit

    a. Build an advanced analytics infrastructure to align block time and surgeon demand to track staffing models, block scheduling, heatmaps, block utilization, etc.

    b. Strengthen OR governance by enforcing proactive block release policies and utilization thresholds in a fully transparent manner to maintain blocks and credibility.

    c. Simulate the effects of how efficient proactive release would impact overall block utilization.

    d. Design in close concert with CIO/CMIO.

III. Create the surgical services improvement team

    a. Physician/surgeon leader(s)—internal, external

    b. Anesthesiologist leader

    c. Ancillary service representatives (e.g., imaging, lab, cardiology)

    d. Nursing representative

    e. Performance improvement leader

    f. Infection control

    g. Environment services

    h. Data analytics

    i. Others

IV. Dashboard metrics

    a. Time based

        a. OR arrival to surgery start cycle time

        b. Surgery start to surgery finished cycle time and variance

            i. Percentage of first and subsequent on-time starts (wheels in room, physician in room, anesthesiologist in room, staff in room, equipment ready to go, patient already prepped)

            ii. Given 30%—40% late first case MH starts, and that the cost of operating room time nationally averages \$36—37/minute, create and widely report on how much the late first cases cost MH in lost revenue and opportunities.

                1. Comparison by type of surgery, add-on versus scheduled, physician/physician group, location

        c. OR room turnaround time

            i. Turnover minutes are credited for sequential cases in the same room for the same block owners (accounts for surgeon, group, and service blocks alike)

        d. Smart, transparent block time policies

            i. Improve average block utilization by >8% Year on Year (YoY)

            ii. Partial block release was not permitted

            iii. Increase surgeon access by providing a transparent way for surgeons to see all of their surgical data and to schedule proactively released "open" times

            iv. Develop and use interactive dashboards that provide granular insights about how blocks are being used and managed throughout MH.

            v. Provide block utilization rates, block utilization report, OR usage by block owner that reflects the day of week usage by block owner and shows which members are contributing to the block utilization.

            vi. Unused days that are not actively being used contribute to poor overall utilization.

      vii. Lack of proactive release was a major factor contributing to low OR utilization.

     viii. Surgeons, staff, and administration all benefit as promotes responsible scheduling practices and allows for sufficient lead time when booking cases.

      ix. Creates a "load balancing" effect, permitting more efficient accommodation of urgent and emergent cases

b. Quality based

  a. Infection control measures

    i. with active involvement and oversight with infection control and environmental services (ES) expertise

      1. First incisions starting with patients not having received antibiotics within previous 60 min

      2. Engage ES for ALL cleaning for preparation of surgical suites, between cases and terminal cleaning

      3. Avoidance of walking between cases unless absolutely necessary, consider door counters to avoid opening and closing surgical suite doors

      4. Deploy stringent access control and stop all potential causes of infection such as walking into the surgical suite in street clothes

  b. Waivers of recommended sterilization times or methods

    i. With active involvement by MH supply chain expertise

  c. Patient safety issues

    i. Design and work closely with director of risk management and patient safety

      1. Review and control the number of individuals entering during surgery

      2. Document the number of individuals entering surgery not properly garbed and prepped (e.g., wearing street cloths)

      3. First incisions starting with patients not having received antibiotics within previous 60 min

      4. Physician, anesthesiologist, and nurse not together at patient induction time

i. Three-time outs completed and documented

    d. Near misses, adverse events reporting, and learning

      i. Work closely with active oversight by risk management

        1. Examples—Instruments or materials potentially left behind, how documented, discussed and reported to hospital risk management for learning

        2. Wrong-sided/level/patient anesthesia blocks/surgical procedures/device implant

c. Cost based

  a. Work closely with CFO

    i. Higher cost supplies/instruments substituted for less costly version

        ii. Pharmacy costs
           1. Comparison by type of surgery, add-on versus scheduled, physi-cian/physician group, location

V. Quality feedback cycles (QFCs)
    i. Establish daily huddles, guided by the improvement team, to huddle at least twice a day.
    ii. Feedback loops serve as a way to increase productivity in an individual's performance, surgery teamwork, or process. Through feedback loops, we are capable of identifying areas in surgical services for improvement regularly.
    iii. Feedback loops help surgical teams to have more coordinated, collabora-tive, and committed service, quality, cost deliverables. They can also encourage more proactive and shared ownership within the team, improved team, and hospital performance.

Recommendations for the after surgery processes

I. Create the after surgery improvement team
    a. Nurse leader (PACU)
    b. Bed mgt. representative
    c. Admissions/finance representative
    d. Transportation
    e. Hospitalist representative
    f. Performance improvement leader
    g. Infection control
    h. Data analytics
    i. Others

II. Dashboard metrics
    a. Time based
        a. OR surgery complete to OR depart cycle time
        b. OR depart to PACU arrival cycle time
        c. PACU arrival to PACU depart cycle time
        d. PACU depart to patient depart cycle time
    b. Quality based
        a. Number/percentage of inpatients crashing (e.g., unexpected need to go to ICU or observation instead of their room)
        b. # Outpatients admitted rather than discharged
        c. Infection control audits with weekly reports
        d. Risk management data on transitions out of postsurgery, bounce back to OR, and to ICUs
    c. Cost based
        a. Length of stay in PACU
        b. Staffing levels for monitored beds, transporters

Appendix VIII. Analyzing add-on surgical cases deep dive (pg. 309–323)

Background

The perioperative system is a primary source of revenue for hospitals and clinics, which makes it a key opportunity for improvement in efficiency. Surgery schedules at MH drive the department and affect the operations of many other departments. The three most significant challenges to creating an efficient surgery schedule are as follows:

- Estimating the duration of surgery
- Scheduling cases to minimize the time a surgery is off schedule and maximize utilization of resources.
- Clearing patients for surgery

The operating room (OR) is at the heart of hospital care and surgery scheduling affects expensive resources within the postanesthesia care unit (PACU), intensive care unit (ICU), and ORs. Surgeries alone at MH Care account for more than 60% of MH hospital's total profits. The schedule of the OR affects many additional hospital departments, such as nurse schedules and inpatient bed capacities. We have seen that numerous demands like surgeon requests, changing staffing requirements, and capacity issues compete for OR time and space, challenging the surgical schedule.

Scheduling surgeries is a complicated process. Variability among surgery, anesthesia, and cleanup durations definitely affect the OR schedule. Surgery schedulers must also take into account varying priorities in the schedule. The OR managers want to keep the surgeons satisfied and have high utilization of the rooms. The surgeons do not want downtime between surgeries and prefer to be scheduled at times that work around their clinic schedules. On the other hand, surgeons need to be on time for the scheduled surgeries or it can cause rippling delays throughout the day. In addition, add-ons can also impact the schedule and available resources. Nurses want evenly dispersed patient flow so there are not peaks where are they are busier. Patients want minimal indirect and direct delays. These varying priorities are difficult to balance when scheduling surgeries, as they often conflict. Our goal is to propose a more effective surgical scheduling process in which schedulers consider five key guiding principles: patient safety, access, OR efficiency, patient service, and physician satisfaction. Finally, timely patient clearance is important because patients that arrive at preop without H&P's, testing, preop orders, and/or consents add time to the preop schedule.

This report contains a descriptive analysis of data that MH is currently collecting in various databases. The different charts and tables will show patterns and signals in the data that will prompt follow-up questions from key stakeholders and subject matter experts. Important answers will often emerge from closer examinations of the who, what, when, and where variables.

Patient clearance

The following table is based on data received from MH IT team (J.L.) reveals issues for the time period of October 2019 through September 2020:

Patient clearance item	Average monthly completion
H&P's	44%
Surgical consents	12.9%
Preop orders	71.3%

Busy nurses have to correct these deficiencies and that can lead to late or inappropriate administration of antibiotics and delayed hand-offs to the OR. There can also be problems with the hand-offs (transitions) from preop to the OR. Nurses who rush to ready patients for surgery can also pass on incorrect or incomplete information to the OR staff.

Antibiotic administration

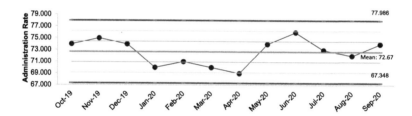

1. Consider the clinical implications for surgical site infections (SSI) or other adverse events if the average for this antibiotic administration time period was 72.7%. On average across this 12-month time period, 27.3% of the preop patients did not receive correctly administered antibiotics. This individual control chart shows that the rates range from 69 to almost 77. The process is stable and predictable and there is no special cause variation. There is variation, but there are no extreme high or low data points; no significant trends; and no major data shifts. However, questions still need to be asked about the overall low performance and the below average months from January to April. Finally, why did performance improve starting in May and then decrease again in July?

First start surgical delays

Surgical delays are a serious problem and this is especially true when it occurs for the first scheduled surgeries of the day. That can disrupt the rest of the schedule for that day. Delays are very expensive in the OR, estimated at $66/minute loss to MHC.

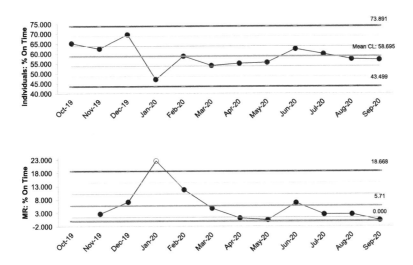

This individual and moving range chart reveals that the first surgery on-time percentages ranges from 47% to 69% with an average on time performance of 58.9%. This process is not stable and or predictable. These individual chart data points are not significantly distant from the mean, but the moving range between December 2019 and January 2020 shows significant special cause variation. Why did such a major decrease occur in January 2020? Finally, is the overall process performance acceptable?

Why was January so much lower than December?

Surgery scheduling process

Surgery scheduling at MCHC is the process by which the surgery case is requested, an estimate of duration is given, the case is tentatively scheduled for the date requested, but a time slot is not assigned. Add-on scheduling is the process of assigning late additions to the surgical schedule. **A "late" addition to the schedule is defined at Muda Health Care as one that is scheduled after 1 PM on a weekday before surgery.** The standard procedure for accommodating emergency cases is to keep at least one operating room open at all times, and the add-on schedulers take care of scheduling within that limitation for those scheduled for the next weekday or for weekends. Accidents may often result in more than one patient needing emergency surgery. Mass casualty events (e.g., bus accident, multiple car crash) may require coordination with other hospitals in the system to route patients to places with openings.

The hospital operates using a master surgical schedule, which allocates certain surgeons or groups of surgeons, blocks during the week. A block is a space of time in a given OR on a given day of the week. The schedule is cyclical, and is repeated every week, with the exception of certain groups who trade-off periodically. The blocks occupy an OR for the entire day, as it is difficult to plan an exact start in the middle of the day following other surgeries.

A surgery can be requested days or months in advance, by one of three methods: (a) electronically via the scheduling software, (b) phone, or (c) fax. The requests come from the physician's offices and outpatient clinics. When the request for surgery is received, it is printed, and verification is sent to the doctor's office. The patient and case information are recorded, and the surgery will tentatively be scheduled on the day requested. A part of the case information recorded is estimated surgery duration. When recording this, the scheduler compares the estimate given by the doctor and compares it to the estimate given by the software. This is the case for surgeries scheduled in advance and perhaps a portion of add-ons although it may be that add-ons do not conform to block schedule processes, test and treatment presurgery processing, and may not be synergistic with the ongoing scheduling (Figs. 15.37 and 15.38).

It must be noted that this is a very elaborate and complicated process. The number of process steps adds time, cost, and increases the likelihood that more errors will be made. The rework adds more time, confusion, and cost to the process. In addition, each surgical service has a different process.

Add-on surgery cases

Muda Health Care continuously reports high add-on surgical cases that range from 40% to 55% of all cases, whereas hospitals of similar size and case acuity will have add-on cases in the range of 15% of their surgical cases. A problem that operating room managers face in running an OR suite on the day of surgery is to identify "holes" in the OR schedule in which to assign "add-on" cases. This process necessitates knowing the typical and maximum amounts of time that the case is likely to require. This process necessitates knowing the distribution in length of surgery times that the case may likely require. "ADD-ON" surgical cases usually are scheduled individually.

We are not confident MHC has established an appropriate operational definition of "add-on" cases. The current operational definition of add-on cases may lead to less-than-optimal surgical case preparation and scheduling.

The before surgery team (BST) was assigned the responsibility to improve the OR scheduling by exploring the effectiveness of the add-on measures as late additions to schedule impact presurgical processing time. Nonetheless, add-ons do impact the perioperative service flow from *before to during to after* surgery activities. For example, add-ons may impact staffing schedules, bed capacity utilization, sterilization staffing and sterile kit readiness, and ability to turn over rooms effectively that in turn may impact surgical site infection rates.

This analysis of surgical add-ons was based upon data from EPIC that was obtained from MH. It covers the time period from October 2019 to November 2020. It includes information on 134 listed surgeons and a total of 8779 surgical patients.

Questions to explore relative to an effective choice of operational definition of an "add-on" case

1) Is the choice of 1 p.m. as the cutoff between scheduled and add-on operations optimal?

2) Is an add-on case accepted whether or not there is sterilized equipment available and ready (e.g., some specific sterilized equipment is brought in by vendors before the day of surgery as this equipment may not be held in inventory at Muda Health)?

3) Is an add-on accepted whether or not there are appropriate staff (e.g., techs, anesthesiologists, nurses, room turnover staff) available to handle the surgery?

4) Are add-ons accepted whether or not the labs are in the system, consents signed, and H&Ps done? If so, is there any opportunity to enforce that they be completed before 6 a.m. the day of surgery?

Definitions

It is important to define "add-ons" more precisely before analyzing the data. Josh L provided the following definitions:

1) "A case is considered an add-on if it is added to a day's schedule after that day's schedule has been finalized. We currently finalize schedules at 13:00 on the day prior, or at 13:00 on Friday for Monday's schedule. All cases performed on weekends and holidays are considered add-ons."

2) "Moving the room that a case is scheduled to be performed in, changing the time of the case, or adding/removing procedures from the case DOES NOT affect the case's add-on status. For example, if I have a non—add-on case on today's schedule for 07:00 in OR1 and decide to bump it back to 09:00 in OR2, that case will remain a non—add-on."

3) "A case that was not scheduled as a non—add-on can become an add-on if it is added to the day's schedule after that day's schedule was finalized. For example, I schedule a case for 12/17 on 12/14 as a non—add-on, but on 12/15 there is an opening in the schedule, so we decide to fit that surgery in. Because the case will then be added to the day's schedule after the schedule had been finalized, that case is now classified as an add-on. This type of add-on is not very common (<5% of the add-ons that I sampled)."

It would be expected that trauma/emergency department cases may be add-on cases. We did not anticipate that the percentage of inpatient add-on cases would be over 75% of all inpatient cases. What can be done to lower the percentage of inpatient add-on cases of the total add-on cases?

Overall surgical add-ons

Add-on	Count	Percentage
No	4783	54.48%
Yes	3996	45.52%
Grand total	**8779**	

This table indicates that there were 3996 add-ons during the study time period, and this accounted for over 45% of the total cases. Is this not relatively high?

Now let us examine some of the factors that may help explain this situation.

Pareto chart for surgeries stratified by month and year

It is common practice to examine an issue by seeing if a "few of the causes account for most of the problem." More specifically, researchers will drill down into data to see if "when, where, who, and what" categorical variables can better explain higher level data such as the number of surgical add-ons.

Let us begin with months of the year and then days of the week.

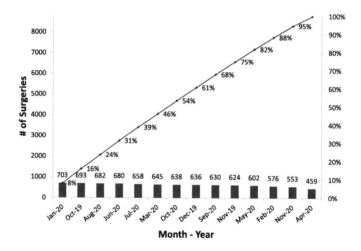

This chart reveals that the most surgeries were conducted in January 2020 (703 or 8%) and the least occurred in April of 2020 (459 or 5%) for a difference of 244 cases. There was very little variation in the other months.

Row labels	Count of year–month
2019	**1953**
10	693
11	624
12	636
2020	**6826**
1	703
2	576
3	645
4	459
5	602
6	680
7	658
8	682
9	630
10	638
11	553
Grand total	**8779**

Pareto chart and tables for surgery cases by days of the week

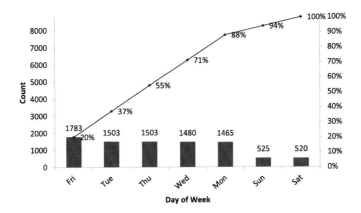

These charts demonstrate that 1783 surgical cases (20%) occurred on Fridays and the fewest cases were scheduled for Sunday (525) and Saturday (520).

Row labels	Count of months
Sun	525
Mon	1465
Tue	1503
Wed	1480
Thu	1503
Fri	1783
Sat	520
Grand total	**8779**

Number and percent of add-ons by days of the week

DOW	Add-on No	Add-on yes	Grand total	Add-on %
Sun		525	525	100.0%
Mon	861	604	1465	41.2%
Tue	928	575	1503	38.3%
Wed	880	600	1480	40.5%
Thu	908	595	1503	39.6%
Fri	1206	577	1783	32.4%
Sat		520	520	100.0%
Grand total	**4783**	**3996**	**8779**	**100.0%**

J.L. indicated that this table verifies that all weekend cases were add-ons. Most of the add-on cases happened on Monday (604 or 41%) and Wednesday (600 or 40%). As indicated, Monday's scheduled surgeries must be scheduled by 1:00 p.m. the Friday before to not be considered an add-on case. Any cases scheduled for Monday after 1:00 p.m. on Friday through the weekend are considered add-on cases on Monday. Interestingly, there is a lower percentage of add-on cases handled on Friday.

Pareto chart for the number of surgeries by patient class

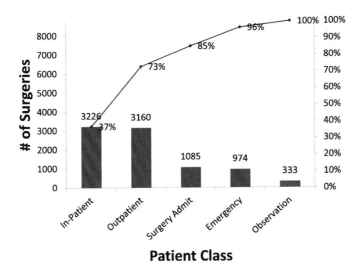

By far, most of the surgeries (73% combined) occur in the inpatient and outpatient classes.

Pareto chart for the number of surgical add-ons by patient class

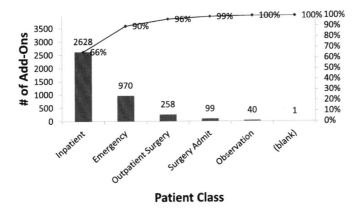

Number and percent of add-ons within each patient class

Row labels	Count of patient class			
	Column labels			
	No	Yes	Grand total	% add-on
Emergency	4	970	974	99.6%
Inpatient	598	2628	3226	81.5%
Observation	293	40	333	12.0%
Outpatient surgery	2902	258	3160	8.2%
Surgery admit	986	99	1085	9.1%
Grand total	**4783**	**3995**	**8778**	45.5%

It is also important to define "patient classes," and Josh L offered the following definitions:

- **Emergency**: A patient who is coming directly from the emergency department to surgery.
- **Inpatient:** A patient who is currently admitted.
- **Observation:** An outpatient who is coming in for surgery and is expected to be admitted for a short period of time (potentially overnight), but whose length of stay is not expected to exceed 24 h.
- **Outpatient Surgery:** An outpatient who is coming in for surgery and is expected to be discharged directly from PACU without requiring a hospital admission.
- **Surgery Admit:** An outpatient who is coming in for surgery and is expected to be admitted to the hospital for more than 24 h postsurgery.

The Pareto chart and table above reveal that most of the add-ons are either emergencies (970) or inpatients (2628). Inpatient add-ons account for 65.8% of the total add-ons (i.e., 2628 add-ons out of 3995 total add-ons) and 81.5% of the total of inpatient cases. This should be a primary focus of any investigation because this patient class accounts for about 2/3 of the cases. How are these cases scheduled? Do scheduling practices differ by who does the scheduling (e.g., hospitalists, nursing managers)?

Saturday and sunday add-on cases

Saturday add-ons

Row labels	Column labels	
Patient class	Yes	Grand total
Emergency	144	144
Inpatient	348	348
Observation	7	7
Outpatient surgery	17	17
Surgery admit	3	3
(Blank)	1	1
Grand total	**520**	**520**

Sunday add-ons

Row labels	Column labels	
Patient class	Yes	Grand total
Emergency	143	144
Inpatient	364	348
Observation	2	7
Outpatient surgery	10	17
Surgery admit	6	3
Grand total	**525**	**525**

The number of surgeries by service and patient class

Surgery by service and patient class

Row labels	Column labels						
Service	Emergency	Inpatient	Observation	Outpatient surgery	Surgery admit	(Blank)	Totals
Anesthesiology		2		8			**10**
Cardiothoracic	15	101			47		**163**
Cardiovascular	10	26	1	3	20		**60**
Dentistry	1	5		68			**74**
Endoscopy	6	17					**23**
ENT	29	63	11	70	18		**191**
General	579	1032	99	1106	479		**3295**
Gynecology	27	61	44	20	31		**183**
Neurosurgery	40	196	24	50	143		**453**
Obstetrics	13	32		5	2		**52**
Oncology				25	18		**43**
Ophthalmology	3	3		1			**7**
Oral surgery	33	47	1	293	1		**375**
Orthopedics	133	987	40	230	130	1	**1521**
Plastics	3	93	3	52	31		**182**
Podiatry	2	201	5	59	2		**269**
Urology	72	316	105	1156	131		**1780**
Vascular	8	44		14	32		**98**
Grand total	**974**	**3226**	**333**	**3160**	**1085**	**1**	**8779**

A review of the above table shows that the general, orthopedic, and urology surgeons had the most emergency and inpatient cases.

The busiest surgeons by service

Surgeons by service			
Row labels	Column labels		
Surgeons	General	Urology	Orthopedics
R.S–C.		692	
J.L.			587
R.H.		539	
M. W.	451		
I.S.	440		
R. M.	371		
B.A.		353	
P.K.	321		
M.S.	318		
J.W.	308		
D.F.	299		
T.B.	271		
Totals	2779	1584	587

The surgeons listed above performed the most surgeries in the three surgical service areas that comprise most of the cases that come from the inpatient class. These 12 surgeons were selected because they all performed at least 200 surgeries. They accounted for 56.4% (4950) of the 8779 total surgeries performed.

Most of the high-volume surgeons are "general" but so are most of the surgeries. How do these busy surgeons do with add-on numbers?

(Note: Dr. B.A. performs surgeries approximately only 2 weeks per month. If that is the case, then perhaps his case volume per week is higher than the others. The next few charts may not be indicative of the weekly volume of add-on cases he performs.)

Add-ons for the busiest surgeons by patient class

Row labels	Column labels			
Surgeons	**Emergency Add-ons**	**Inpatient Add-ons**	**Outpatient Add-ons**	**Totals for all surgeries**
R.S–C.	4	58	32	695
J.L.	10	494	12	587
R.H.	45	118	16	539
M.W.	67	132	21	451
I.S.	76	112	8	441
R.M.	64	92	12	371
B.A.	8	23	8	353
P.K.	42	64	14	322
M.S.	59	68	15	331
J.W.	52	71	7	309
D.F.	45	75	8	301
T.B.	63	79	13	271
Totals for the 12 surgeons	**535**	**1386**	**166**	**4971**
Totals for all surgeons	**970**	**2628**	**258**	**8779**
Percentages for the 12 surgeons	**55.2%**	**52.7%**	**64.3%**	

(Add-ons for surgeons by patient class)

This small subgroup of surgeons scheduled a higher percentage (55% and 52%) of the add-ons in these two busy classes. They also were responsible for 64% of the outpatient surgery add-ons.

Some surgeons commented that there are several problems with the "inpatient" category that may explain its size:

1. The breakdown of patient class by inpatient, emergency, outpatient, surgery admit, and observation is somewhat artificial. It is generated by Epic during our case request, which is often placed while the patient is still in the ER, before a disposition has been made. He suspects it defaults to inpatient, unless we specify otherwise.

2. Many of the inpatient cases are performed on recent ER patients. If a patient is admitted overnight through the ER with bowel obstruction or gallstone pancreatitis, and we operate on them the next morning, they are now considered inpatient, because an admit order has been placed. Functionally, these are more similar to ER cases or surgery admits, as they are generated by being on call.

3. Two categories of actual inpatient surgeries that I think we do need to identify are hidden within this breakdown:

   i. those who came to the hospital, then got sick and required surgery (GI bleed after orthopedic procedure, pressure ulcer after prolonged stay, trach and PEG for COVID-19 patients)

   ii. planned or unplanned reoperations on surgical patients (reopening laparotomy for anastomotic breakdown, takeback for bleeding, wound vac changes for NSTI).

Busiest surgeons by add-ons

Add-ons for surgeons				
Row labels			**Column labels**	
Surgeons	**No**	**Yes**	**Total cases**	**Percent of add-ons**
R. S–C.	592	103	695	14.8%
J.L.	62	525	587	89.4%
R.H.	358	181	539	33.6%
M.W.	229	222	451	49.2%
I.S.	241	200	441	45.3%
R.M.	195	176	371	47.4%
B.A.	310	43	353	12.2%
P.K.	194	128	322	39.8%
M.S.	178	153	331	46.2%
J.W.	176	133	309	43.0%
D.F.	167	134	301	44.5%
T.B.	109	162	271	59.8%
Totals	**2811**	**2160**	**4971**	

The highest percentages of add-ons cases come from the eight general surgeons with the one orthopedic surgeon being the exception. The three urologists have the lowest percentages.

Next steps

1. Finalize definitions for add-ons and patient classes.

   a. Create and implement a new, standardized operational definition of surgical "add-ons" and collect that revised data starting on January 1, 2021.

   b. Spell out what are appropriate and in-appropriate add-ons.

2. Conduct a deeper dive on surgical add-ons to help explain possible causes and consistent variation.
   a. How are "direct admits" handled?
   b. Review these preliminary findings with surgical leadership.
   c. Discuss these findings with all surgeons.
   d. Get input from anesthesiologists and CRNAs.
   e. Discuss the inpatient add-ons with identified hospitalists and nurse managers.
   f. Sample some inpatient patients' records for possible explanations.
   g. Explore whether the existing surgical scheduling processes may contribute to the number of and variation in add-ons.
   h. Review the connection between block time availability and the number of add-ons.
3. Implement a general trauma and/or ortho trauma room into which patients can be booked, both during the week and with at least one catch-all trauma room on Saturday into which all surgeons could book semiurgent cases.
4. Simplify and standardize the different scheduling processes that exist for each surgical service.
5. Explore the connection between patient clearance and scheduling. How does this impact OR scheduling and surgical site infections (SSI)?
6. Examine and improve first time surgical starts.
7. Communicate findings and changes to all staff.

Appendix IX. Kaizen training to ready the MH staff and clinicians for the project

Program description

The topics listed below were designed to facilitate upskilling of MH surgical teams using adult learning principles and deep reflective practices. The training modules are short, relevant, practical and are designed to be viewed many times over the course of the project. The training materials included PowerPoint slides, videos, and articles that were posted on the MH Surgical Improvement Training Program Intranet site for easy access and to support deeper learning and mastery of the curriculum. We designed the training with a "bias toward action" approach and it was conducted "just in time" for MH and BDA teams to apply the new knowledge and skills as they lead the improvement work. The training was a resounding sucess based on staff feedback and was felt to be huegly contibutory to the project's overall success and sustainability.

Program objectives

The objectives of the training program were to familiarize MH surgical teams—clinicians, nonclinicians, and management with both the present state of substantive knowledge in the field of surgical safety, quality, and efficiency and to support implementation of these ideas and methods of organizational improvement at MH. See below for list of seminars.

Champion training for the LST and PI team

- Senior leadership involvement is essential for any successful organizational improvement implementation. We developed and delivered two dedicated sessions to the project champions. Project champions were the identified LST leaders who will provide direct support and advocacy for each of the BDA teams. This brief, basic training will help the LST understand the crucial role of the designated champions and learn how the consultants plan to begin work with the BDA teams.

We began with modules that are related to the ADAMS activities: "Month 0" Training Schedule

Week one

- Introduction to lean six sigma
- Seeing value through the eyes of MH patients—the voice of the customer (See figure below for the PICK chart and POP-Points of Pain)

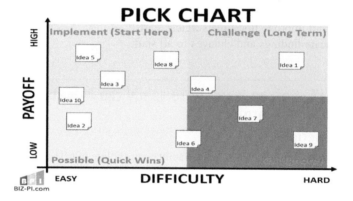

- Developing eyes for waste (waste walks)
- Process mapping: understanding and mapping the value stream mapping, SIPOC-R, and swim lanes
- Project charters and plans
- Simple Kaizens and rapid improvement events

Week two

- Understanding creating flow and establishing pull
- Demand, take time and work leveling
- Waste analysis
- Failure Modes and Effects Analysis (FMEA)

- Fishbone and five whys

Week three

- Breakthrough equation
- Introduction to measurement
- Types of data
- Stratification
- Basic data collection
- Lean metrics
- Lean management

Week four

- Daily management systems

Training seminars

Definitions in patient safety and quality improvement: an overview

In this module, you will be reviewing several key terms and tools that are used in patient safety and quality improvement. This will allow you to begin to develop the common language used among patient safety and quality improvement experts and practitioners. By the end of this module, you will be able to (1) differentiate between the terms harm, hazard, error, and risk within a patient safety and quality improvement framework, (2) describe how quality and safety overlap and how they are different, and (3) differentiate between root cause analysis and a failure mode and effects analysis.

Approaches to measuring healthcare quality and performance

In this module, we will review standardized, replicable, and comparable metrics for quality of medical care, and explore the highly variable implementation of these practices. Poor quality is often attributed to lack of resources; however, high variation in processes of care has been observed within and between states and healthcare systems. Available data mostly consider aspects of healthcare infrastructure, availability of human resources, equipment and supplies, services provided, coverage, and outcomes. We will explore quality perspectives from users and patients. We will review the three categories described by Donabedian (structure, process, and outcome) as fundamental for the performance of processes of care. Adequate healthcare is as much about process as it is about outcome.

High reliability organizing and why it matters

In this module, you will learn the fundamental principles of high reliability organizing. At the end of this lesson, you will also be able to: (1) describe the sociocultural characteristics of high reliability organizations (HROs), (2) compare and contrast healthcare with high reliability organizations, and (3) identify three improvement tools for high reliability organizing.

Applying a systems and human factors lens to healthcare

In this module, you will learn the basics of systems thinking and human factors and then apply these to a healthcare setting. At the end of this module, you will be able to (1) explain the basic components of a system, (2) differentiate first-order problem solving and second order problem solving, and (3) explain the benefits of having strategies for both proactive and reactive systems thinking.

Systems of care—surgical clinical microsystems

This module will explore surgical microsystems—a small, interdependent group of people who work together regularly to provide care for specific groups of patients. This small group is often embedded in a larger organization. A general clinical microsystem includes, in addition to surgeons/anesthesiologists, and nurses, other clinicians, some administrative support, and a small population of patients as critical "participants."

Recognize the importance of collaboration and effective communication and patient handoffs

This module will review the patient handoff—the transfer of a surgical patient from one caregiver to another—has come under increased scrutiny in recent years. This is due to many factors including high-profile and well-documented incidents of medical errors. As surgical care becomes more specialized and increasingly fragmented, handoffs are necessary in order to maintain consistency of information and plans of care. However, despite this increased focus, errors in transferring medical information are still common. We will (a) Describe when a handoff occurs in patient care; (b) Discuss the potential sources of errors for patient handoffs; (c) Identify mechanisms for safe and effective patient handoffs; (d) Learn to utilize SBAR and other communication tools for effective patient handoffs.

Assessing and improving teamwork performance/introduction to TeamSTEPPS

This module will address the key factors of teams as the cornerstone for health systems resilience. Human factors research has shown that even highly skilled, motivated professionals are vulnerable to error due to human limitations. Health care teams that communicate effectively and have mutual support reduce the potential for error, resulting in enhanced patient safety and improved clinical performance. However, teamwork is not innate; it must be learned. Over the course of the project, we will introduce TeamSTEPPS, a nationally acclaimed framework, specifically designed as a resource for healthcare providers to improve patient safety through effective communication and teamwork skills.

Identify the characteristics of a just culture

People make errors. Errors can cause accidents. In healthcare, errors and accidents result in morbidity and adverse outcomes and sometimes in mortality. In this module, we will review the just culture, one that balances the need for an open and honest reporting environment with the end of a quality learning environment and culture. While the organization has a duty and responsibility to employees (and ultimately to patients), all employees are held responsible for the quality of their choices. Just culture requires a change in focus from errors and outcomes to system design and management of the behavioral choices of all employees. The just culture is a learning culture that is constantly improving and oriented toward patient safety.

Successful surgical event investigation and analysis

Surgical adverse events (AEs), events in which care causes harm, have been recognized as a leading cause of death and injury since at least the late 1990s. This module will (a) Review and assess the strength of root cause analysis tools, and other methods, and recommendations and their perceived levels of effectiveness and sustainability; (b) Explore the spaces for innovation, culture building, and learning from using RCA more effectively. (c) Review how RCAs should remain relentlessly focused on how to make improvements, and how to help build trust, truth telling, and culture change. (d) Review how corrective actions need to be congruent to the causal factors they are trying to address and monitored for successful implementation and risk mitigation. (e) Gain an appreciation that the most important part of the RCA investigation is follow-up, support and maintaining sense-making solutions.

Critical open disclosure skills after surgical adverse events

A variety of psychological and cultural factors may make clinicians and organizations reluctant to disclose adverse events to patients. This module will review how hospitals should develop clear policies supporting disclosure after patient harm and should create supportive environments that enable clinicians to meet their ethical obligations to disclose adverse events to patients and families. Disclosure is required when the adverse event (1) has a perceptible effect on the patient that was not discussed in advance as a known risk; (2) necessitates a change in the patient's care; (3) potentially poses an important risk to the patient's future health, even if that risk is extremely small; and (4) involves providing a treatment or procedure without the patient's consent.

Process improvement in health care

Lean six sigma (LSS) is one of the most widely used and effective comprehensive process improvement approaches. It includes both quantitative and qualitative methodologies and it is organized around a problem-solving model called the DMAIC (Define, Measure, Analyze, Improve, and Control). The PDSA model can also be used. This approach incorporates hundreds of tools borrowed from many disciplines, but we limit them to the most useful for this MH implementation project.

References and Resources

Books

1. Learning to see: value stream mapping to add value and eliminate MUDA, Book by John Shook and Mike Rother.
2. The improvement guide: a practical approach to enhancing organizational performance by Ronald D. Moen, Clifford L. Norman, Kevin M. Nolan, et al..
3. The goal: a process of ongoing improvement by Eliyahu M. Goldratt.
4. Quality by design: a clinical microsystems approach 1st edition by Nelson EC, Batalden PB, Godfrey MM, editors.
5. Weick KE, Sutcliffe KM, editors. *Managing the unexpected: sustained performance in a complex world*; 2015.
6. Johnson JK, Haskell HW, Barach PR, editors. *Case studies in patient safety: foundations for core competencies*; 2017.
7. Sanchez JA, Barach P, Johnson JK, Jacobs JP, editors. *Surgical patient care: improving safety, quality and value*; 2017.
8. The lean Six Sigma pocket toolbook: a quick reference guide to 100 tools for improving quality and speed 1st ed., George ML, Maxey J, Rowlands D, Price M authors.

Other References

9. Wachter R. *The end of the beginning: patient safety five years after: to err is human.* Health Affairs; 2004.
10. Thomas E, Peterson L. Measuring errors and adverse events in health care. *J Gen Intern Med* 2003;(18):61−7.
11. Leape LL, Berwick DM, Bates DW. What practices will most improve safety? Evidence-based medicine meets patient safety. *JAMA* 2002;**288**(4):501−7.
12. Amalberti R, Auroy Y, Berwick DM, Barach P. Five system barriers to achieving ultra-safe health care. *Ann Intern Med* 2005;**142**(9):756−64.
13. Marcus LJ, Dorn BC, Henderson J, Eric J, Nulty MH. *Meta-leadership: a framework for building leadership effectiveness: a working paper.* National Preparedness Leadership Initiative Harvard School of Public Health; 2015.
14. Dekker SW, Leveson NG. The systems approach to medicine: controversy and misconceptions. *BMJ Qual Saf* 2015;**24**:7−9.
15. Barach P, Kleinman L. Measuring and improving comprehensive pediatric cardiac care: learning from continuous quality improvement methods and tools. *Prog Pediatr Cardiol* 2018;**48**:82−92.
16. Lilford R, Chilton PJ, Hemming K, Brown C, Girling A, Barach P. Evaluating policy and service interventions: framework to guide selection and interpretation of study end points. *BMJ* 2010;**341**:c4413.
17. Bognar A, Barach P, Johnson J, Duncan R, Woods D, Holl J, Birnbach D, Bacha E. Errors and the burden of errors: attitudes, perceptions and the culture of safety in pediatric cardiac surgical teams. *Ann Thorac Surg* 2008;(4):1374−81.
18. Salas E, Baker D, King H, Battles J, Barach P. On teams, organizations and safety. *Joint Comm J Qual Saf* 2006;**32**:109−12.
19. Baker D, Battles J, King H, Salas E, Barach P. The role of teamwork in the professional education of physicians: current status and assessment recommendations. *Joint Comm J Qual Saf* 2005;**31**(4):185−202.

20. Wahr JA, Prager RL, Abernathy JH, et al. Patient safety in the cardiac operating room: human factors and teamwork: a scientific statement from the American Heart Association. *Circulation* 2013;**128**.

21. Schraagen JM, Schouten T, Barach P. Assessing and improving teamwork in cardiac surgery. *Qual Saf Health Care* 2010;**19**:e29.

22. Cassin B, Barach P. Making sense of root cause analysis investigations of surgery-related adverse events. *Surg Clin* 2012;**92**:101–15.

23. Schraagen JM, Schouten A, Smit M, van der Beek D, Van de Ven J, Barach P. A prospective study of paediatric cardiac surgical microsystems: assessing the relationships between non-routine events, teamwork, and patient outcomes. *BMJ Qual Saf* 2011. https://doi.org/10.1136/bmjqs2010.048983.

24. Popovich E, Wiggins H, Barach P. The patient flow Physics framework. In: Sollecito W, Johnson J, editors. *Continuous quality improvement in health care: theory, implementations, and applications*. 5th ed. Jones and Bartlett; 2019. p. 143–74. ISBN 978-1-284-12695-4.

Index

Printed and bound by CPI Group (UK) Ltd, Croydon, CR0 4YY

03/10/2024

01040300-0009